GERIATRICS, GERONTOLOGY AND ELDERLY ISSUES

GERIATRIC PSYCHODERMATOLOGY

PSYCHOCUTANEOUS DISORDERS IN THE ELDERLY

GERIATRICS, GERONTOLOGY AND ELDERLY ISSUES

Additional books in this series can be found on Nova's website
under the Series tab.

Additional e-books in this series can be found on Nova's website
under the e-book tab.

GERIATRICS, GERONTOLOGY AND ELDERLY ISSUES

GERIATRIC PSYCHODERMATOLOGY

PSYCHOCUTANEOUS DISORDERS IN THE ELDERLY

MOHAMMAD JAFFERANY, M.D.
AND
KATLEIN FRANÇA, M.D.
EDITORS

NOVA BIOMEDICAL

New York

Library of Congress Cataloging-in-Publication Data

ISBN: 978-1-63463-853-1
Library of Congress Control Number: 2014959216

Published by Nova Science Publishers, Inc. † New York

"I dedicate this book to Professor Tahir Saeed Haroon, who taught me the first lesson of dermatology. I also dedicate this book to my two beautiful daughters Maha and Yusra who inspired me to edit this book."

Mohammad Jafferany

"I dedicate this book to my father and mother, Reginaldo and Aparecida França, who have encouraged and guided me in my professional and personal evolution.
I dedicate this book to my sisters, nephew and niece and to the rest of my lovely family.
I am very fortunate to have you all.
I dedicate this book to my patients, professors, mentors and friends.
Thank you for the inspiration and support"

Katlein França

Contents

Foreword

Caroline S. Koblenzer, M.D.

The entire field of psychodermatology has been rather slow to take hold in a meaningful way, in recent years, in the United States. This is perhaps surprising, because in the first four decades of the last Century significant work was underway. John Stokes, of Philadelphia, made reference to the importance of psychological factors in skin disease and indeed made many contributions to the field [1-3], while in 1925 Klauder noted that "the psychological phase of certain skin disease should not be neglected" [4]. In similar mode, in 1979, Rook and Wilkinson reported that "emotional factors" are significant in 40% of patients attending departments of dermatology [5], and two years later Medansky and Handler increased that number to 80% [6]. Today somewhat similar figures are reported. So it is evident that frustrating chronic and persistent clinical conditions in this genre still haunt us. While some of these conditions have their genesis in the psyche, some arise in the skin and are negatively affected by the psyche, while yet others, by their very nature, have a negative impact on the quality of life of the sufferer, and this in turn may strongly affect the psyche [7].

No one of these three clinical situations is a respecter of age, and it is important that we address the presentations that we meet in each of these three groups in our geriatric patients, and that we apply, as effectively as we can, the information that we have as to how best to handle these very difficult disorders.

Ours is a culture of youth, and advancing age is generally perceived to be a disadvantage both by society and within the self — hence the ever-increasing literature and the funding that is devoted to every aspect of cosmesis. Psychodermatologic issues, though perhaps latterly receiving token lip-service, unfortunately still tend to be given short-shrift at a therapeutic level — for example there are very few clinics solely devoted to clinical psychodermatology currently in the U.S — so that texts that address these issues can be of enormous value to the practicing dermatologist. In the elderly, the clinical situation may also be complicated by psychosocial factors, factors that to date have had little specific focus in dermatology texts.

To put this current text in perspective it is important to note that in the the years between the Second World War and the 1980's, a number of relevant papers and comprehensive monographs were published in the English language [8-120]. These began to tie together in a meaningful way, the crucial interactions between skin and psyche. Much of this work followed upon a more profound recognition of the importance of skin in our emotional lives

— a recognition that had been clarified to a large extent by psychiatrists and psychoanalysts who had engaged in infant and child observation [13]. The impact of this work was beautifully illustrated by Musaph, in 1964 [14].

As we know, the skin and the psyche are derived from the same embryonic layer, the ectoderm, and that touch, the first of our senses to develop, remains perhaps the most important of those senses. We know also that there is crucial and close communication between the two, the skin and the psyche, that is ongoing throughout our lives and into old age. How we look to others, how we feel about how we look, and the complexities of the sensation of touch, all contribute to our feeling of physical and emotional well-being. [15]

In the past two or three decades, an overwhelming amount of exciting scientific information has emerged, that helps us to understand at a cellular level, some of the chemical, neurologic, psychoneurologic and immunologic interactions that take place between skin and psyche [16], and that are involved in the clinical representations of psychodermatology. It had seemed, at first that perhaps these advances could answer all our questions about the pathophysiology of diseases of the skin, and so psychological issues tended to be pushed into the background during those years.

However, despite this emerging and ever-increasing, important scientific information, the frustrating chronic and persistent clinical examples of psycho – dermatologic interaction continue to haunt us. Many of these very difficult patients are in their later years, and in order to work effectively with these older patients, it is important to bring both dermatologic and psychiatric knowledge and experience to bear. Happily, it is gradually becoming more usual to have input from both specialties in the same facility, a situation that has been common in a number of European countries for several decades. This arrangement may entail a psychiatrist who is available in the dermatology clinic on certain days, or a specialty clinic that treats only patients with psychodermatologic disorders.

As I have noted, these problematic conditions are frequently encountered in the geriatric patient population. In addition to addressing the better known dermatologic aspects of these disorders, a text devoted to geriatric psychodermatology should help us to understand the psychological underpinnings that we encounter in the elderly. It is important to explore the psychiatric diagnostic features, together with the appropriate use of psychotropic medications, and the forms of psychotherapy that are available. Ways of handling psychosocial issues, not uncommon in this group, are discussed, and — most importantly, something that is all too often neglected in to-day's culture, where speed is of the essence — attention is given to the doctor-patient relationship. Recognition of the value and therapeutic importance of a trusting relationship, and ways in which such a relationship may be developed is also clearly of great importance.

So, in summary, this is a text designed to address important issues related to psychodermatologic disorders in the geriatric patient population, a group that is not often distinguished separately. That there is international authorship is of interest, as it adds a perspective from other countries in which psychodermatology has already become a more integral part of our field.

References

[1] Stokes JH. Effects on the skin of emotional and nervous states – part one. *Arch. Derm. Syph.* 1930. 22 (6): 803-810.

[2] Stokes JH. Effects on the skin of emotional and nervous states – part two. *Arch. Derm. Syph.* 1932. 26 (3):478-494.

[3] Stokes JH. Effects on the skin of emotional and nervous states – part three. *Arch. Derm. Syph.* 1935. 31 (4): 470-499.

[4] Klauder JV. The cutaneous neuroses. JAMA. 1925. 1925. *JAMA* 85: 1683-1690.

[5] Rook AJ, Wilkinson DS: in Rook AJ, Wilkinson DS. Ebling FJG. (eds) *Textbook of Dermatology* (3rd ed), Boston 1979, pp 2023-2035.

[6] Medansky RS, Handler RM: Dermatopsychosomatics: classification, physiology, and therapeutic approached. *J. Am. Acad Dermatol* 1981; 5:125-126.

[7] Koblenzer CS. The emotional impact of chronic and disabling skin disease: a psychoanalytic perspective. *Dermatolog Clin.* 2005;23: 619-627.

[8] Wittkower E, Russell, B. *Emotional Factors in Skin Disease New York*, 1953. Harper and brothers, New York.

[9] Obermeyer ME. *Psychocutaneous Medicine*. Springfield Il. 1955. Charles C.Thomas.

[10] Whitlock FA. *Psychophysiologic Aspects of Skin Disease*. Philadelphia.1976. WB Saunders.

[11] Panconesi E. Stress and Skin Disease. Psychosomatic Dermatology. *Clinics in Dermatology,* Philadelphia. 1984.

[12] Koblenzer CS. *Psychocutaneous Disease*. New York, 1987. Grune and Strattan.

[13] Spitz RA, *The First Year of Life*. New York. 1965, International Universities Press.

[14] Musaph, H. *Itching and Scratching*. Philadelphia. 1964. F.A. Davis Company.

[15] Millard LG, Millard J. Psychocutaneous disorders, in *Rook's Textbook of Dermatology.* 8th Ed. Barnes T, Breathnach S, Cox N, Griffiths C. (eds), Oxford. 2010, Wiley-Blackwell, pp 64.1-64.55.

[16] Ader R. *Psychoneuroimmunology*. 4th Ed'n. Amsterdam 2007. Elsevier Academic Press.

Preface

Eric Sorenson, BS and John Koo, M.D.

This volume on psychodermatology is unique because it is devoted specifically to the management of psychodermatological issues in the elderly. Today, the elderly are the fastest growing segment of the population in many parts of the world including countries like the United States and Japan. Geriatric patients have special needs related to issues such as concurrent comorbidities, social isolation, and logistical limitations including difficulty with transportation or even basic activities of daily living. Therefore, it is helpful to have a book that discusses psychodermatological management in the face of these special concerns, as well as other important topics such as chemotherapy and other oncologic complications, the influence of systemic disease on the skin, infectious complications in the elderly, and psychopharmacologic management. Moreover, beyond technical aspects of the provision of medical care, there are a number of unique considerations for the geriatric population, such as bioethical and medico-legal issues, a clinician needs to understand in order to optimize the physician-patient relationship. This book is the only volume of which I am aware that addresses each of these issues in depth.

In addition, a number of dermatological disorders are associated with well-established propensities to cause significant negative consequences on psychological wellness and quality of life, such as hair disorders and nail disorders, and these warrant special consideration among the elderly. These disorders are similarly well discussed in this volume. Lastly, more than any other age group or ethnic subgroup, elderly patients are more likely to suffer from cutaneous sensory syndrome ranging from chronic intractable pruritus of unknown etiology, which may be localized only to areas such as the scalp or involve the whole body, to formication which may even be associated with delusional ideation. These highly relevant topics are also discussed in detail in this book.

In short, this volume is not only timely in meeting the challenges of a growing geriatric population, but the detailed information included in it is critically needed to optimize psychodermatological management of the elderly. In view of the tragic reality that geriatric patients often “fall through the cracks ” and are at great risk for suboptimal care, which may even border on neglect, I recommend this volume to all health care providers so that we can be part of the solution for the elderly with psychodermatological disorders and not part of the problem.

Acknowledgments

"If I have seen further it is by standing on the shoulders of giants"

(Isaac Newton)

We sincerely thank all the authors of this book, whose untiring efforts in writing chapters are highly appreciated. Without your help and contribution, the production of this book would not have been possible.

We are also inspired with the work of Association of Psychocutaneous Medicine of North America (APMNA), European Society of Dermatology and Psychiatry (ESDaP), Psychodermatology Group of the Brazilian Society of Dermatology, Japanese Society of Psychosomatic Medicine, British Association of Dermatology (BAD), efforts to launch a website for psychosocial comorbidities in patients with skin diseases, the online community for practitioners and patients for atopic eczema in United Kingdom. All these organizations, societies and groups have inspired us tremendously to edit a book on this important forgotten topic. We are also thankful for the Department of Dermatology & Cutaneous Surgery at University of Miami Miller School of Medicine and especially to Dr Keyvan Nouri for his unconditional support.

Our fellows, residents and medical students at University of Miami School of Medicine and Jafferany Psychiatric Services PLC in Saginaw, Michigan, Including Shailee Patel, Tulsie Patel, Mariam Mahmud and Sehrish Khurram.

We are also indebted to our families for their patience and support during the entire time we were working on editing of this book. Our geriatric patients who suffered psychocutaneous diseases also inspired us and gave us a new perspective of diagnosis and treatment in more holistic way.

We are also thankful to NovaScience Publishers for providing the opportunity to bring this book for the readership. It has been a pleasure working with them in this inspiring project.

Mohammad Jafferany
Katlein França

About the Editors

Mohammad Jafferany, M.D.

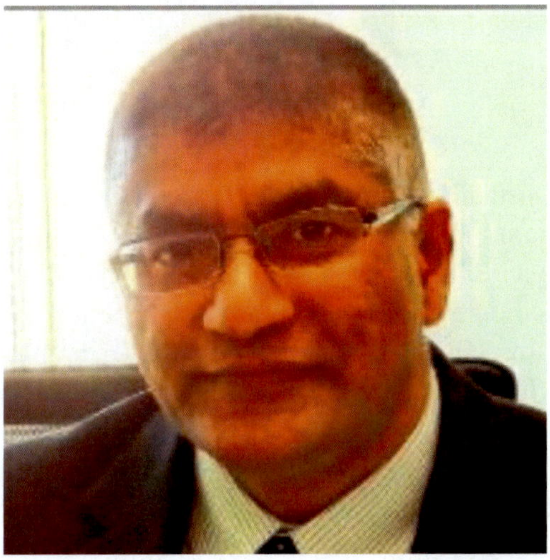

Dr. Jafferany is a board certified Psychiatrist who practices in Saginaw, MI. He is Director Psychodermatology clinic at Jafferany Psychiatric Services, PLC. He is also Adjunct Assistant Professor in Psychiatry at Michigan State University and Central Michigan University. He did his adult Psychiatry residency at Hennepin County Medical Center in Minneapolis, MN and fellowship in Child & Adolescent Psychiatry at University of Washington in Seattle, WA. Skin picking, trichotillomania and other psychocutaneous disorders are his particular interest. He is also the Executive Secretary of Association of Psychocutaneous Medicine of North America, the national association for these disorders. He has numerous publications to his credit on various psychodermatological topics. He is the co-editor of a book on Pediatric Psychodermatology and has written chapters in many books. He is a researcher, writer, lecturer and speaker in national and international conferences on psychodermatology.

Katlein França, M.D., M.Sc.

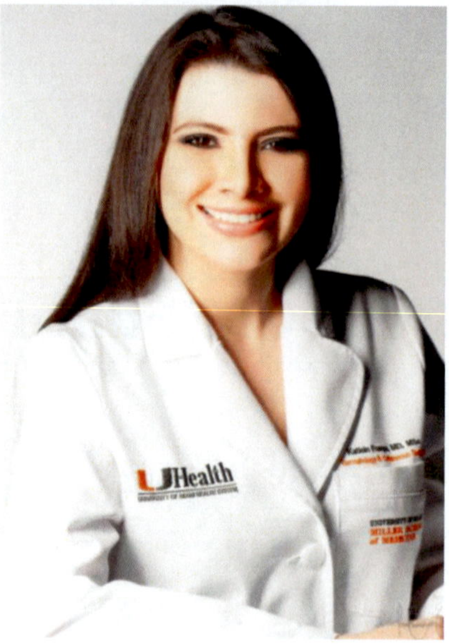

Volunteer Faculty- Assistant Professor at the Department of Dermatology & Cutaneous Surgery, University of Miami Miller School of Medicine. Previously, she has a Research Fellowship in Dermatologic Surgery & Laser at the same University. She also has a Fellowship in Cosmetic Medicine at the Department of Otorhinolaryngology & Facial Plastic Surgery, University of Miami Miller School of Medicine. Dr França has numerous scientific papers to her credit currently published in peer-reviewed journals. She is an author of a book entitled "Dermatology and Doctor-Patient Relationship" and the editor of "New Treatment Approaches to Management of Alopecia". She has contributed chapters on dermatology in various books. She is currently a member of the executive committee of the Association of Psychoneurocutaneous Medicine of North America. Researcher, lecturer, writer. Reviewer and regular speaker in international dermatology and psychodermatology conferences.

Contributors

İlknur K. Altunay, M.D.
Dermatology and Venereology Clinic
Şişli Etfal Training and Research Hospital
Istanbul, Turkey

Christopher Bridgett, M.D.
Consultant Psychiatrist
London, United Kingdom

Gabrielle Brown, MSc
Department of Dermatology
University of California - San Francisco
San Francisco, CA, US

Susana Coimbra, Ph.D.
Instituto de Biologia Molecular e Celular
Universidade do Porto
Porto, Portugal

Instituto de Investigação e Formação
Avançada em Ciências e Tecnologias
da Saúde
Gandra-PRD, Portugal

Américo Figueiredo, M.D., Ph.D.
Department of Dermatology
Faculdade de Medicina
Universidade de Coimbra
Coimbra, Portugal

Aparecida Porto França, MSc
Bioethics Master's Degree Program
Universidad del Museo Social Argentino
Buenos Aires, Argentina

Facultad de Derecho
Universidad de Buenos Aires
Buenos Aires, Argentina

Katlein França, M.D., MSc
Department of Dermatology &
Cutaneous Surgery
University of Miami Miller School
of Medicine
Miami, FL, US

Reginaldo de França, MSc
Facultad de Derecho
Universidad de Buenos Aires
Buenos Aires, Argentina

Zeba Hasan Hafeez, M.D.
Kaiser Permanente Medical Group
Santa Rosa, CA

Touro University,
Vallejo, CA, US

Josie Howard, M.D.
Department of Dermatology
University of California - San Francisco
San Francisco, CA, US

Mohammad Jafferany, M.D., FAPA
Department of Psychiatry
Central Michigan University
Jafferany Psychiatric Services, PLC
Saginaw, MI, US

Jonette Keri, M.D., Ph.D.
Department of Dermatology &
Cutaneous Surgery
University of Miami Miller School
of Medicine
Miami, FL, US

Thelda Kestenbaum, M.D.
Department of Dermatology
University of Kansas Medical Center
Kansas, KS, US

Caroline Koblenzer, M.D.
Consultant Dermatologist
University of Pennsylvania
Philadelphia, PA, US

John Koo, M.D.
Department of Dermatology
University of California - San Francisco
San Francisco, CA, US

Mariam Mahmud, BSc
Research Assistant
Jafferany Psychiatric Services, PLC
Saginaw, MI, US

Mona Malakouti, MSc
Department of Dermatology
University of California - San Francisco
San Francisco, CA, US

Servando E. Marron, M.D.
University of Zaragoza
Aragon Health Sciences Institute,
Zaragoza, Spain

Sibel Mercan, M.D.
Department of Psychiatry,
Sisli Etfal Education and Research Hospital
Istanbul, Turkey

Peter Norén, M.D.
Consultant Dermatologist
Uppsala, Sweden

Keyvan Nouri, M.D.
Department of Dermatology &
Cutaneous Surgery
University of Miami Miller School
of Medicine
Miami, FL, US

Malgorzata Olszewska, M.D.
Department of Dermatology
Medical University of Warsaw
Warszawa, Poland

Shailee Patel, BS
Department of Dermatology &
Cutaneous Surgery
University of Miami Miller School
of Medicine
Miami, FL, US

Tulsie Patel, BS
Department of Dermatology &
Cutaneous Surgery
University of Miami Miller School
of Medicine
Miami, FL, US

Adam Reich, M.D.
Department of Dermatology,
Venereology and Allergology
Wroclaw Medical University
Wroclaw, Poland

Rafael Henrique Rocha, M.D.
Department of Dermatology
Resident
Universidade Federal do Espírito Santo
Vitória, Brazil

Tania Nely Rocha, M.D.
Diversitá Dermatologia Ltda
Dermatologist & Integrative
Psychotherapist
Belo Horizonte, Brazil

Lidia Rudnicka, M.D., Ph.D.
Department of Dermatology
Medical University of Warsaw
Warszawa, Poland

Maria Helena Lesqueves Sandoval, M.D.
Department of Dermatology –
Cosmiatric Clinic
Hospital Universitário Cassiano
Antonio Moraes
Vitória, Brazil

Alice Santos-Silva, Ph.D.
Instituto de Biologia Molecular e Celular
Universidade do Porto
Porto, Portugal

Departamento de Ciências Biológicas,
Faculdade de Farmácia
Universidade do Porto
Porto, Portugal

Anna Skrok, M.D.
Department of Dermatology
Medical University of Warsaw
Warszawa, Poland

Eric Sorenson, BS
Department of Dermatology
University of California - San Francisco
San Francisco, CA, US

Jacek C Szepietowski, M.D.
Department of Dermatology, Venereology
and Allergology
Wroclaw Medical University
Wroclaw, Poland

Kinza Nisar Tareen, BS
College of Human Medicine
Michigan State University
Lansing, MI, US

Ruqiya Shama Tareen, M.D.
Department of Psychiatry,
Western Michigan University School
of Medicine
Kalamazoo, MI, US

Lucia Tomas-Aragones, Ph.D.
University of Zaragoza
Aragon Health Science Institute
Zaragoza, Spain

Eva Wang, BS
Department of Dermatology
University of California - San Francisco
San Francisco, CA, US

Part I. Basics of Psychodermatology

In: Geriatric Psychodermatology
Editors: Mohammad Jafferany and Katlein França

ISBN: 978-1-63463-853-1

Chapter 1

The Interface between Geriatrics, Psychiatry and Dermatology

Mohammad Jafferany, M.D, FAPA*
and Katlein França, M.D., MSc

To hypothesize the validity of connection between mind and skin, we trace the origin of each. Human embryogenesis involves the development of both the progenitors of nervous system as well as the skin from the ectoderm primary germ cell layer. Neural crest cells pigmentize the skin via melanocytes while simultaneously shaping the connections of the central and peripheral nervous systems via ganglia. Similarly, the epidermis of the skin as well as the epithelia of the pineal and pituitary glands share a common progenitor in the form of surface ectodermal cells.

On the foundation of this primordial relationship does the field of psychodermatology arise, placing emphasis on the interaction between the psyche, or human mind in its entirety and the dermis or skin, ensheathing the carrier of the psyche. The psyche encompasses both the conscious and the unconscious and as such, either component may arouse dermatological disorders. Both neuroendocrine and immune systems interact in a complex pattern with a disturbance in equilibrium of either component of the neuro-immuno-cutaneous system [1] (NICS) resulting in a plethora of dermatological manifestations. It is therefore not surprising to unearth psychological problems in over 30% of patients presenting with a primarily dermatological complaint. [2]

This book presents the most important psychodermatological disorders of the elderly- an age group already at increased susceptibility to both psychiatric as well as dermatological ailments owing to a variety of factors including immunocompromise, lifestyle, chronic diseases such as diabetes mellitus and rheumatoid arthritis, polypharmacy, as well as financial and social adjustment among others.

The decisive objective here would be to enhance the interaction between the fields of primary care, geriatrics, dermatology, and psychiatry (Table 1) such that the diagnosis,

* Corresponding author: Mohammad Jafferany. Email: mjafferany@yahoo.com.

referral and ultimately treatment of the needy are superlative- a synergy that is at present sorely lacking. [3, 4]

Table 1. Classification of Geriatric Psychodermatological Disorders

Classification	Age of presentation (in years)
Psychophysiologic disorders	
Psoriasis	20-30 and 50-60+
Atopic dermatitis	<5
Hyperhidrosis	25
Urticaria	All age groups
Herpes simplex virus infection	14-49
Seborrheic dermatitis	2 weeks-12 months and 30-40+
Aphthosis	<30
Rosacea	>30
Pruritus	All age groups
Psychiatric disorders with dermatologic symptoms	
Dermatitis artefacta	18-60
Delusion of parasitosis	50+
Trichotillomania	9-13
Obsessive compulsive disorder	Juvenile: 10 and Adult: 21
Phobic states	20
Neurotic excoriation	30-45
Psychogenic pruritus	64
Dermatologic disorders with psychiatric symptoms	
Alopecia areata	<30
Vitiligo	20-30+
Generalized Psoriasis	20-30 and 50-60+
Chronic Eczema	20
Rhinophyma	30-50
MISCELLANEOUS	
Glossodynia	55-60
Vulvodynia	25
Chronic itching in scalp	30-50+
Psychogenic purpura syndrome	14,40
Pseudopsychodermatologic disease	21,68

Note: Mean age of presentation does not exclude incidence in geriatric population.

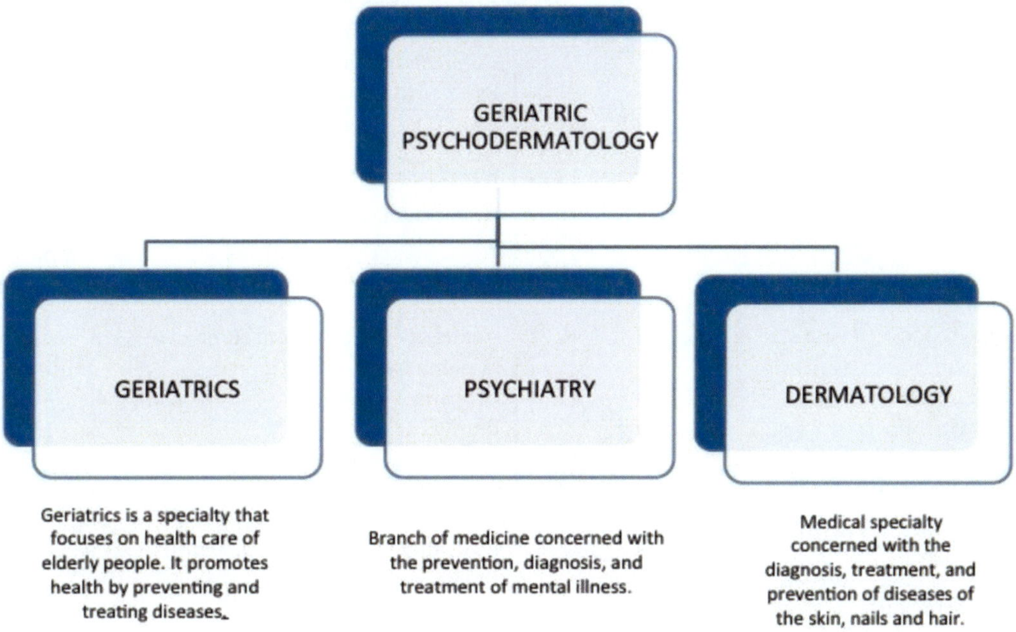

Chart 1. Geriatric Psychodermatology: Connecting Geriatrics, Psychiatry and Dermatology.

Aging Population and Geriatric Psychodermatology

Statisticians point out that the rate of population aging in the near future will exceed one seen in the past century. The United Nations report on World population ageing states this trend towards older populations is largely irreversible. Over one-fifths of society, some two billion people, will fall in this demographic by the year 2050. [5] Geriatric psychodermatology is already complicated by pre-existing age -related decline in cognition, decreased physical capabilities activities of daily living, and disabilities among others. Multiple morbidities along with their medications and treatment plans as well as complex social and financial relationships add numerous variables to this already challenging field. With other avenues of communication inhibited, the elderly patient may use the skin as a heliograph for elevated psychological distress. It is therefore imperative that clinicians understand, diagnose and treat this impending deluge of humanity in an integrative and holistic manner. Further categorization can be done in the form of psychophysiologic, primary psychiatry and secondary psychiatric disorders. [6] Koo and Lee's widely accepted classification [7] of dermatological disorders with underlying psychiatric component is displayed in Table 2. Real world data is seen in two Washington state surveys [3,4] highlighting the cross-pollination of psychiatric and dermatological referrals in Table 2. With over a third of patients with dermatological complaints having psychiatric comorbidities, [8, 9] effective diagnosis and ultimately management of underlying psychiatric stressors assumes an even greater importance as compared to the general population. [10]

Table 2. Commonly Referred Psychodermatological Disorders

Common Diagnoses Referred by Dermatologists to Psychiatrists	N	(%)	Common Diagnoses Referred by Psychiatrists to Dermatologists	N	(%)
Delusion of parasitosis	42	(41.1)	Drug-related rash	61	(27.4)
Neurotic excoriation	24	(23.5)	Acne	31	(13.9)
Trichotillomania	17	(16.6)	Psoriasis	28	(12.6)
Depression associated with chronic skin disease	11	(10.7)	Atopic dermatitis	28	(12.6)
Skin-related obsessive-compulsive behavior	11	(10.7)	Alopecia areata	11	(4.9)
Anxiety associated with skin disease	9	(8.8)	Anxiety/depression from chronic skin disease	8	(3.6)
Acne excoriée	8	(7.8)	Urticaria	8	(3.6)
Psoriasis	6	(5.8)	Pruritus	8	(3.6)
Alopecia areata	5	(4.9)	Delusion of parasitosis	7	(3.1)
Prurigo nodularis	5	(4.9)	Skin picking	6	(2.7)
Body dysmorphic disorder	5	(4.9)	Factitious dermatitis	5	(2.2)
Factitious dermatitis	4	(3.9)	Evaluation for obsessive thoughts about suspected skin cancer	5	(2.2)
Atopic dermatitis	3	(2.9)	Trichotillomania	4	(1.8)
Miscellaneous	4	(3.9)	Fungal infections	3	(1.3)
			Miscellaneous Conditions	21	(9.4)

Ref: [3, 4].

References

[1] Misery L. [Neuro-immuno-cutaneous system (NICS)]. *Pathol. Biol.* 1996; 44(10):867–74.

[2] Picardi A, Abeni D, Melchi CF, Puddu P, Pasquini P. Psychiatric morbidity in dermatological outpatients: an issue to be recognized. *Br. J. Dermatol.* 2000; 143(5):983–91.

[3] Jafferany M, Stoep AV, Dumitrescu A, Hornung RL. Psychocutaneous disorders: a survey study of psychiatrists' awareness and treatment patterns. *South. Med. J.* 2010; 103(12):1199–203.

[4] Jafferany M, Vander Stoep A, Dumitrescu A, Hornung RL. The knowledge, awareness, and practice patterns of dermatologists toward psychocutaneous disorders: results of a survey study. *Int. J. Dermatol.* 2010; 49(7):784–9.

[5] United Nations Department of Economic and Social Affairs Population Division. World Population Ageing: 1950-2050 [Internet]. New York, NY; 2002. Available from: http://www.un.org/esa/population /publications/worldageing19502050/

[6] Koo J, Lebwohl A. Psycho dermatology: the mind and skin connection. *Am Fam Physician.* 2001; 1;64(11):1873–8.

[7] Koo JYM, Lee CS. *Psychocutaneous medicine.* New York: Marcel Dekker; 2003.

[8] Sandoz A, Koenig T, Kusnir D, Tausk F. Psychocutaneous diseases. In: Burgdorf W, Plewig G, Wolff H, Landthaler M, editors. *Braun-Falco's Dermatology.* 3rd ed. Berlin: Springer Medizin Verlag Heidelberg; 2009. p. 912–26.

[9] Millard LG, Cotterill JA. *Psychocutaneous Disorders.* In: Burns T, Breathnach S, Cox N, Griffiths C, editors. Rook's Textbook of Dermatology [Internet]. 7th ed. Malden, Massachusetts, USA: Blackwell Publishing, Inc.; 2004 [cited 2012 Apr 15]. p. 3095–136. Available from: http://doi.wiley.com/10.1002/9780470750520.ch61

[10] Hughes JE, Barraclough BM, Hamblin LG, White JE. Psychiatric symptoms in dermatology patients. *Br J Psychiatry.* 1983; 143:51–4.

In: Geriatric Psychodermatology
Editors: Mohammad Jafferany and Katlein França

ISBN: 978-1-63463-853-1

Chapter 2

Doctor-Patient Relationship in Geriatric Psychodermatology

Katlein França, M.D., MSc* and Mariam Mahmud, BSc

Introduction

The doctor-patient relationship is the keystone of the entire medical practice [1]. For centuries, this relationship has been studied by different cultures. Hippocrates, considered the father of medicine, developed a code that covers several important ethical issues between doctors and patients [2]. Followed by physicians today, this code was updated with the contemporary behavior, culture and medical practice laws. The number of individuals 65 years of age and older is constantly increasing as well as the life expectancy in many countries. As people age, their chances of developing skin -related disorders increase. Geriatric patients have special physical, emotional, social and psychological needs [3].

Physicians should be prepared to develop the appropriate skills to deal with these patients. The daily work of a dermatologist requires constant concern with the psychological issues of patients. The proper diagnosis and treatment of skin diseases are based on the harmonic interaction between dermatologists and their patients [1]. This chapter will discuss the doctor-patient relationship in geriatric psychodermatology.

Geriatric Patients

As people age, there is an increased risk for illnesses and injuries. Health problems related to cardiovascular system, bones and muscles are common among geriatric patients [4]. Studies have shown that older patients are more satisfied with patient-centered encounters but have a lower tendency to be involved in medical decision-making [5, 6, 7].

* Corresponding author: Katlein França. E-mail: k.franca@med.miami.edu.

The geriatric healthcare professional must carefully consider the patient's life history and social and psychological characteristics [4]. These characteristics may vary. Geriatric patients may be socially isolated or have the constant presence of family members interfering in their autonomy. These patients usually come to appointments accompanied by family members. Working with the patient's family is a key part of this relationship [8].

Elderly patients have an increased risk for mental illness es such as depression; biological changes such as diabetes and hypertension can also lead to depression [9]. Alzheimer's disease and other dementias are more prevalent in this population as well [10]. The communication between physicians and geriatric patients may be complex considering these scenarios. Difficult geriatric patients can also be challenging.

Some patients are "difficult" based on the feelings that they invoke in their doctors, such as frustration, anger and dread [11].

The next session will discuss the characteristics and management of difficult patients.

Difficult Patients

Difficult patients can take up the doctor's time and physical and emotional energy. In a study performed by Hahn and colleagues, physicians rated 15% of their patients as difficult. These patients are more likely have mental disorders when compared with non-difficult patients. The authors found that difficult patients had lower satisfaction rates, more functional impairment and used the health care system more often. Demographic characteristics and physical illnesses were not associated with difficulty [12]. The following table shows some characteristics of patients that are labeled "difficult" by clinicians.

Table 1. Characteristics of difficult patients

Angry
Anxious
Depressed
Feeling Guilty
Frustrated
Helpless
Hostile
Self-loathed
Uncooperative
Ungrateful
Unpleasant

Managing Difficult Patients

Managing difficult patients can be a challenge for many doctors. Learning how to manage these patients is very important for any successful practice. Some tips and practical guidelines are presented below:

- SHOW EMPATHY: Empathy refers to the ability of sharing feelings and understanding another person. Showing empathy to patients can motivate them to pursue the treatment, improve their satisfaction and lower malpractice complaints [13]. Most "difficult" patients have experienced adversities and frustration in their lives. Being an empathic and compassionate doctor may help these patients to overcome any new obstacle [13, 14, 15].
- LISTEN CAREFULLY: Listening is a very important skill for any doctor, especially those dealing with difficult patients. Paying attention to vocal inflections can help the doctor understand the patient's state of mind [16].
- INVOLVE THE PATIENT AND THE FAMILY: When patients feel responsible for their choices and treatment, there is an increased chance of success. Family members can sometimes be very helpful when it comes to improving the connection between the doctor and the difficult patient [17].
- VERBALIZES THE DIFFICULTY: Mentioning the problem or difficulty to the patient creates a sense of shared ownership. The patient may or may not agree with the problem presented, but it is an important step to try to solve difficult situations in clinical interaction [18].
- STAY POSITIVE, FOCUS ON FINDING SOLUTIONS: All patients need encouragement and a positive environment. They should feel that the doctor is working with them as a team. Focus on possible solutions rather than areas of disagreement [19].

The Importance of a Physician Being a "Good Psychologist"

In regard to the patient's overall health, the patient's mental state should never be ignored. Thus, it is imperative that geriatric physicians and dermatologists take note of the patient's mental health and act accordingly. In addition to their physical diagnosis, geriatric patients have emotional and psychological needs that also require the steadfast observation of their physician. Every doctor-patient relationship could largely benefit from employing certain tools used by a physician who is always keen to look into the emotional aspect of the diagnosis. These tools include those such as effective communication, listening, and making oneself approachable. Effective communication ensures not only that the patient is heard, but also that the physician's professional opinion is conveyed to the patient in a good-natured, effective and comprehensible manner. Good listening skills assure that the patient's background and full situation is well understood, as this can also contribute to their current mental state. Furthermore, making oneself approachable is of utmost importance.

The patient must feel comfortable enough to be able to share personal details with their physician, and this is much easier done when the physician comes across as open, friendly, and understanding. Additionally, expressing concern and respecting the patient's concerns and worries is much appreciated by the patient. All of these characteristics contribute to the level of comfort the patient feels with his or her physician, which in turn leads to a stronger doctor-patient relationship and an effective bond between them.

Conclusion

In this chapter we discussed several aspects of the doctor patient-relationship in geriatrics, as well as its importance in the treatment model. The doctor-patient relationship is a vital part of any medical practice. Geriatric patients have notable emotional, social, physical and psychological needs that can differ from those of younger patients, and also have an increased risk of emotional repercussions. "Difficult" geriatric patients will be encountered as well, and typical characteristics of a difficult patient include anger, anxiety, depression, and feelings of guilt, helplessness, hostility, and frustration amongst others. When dealing with these types of patients, it can be helpful to utilize certain strategies such as empathizing with the patient, listening carefully, and involving the patient and their family in medical decisions and all aspects of the treatment process. Verbalizing the problem as well as conveying a positive attitude by focusing on solutions as opposed to disagreements can also be effective techniques. It is also noteworthy that harnessing the tools of an effective "psychologist" can significantly improve the doctor-patient relationship. Methods such as being open and friendly and expressing concern may go a long way with the patient, and may also help improve the doctor-patient relationship. A favorable correspondence between dermatologists and their patients contributes to achieving the correct diagnosis and treatment of disease.

References

[1] França, K. *A Dermatologia e o relacionamento médico-paciente: aspectos Psicossociais e Bioéticos*. Brasil: Ed. Juruá; 2012.

[2] Popović, M. [Hippocratic Oath: professional or ethic code?]. *Acta Chir. Iugosl.* 2011; 58(3):9-14; discussion 14.

[3] Norman, R. A. Geriatric dermatology. *Dermatol. Ther.* 2003;16(3):260-8.

[4] Sleeper, R. B. Geriatric primer - common geriatric syndromes and special problems. *Consult. Pharm.* 2009 Jun.; 24(6):447-62.

[5] Swenson, S. L., Buell, S., Zettler, P., White, M., Ruston, D. C., Lo, B. Patient-centered communication: do patients really prefer it? *J. Gen. Intern. Med.* 2004;19:1069–79.

[6] Hibbard, J. Moving toward a more patient-centered health care delivery system. *Health Affair* (Millwood) 2004:133–5.

[7] M. G. Greene, R. D. Adelman, E. Friedmann, and R. Charone, "Older patient satisfaction with communication during an initial medical encounter," *Social Science and Medicine*, vol. 38, no. 9, pp. 1279–1288, 1994. View at Publisher View at Google Scholar View at Scopus.

[8] Rosin, Dijk, J. Subtle ethical dilemmas in geriatric management and clinical research. *Med. Ethics* 2005;31:355-359 doi:10.1136/jme.2004.008532.

[9] Alexopoulos, G. S. Depression in the elderly. *Lancet.* 2005 Jun. 4-10;365(9475):1961-70.

[10] Fratiglioni, L. 1., Grut, M., Forsell, Y., Viitanen, M., Grafström, M., Holmén, K., Ericsson, K., Bäckman, L., Ahlbom, A., Winblad, B. Prevalence of Alzheimer's disease and other dementias in an elderly urban population: relationship with age, sex, and education. *Neurology.* 1991 Dec.;41(12):1886-92.

[11] Wasan, A. D., Wootton, J., Jamison, R. N. Dealing with difficult patients in your pain practice. *Regional Anesthesia and Pain Medicine.* 2005; 30: 184-192.
[12] Hahn, S. R., Kroenke, K., Spitzer, R. L., Brody, D., Williams, J. B., Linzer, M., et al. The difficult patient: prevalence, psychopathology, and functional impairment. *J. Gen. Intern. Med.* 1996;11:1-8.
[13] *Canadian Medical Association Journal.* "Showing empathy to patients can improve care." *ScienceDaily. ScienceDaily*, 24 January 2011. <www.sciencedaily.com/releases/2011/01/110124121543.htm>.
[14] Krebs, et al., 2006; Wasan, et al., 2005; Elder, et al., 2006; Hass, et al., 2005.
[15] Haslam, N. Humanizing medical practice: the role of empathy. *Med. J. Aust.* 2007 Oct. 1;187(7):381-2.
[16] Lester, G. W., Smith, S. G. Listening and talking to patients. A remedy for malpractice suits? *West J. Med.* 1993;158(3):268–272.
[17] Martire, L. M. 1., Lustig, A. P., Schulz, R., Miller, G. E., Helgeson, V. S. Is it beneficial to involve a family member? A meta-analysis of psychosocial interventions for chronic illness. *Health Psychol.* 2004 Nov.;23(6):599-611.
[18] Davies, M. *Managing challenging interactions with patients.* Available at: http://careers.bmj.com/careers/advice/view-article.html?id=20013822.
[19] Jackson, J. L., Kroenke, K. Difficult patient encounters in the ambulatory clinic: clinical predictors and outcomes. *Arch. Intern. Med.* 1999;159:1069-75.

In: Geriatric Psychodermatology
Editors: Mohammad Jafferany and Katlein França
ISBN: 978-1-63463-853-1

Chapter 3

Pharmacologic Management in Geriatric Psychodermatology

Eric Sorenson, BS*[*]*, Gabrielle Brown, M.D., Mona Malakouti, M.D., John Koo, M.D. and Josie Howard, M.D.

Introduction

Psychotropic medications play an important and frequently essential role in the treatment of psychodermatologic conditions in the geriatric population.

In many cases, pharmacologic management ideally involves coordination of care with a psychiatrist and concurrent nonpharmacologic treatment.

Psychodermatology patients often decline psychiatric referral, however, because they may present with limited insight into the psychological component of their dermatological symptoms. Therefore it is helpful for the practicing dermatologist to be knowledgeable about the characteristics of psychotropic medications and their use in elderly patients.

The use of pharmacologic management in geriatric patients requires individualized consideration due to the unique characteristics of this population. Geriatric patients are more likely to have complex medical histories and be prescribed multiple medications than younger patients (Table 1). Physiologic changes associated with aging, such as changes in hepatic metabolism, renal clearance, and body composition, are likely to affect the pharmacokinetics and pharmacodynamics of drugs and may increase the sensitivity of elderly patients to the side effects of psychoactive medications.

Further, the dermatologist should be aware that geriatric patients are at an increased risk of falls, particularly if prescribed sedating medications.

[*] Corresponding author: Eric Sorenson. E-mail: ericsorenso@usc.edu.

Adhering to a few general principles of evaluation and management can allow the clinician to safely and effectively utilize psychotropic medications in geriatric patients. The basis of this approach is individualized management.

Table 1. CYP Inhibitors and Inducers

Enzyme	Substrates	Inhibitors (increase plasma levels)	Inducers (reduce plasma levels)
CYP1A2	Antipsychotics: olanzapine	Fluvoxamine	Tobacco
		Ciprofloxacin	Barbiturates
			Phenytoin
			Carbamazepine
			Rifampin
CYP3A4	Antidepressants: escitalopram Anxiolytics: buspirone, alprazolam	Ketoconazole, itraconazole, fluconazole	Barbiturates Phenytoin
	Antipsychotics: risperidone, quietapine, pimozide	Erythromycin, other macrolide antibiotics	Carbamazepine, oxcarbazepine Topiramate, felbamate
		Fluvoxamine, nefazodone Cimetidine	Rifampin St. John's wort
		Grapefruit juice	
CYP2D6	Antidepressants: fluoxetine, escitalopram	Fluoxetine, paroxetine Thioridazine, perphenazine	No known agent
	Antipsychotics: risperidone, olanzapine, aripiprazole, pimozide	Quinidine, propafenone	

First, each patient should provide a detailed medical history with special consideration for cardiovascular disease, cerebrovascular disease, diabetes mellitus, and falls. The clinician should elicit a comprehensive list of all concurrent medications and past psychotropic medications. Additionally, a complete physical exam and laboratory analysis may be considered if indicated. Second, the physician should be comfortable "starting low and going slow," with the knowledge that doses of psychotropic medications necessary for clinical efficacy are often lower in psychodermatology patients than in typical psychiatric practice, and effective doses may be even lower still in geriatric patients.

Further, prescribing treatment with the lowest effective dose for the shortest period of time will optimize safety because the risk of adverse effects is often dose dependent. After proper evaluation and the initiation of treatment, the clinician should consider conducting face-to-face monitoring visits 2 to 4 weeks after the initiation of therapy or modification of dose and every 3 months or more frequently once a stable regimen is achieved.

In this chapter, we aim to provide a guide for the practicing dermatologist to select the appropriate medication for each geriatric psychodermatology patient. Characteristics of and general considerations for each class of medications will be provided. Each medication will then be described with reference to dose, common and serious adverse effects, contraindications, important drug interaction s, and monitoring recommendations.

Delusional Infestation

Pharmacologic therapy is often essential in the successful treatment of patients with delusional infestation (DI) because delusional patients by definition cannot be convinced to abandon their unsubstantiated beliefs with reason alone. Both conventional antipsychotics, such as pimozide, and atypical antipsychotics can be effective in the treatment of DI. However, due to an increased risk of cardiovascular events and a greater number of drug interactions associated with pimozide, atypical antipsychotics should be considered first-line medications for geriatric patients with DI [1].

Atypical Antipsychotics

Atypical antipsychotics function through the antagonism of dopaminergic D_2 receptors and serotonergic $5\text{-}HT_{2A}$ receptors. Atypical antipsychotics carry a decreased risk of QT_c prolongation and extrapyramidal symptoms (EPS) compared to conventional antipsychotics like pimozide. It should be noted that in 2005, the US Food and Drug Administration (FDA) issued a boxed warning for the use of all atypical antipsychotics in elderly patients with dementia due to an increase in all-cause mortality, which was later expanded to include conventional antipsychotics. Because this warning was directed specifically towards patients with dementia, the use of atypical antipsychotics in elderly patients not suffering from dementia may be considered on a case-by-case basis as long as it is clinically indicated, an appropriate evaluation is performed, and informed consent is obtained (Table 2).

Table 2. Assessment of cardiac and neurological risk for antipsychotic use in the elderly

Assessment of cardiac risk Known cardiac disease, including long QT syndrome Family history of arrhythmia or sudden cardiac death Cardiac symptoms: syncope, palpitations, dyspnea, or angina Other QT prolonging or interacting drugs Hypokalemia ($K^+ < 3.5$ mEq/L) or hypomagnesemia ($Mg^{2+} < 1.7$ mg/dL) ECG: $QT_c > 480$ ms or other abnormalities Age > 70
If yes to any of the above, consider referral to a cardiologist to assess risk and optimize management, or potentially reconsider choice of drug prior to initiation of therapy.
Assessment of neurological risk History of stroke or TIA Uncontrolled hypertension DM Family history of stroke
If yes to any of the above, consider referral to a neurologist prior to initiating treatment or potentially reconsider choice of drug.

*Adapted from Fanoe et al.

The selection of an optimal agent should be based on medication side effect profiles in relation to the individual patient (Table 3). The use of low dosages and short treatment courses (e.g., 6 to 9 months) is likely to reduce the risk of adverse events. It should be noted that therapeutic effect may not be seen until 6 weeks after the initiation of treatment. Pharmacologic therapy can often be tapered and discontinued after 6 months of improved symptoms.

Table 3. Side Effect Profiles of Antipsychotic Medications

Drug	Side effect				
	EPS*	NMS**	QT_c prolongation	Weight gain/diabetes	Orthostatic hypotension
Quetiapine	+/-	+/-	+	++	++
Risperidone	++	+/-	+	++	+
Olanzapine	+/-	+/-	+	+++	+
Aripiprazole	+/-	+/-	+/-	+/-	+
Pimozide	+++	+	+++	+/-	++

+/- = rare, + = lower risk, ++ = medium risk, +++ = higher risk.
*Extrapyramidal symptoms.
**Neuroleptic malignant syndrome.

Quetiapine (Seroquel®)

Quetiapine is FDA approved for the treatment of schizophrenia, bipolar disorder, and major depressive disorder. Although it can cause sedation and orthostatic hypotension, these side effects can be minimized by the use of low doses and slow titration.

Dose

Start at 12.5 mg every evening. Consider titrating slowly to a therapeutic dose of 200 to 600 mg every evening or until significant remission of symptoms is achieved.

Adverse effects

Common: Orthostatic hypotension (can be dose-limiting), sedation, weight gain

Serious: Diabetes mellitus, dyslipidemia, seizures

Contraindications

Arrhythmia, heart disease, electrolyte imbalances, diabetes mellitus, dementia

Drug interactions

Antiarrhythmics, diuretics, macrolides, fluoroquinolones, other antipsychotics, cimetidine

Monitoring

Consider obtaining a complete metabolic panel (CMP), complete blood count (CBC), lipid profile, fasting blood glucose, and weight at baseline. Consider repeating at 3 months, 6 months, and every 6 months thereafter.

Risperidone (Risperdal®)

Risperidone is FDA approved for the treatment of schizophrenia, bipolar disorder, and autism spectrum disorders. Risperidone is the most studied atypical antipsychotic in the treatment of DI, and it is a good choice for the treatment of geriatric patients due to its overall favorable side effect profile [2]. The dermatologist should be aware that risperidone can be associated with weight gain, hyperprolactinemia, and Parkinsonian symptoms and should monitor for these side effects.

Dose

Start at 0.5 mg every night. Consider titrating by 0.5 mg increments every two to four weeks to a therapeutic dose of 1 to 5 mg every night or until significant remission of symptoms is achieved.

Adverse effects

Common: Sedation, orthostatic hypotension, weight gain

Serious: EPS, QT_c prolongation, hyperglycemia, hyperprolactinemia

Contraindications

Arrhythmia, heart disease, electrolyte imbalance s, obesity, diabetes mellitus, Parkinson disease, dementia

Drug interactions

Diuretics, ACE inhibitors, calcium -channel blockers, other antipsychotics

Monitoring

Consider CMP, CBC, lipid profile, fasting blood glucose, prolactin level, weight, and ECG at baseline. Consider repeating at 3 months, 6 months, and every 6 months thereafter.

Olanzapine (Zyprexa®)

Olanzapine is FDA approved for the treatment of schizophrenia and bipolar disorder. It is an effective medication in DI and its use can be appropriate for certain geriatric patients. It is important to note olanzapine is associated with an increased risk for the development of metabolic syndrome, including weight gain, glucose intolerance, and dyslipidemia [3]. It should be avoided in elderly patients with obesity, dyslipidemia, or DM or DM risk factors.

Dose

Start at 2.5 mg daily and consider titrating slowly to a therapeutic dose of 5 to 10 mg daily or until significant remission of symptoms is achieved.

Adverse effects

Common: Sedation, weight gain, hypotension, anticholinergic symptoms

Serious: Hyperglycemia, dyslipidemia, dysphagia, EPS

Contraindications

Arrhythmia, heart disease, electrolyte imbalances, obesity, DM or DM risk factors, dementia

Drug interactions

Other antipsychotics

Monitoring

Consider CMP, CBC, lipid profile, fasting blood glucose, weight, and ECG at baseline. Consider repeating at 3 months, 6 months, and every 6 months thereafter.

Aripiprazole (Abilify®)

Aripiprazole is FDA approved for the treatment of schizophrenia, bipolar disorder, major depressive disorder, and autism spectrum disorders. It is generally well tolerated in elderly patients and has a decreased risk of weight gain, QT_c prolongation, and anticholinergic effects in comparison to other atypical antipsychotics. However, it is less studied in DI and its activating effects, such restlessness and insomnia, are occasionally cause for discontinuation.

Dose

Start at 2 to 5 mg each morning (or evening if sedating) and consider titrating slowly to a therapeutic dose of 10 to 15 mg daily or until significant remission of symptoms is achieved.

Adverse effects

Common: Hypotension, akathisia, sedation

Serious: Seizures

Contraindications

History of seizures, dementia

Drug interactions

No absolute contraindications

Monitoring

Consider CMP, CBC, lipid profile, fasting blood glucose, weight, and ECG at baseline. Consider repeating at 3 months, 6 months, and every 6 months thereafter.

Pimozide (Orap®)

Pimozide is FDA approved for the treatment of Tourette syndrome. It belongs to the family of conventional antipsychotics and functions via the antagonism of dopaminergic D_2 receptors. It is among the most effective medications in DI, although due to safety concerns it may not be the ideal choice for the treatment of geriatric patients. A notable consideration in the use of pimozide is that because it is FDA indicated for the treatment of Tourette syndrome, patients do not perceive it to be an antipsychotic per se and may more readily engage in treatment. Further, pimozide often demonstrates a more pronounced effect on cutaneous dysesthesia symptoms. However, careful risk assessment should be performed prior to initiating therapy with pimozide for the treatment of elderly patients.

Dose

Start at 0.5 mg daily. Can consider increasing every 2 to 4 weeks by 0.5 to 1 mg increments to a therapeutic dose of 2 to 3 mg daily or until significant remission of symptoms is achieved.

Adverse effects

Common: Sedation, akinesia, EPS, anticholinergic symptoms

Serious: Tardive dyskinesia, NMS, arrhythmia

Contraindications

History of heart disease or arrhythmia, electrolyte imbalance, Parkinson's disease, dementia, chronic opioid use (theoretical concern for withdrawal), use of mediations listed under "Drug interactions"

Drug interactions

Antidepressants, antipsychotics, trazodone, doxepin, antiarrhythmics, calcium channel blocker s, cimetidine, macrolide antibiotics, systemic antifungals, HIV medications

Monitoring

Consider CMP, CBC, and ECG at baseline. Consider repeating at 3 months, 6 months, and every 6 months thereafter.

Major Depressive Disorder/ Obsessive-Compulsive Disorder

Geriatric patients with major depressive disorder (MDD) or obsessive-compulsive disorder (OCD) often require pharmacologic treatment due to psychological distress, interference with their daily lives, and, in the case of depression, the risk of self-harm, which is significantly elevated in this age group. It should be noted that, especially in the case of OCD, the use of concurrent behavioral therapy results in higher levels of treatment efficacy.

Selective serotonin reuptake inhibitors (SSRIs) are the class of choice when treating elderly patients with depression or OCD. In all patients with depression, bipolar disorder should be ruled out by careful screening for an underlying predisposition which may be indicated by a history of elevated mood, periods of decreased need for sleep, and/or increased risk taking, as well as a history of substance abuse or a positive family history of bipolar disorder, because antidepressants can trigger manic episodes. The clinician should be aware that improvement of symptoms may require at least 6 to 8 weeks of therapy, so slow titration of dose is warranted. Maintenance therapy should be provided for 12 months after a single episode of depression and for 1 to 3 years for recurrent depression. In the case of OCD, higher doses may be required for successful treatment.

Fluoxetine (Prozac®)

Fluoxetine is FDA approved for the treatment of MDD, OCD, bulimia nervosa, and panic disorder. Fluoxetine has the longest safety record of all SSRIs, demonstrates fewer drug-drug interactions, and is often more activating. Additionally, fluoxetine has a longer half-life than most SSRIs, a characteristic that is beneficial for patients in whom forgetfulness and rapid withdrawal secondary to missed doses may be a concern.

Dose

Start at 10 mg PO daily. Can consider gradually increasing the dose after several weeks to 20 to 60 mg daily or until significant remission of symptoms is achieved.

Adverse effects

Common: Nausea, insomnia, sexual dysfunction

Serious: Serotonin syndrome (if combined with other serotonergic mediations)
Contraindications
Bipolar disorder without presence of mood stabilizer
Drug interactions
Use of MAOIs within 14 days, tricyclic antidepressant s, trazodone, pimozide
Monitoring
Monitor for signs of worsening depression or suicidality.

Sertraline (Zoloft®)

Sertraline is FDA approved for the treatment of MDD, OCD, panic disorder, post-traumatic stress disorder, premenstrual dysphoric disorder, and social anxiety disorder. Sertraline is more sedating on the activation-sedation continuum and can be titrated over a large range of doses, allowing for more precise dose finding. It demonstrates few drug interactions and also has excellent anxiolytic effects.

Dose

Start at 25 mg daily. Can consider increasing by 25 mg increments each week up to 200 mg daily or until significant remission of symptoms is achieved. Taper slowly on discontinuation.

Adverse effects

Similar to fluoxetine but sedation, fatigue, mild weight gain, and GI disturbances are more common

Contraindications, drug interactions, and monitoring

Same as for fluoxetine.

Escitalopram (Lexapro®)

Escitalopram is FDA approved for the treatment of MDD and generalized anxiety disorder. Escitalopram is generally well-tolerated medication with few drug interactions and more activating effects. It is another good option for the treatment of geriatric patients with depression or OCD.

Dose

Start at 5 mg PO daily. May consider gradually increasing to 10 to 20 mg daily after one to two weeks. Taper slowly on discontinuation.

Adverse effects

Similar to fluoxetine but may cause fewer sexual side effects

Contraindications, drug interaction s, and monitoring

Same as for fluoxetine.

Anxiety

Generalized anxiety disorder in geriatric patients is best treated with buspirone and/or SSRIs. Benzodiazepines should be used with caution due to the risk of side effects including sedation, dyscoordination and falls, dependence, withdrawal symptoms, delirium, and decreased functional status with long-term use [4].

Buspirone (Buspar®)

Buspirone is a serotonin 5-HT_{1A} receptor partial agonist that demonstrates anxiolytic and antidepressant effects. It lacks the withdrawal symptoms and addictive potential of the benzodiazepines, is not sedating, and is generally well tolerated in geriatric patients. It should be noted that buspirone must be continued for at least 2 to 4 weeks to achieve therapeutic effect. It should not be used PRN, but instead taken on a regular basis 2 to 4 times per day.

Dose

Start at 7.5 mg twice daily. Can consider increasing by 5 mg per day every 2-3 days to 30 mg daily or until significant remission of symptoms is achieved.

Adverse effects

Usually only mild side effects such as headache and nausea

Contraindications

Use of MAOIs within 14 days

Drug interactions

MAOIs

Monitoring

No routine monitoring recommended.

Escitalopram (Lexapro®)

Escitalopram is also an effective option for the treatment of GAD in the elderly. See description above under Major Depressive Disorder/Obsessive-Compulsive Disorder.

Benzodiazepines

Benzodiazepines potentiate the effects of gamma-aminobutyric acid (GABA) and can play a role in the treatment of panic attacks or other situations requiring acute relief from anxiety. It is recommended that benzodiazepines not be used on a regular, long-term basis in geriatric patients. Although in general lower doses of benzodiazepines are recommended for elderly patients, some patients may require higher dosages, so an individualized approach is indicated. The half-life of benzodiazepines varies widely, and in general shorter-acting medications are preferable.

Lorazepam (Ativan®)

Lorazepam is FDA approved for the treatment of anxiety disorder s, including panic attacks and generalized anxiety disorder. It is also approved for status epilepticus, preoperative sedation, and the short-term treatment of insomnia. It has an intermediate half-life with a short onset of action. Unlike many benzodiazepines, lorazepam does not undergo hepatic metabolism and, for this reason, may result in a more predictable response in geriatric patients. Due to its potential adverse effects, lorazepam therapy should be limited to short courses using as needed dosing.

Dose

Start at 0.5 mg every 4-6 hours as needed, encouraging minimal use given its sedating properties and potential for dependence and abuse. Can consider gradually increasing to no more than 2 mg every 4-6 hours as needed for anxiety with a total dose not to exceed 2 to 6 mg per 24 hours. Taper dose gradually to discontinue.

Adverse effects

Common: Sedation, unsteadiness, confusion

Serious: Delirium, ataxia, respiratory depression, withdrawal symptoms such as seizures, tachycardia, insomnia, and rebound anxiety if abrupt discontinuation

Contraindications

Acute narrow angle glaucoma, sleep apnea and other causes of compromised respiratory function (e.g., COPD), severe hepatic impairment (requires dose reduction)

Drug interactions

Sodium oxybate, other CNS depressants including alcohol

Monitoring

Consider assessing need for continued therapy on a regular basis.

Alprazolam (Xanax®)

Alprazolam is FDA approved for the treatment of panic attacks and generalized anxiety disorder. It has the shortest half-life of all benzodiazepines and a rapid onset of action. At the same time that these characteristics make it particularly useful for patients suffering from panic attacks and reduce the occurrence of morning-after effects, they also contribute to increased potential for abuse and dependence as well as rebound anxiety. It is also important to note that alprazolam demonstrates decreased clearance in elderly patients, and careful titration is necessary to avoid relative overdose. Treatment with alprazolam should also be limited to short courses of therapy using as needed dosing at the lowest possible dose.

Dose

Start at 0.125 mg every 4 hours as needed, encouraging minimal use given its sedating properties and potential for dependence and abuse. Can consider gradually increasing dose to 0.25 to 0.5 mg every 4 hours as needed if clinically indicated with a total dose not to exceed 2 mg per 24 hours. Taper dose gradually to discontinue.

Adverse effects

Similar to lorazepam

Contraindications

Acute narrow angle glaucoma, sleep apnea other causes of compromised respiratory function (e.g., COPD), hepatic impairment (requires dose reduction), use of CYP3A4 inhibitors

Drug interactions

Sodium oxybate, other CNS depressants, CYP3A4 inhibitors and inducers

Monitoring

Consider assessing need for continued therapy on a regular basis.

References

[1] Fanoe, S., Kristensen, D., Fink-Jensen, A., et al. Risk of arrhythmia induced by psychotropic medications: a proposal for clinical management. *Eur. Heart J.* 2014;35: 1306-15.

[2] Freudenmann, R. W., Lepping, P. Second-generation antipsychotics in primary and secondary delusional parasitosis: outcome and efficacy. *J. Clin. Psychopharmacol.* 2008;28:500-8.

[3] Guenette, M. D., Chintoh, A., Remington, G., Hahn, M. Atypical antipsychotic - induced metabolic disturbances in the elderly. *Drugs Aging* 2014;31:159-84.

[4] Peron, E. P., Gray, S. L., Hanlon, J. T. Medication use and functional status decline in older adults: a narrative review. *Am. J. Geriatr. Pharmacother*. 2011;9:378-91.

In: Geriatric Psychodermatology
Editors: Mohammad Jafferany and Katlein França
ISBN: 978-1-63463-853-1

Chapter 4

Psychotherapies for Late Life Psychiatric Issues

Ruqiya Shama Tareen, M.D. and Kinza Tareen, BS*

Interface of Geriatrics and Psychotherapy

Elder adults are less likely to seek psychiatric or psychological help than younger people. A study conducted by Kalp et al. revealed that only 7% of adults age 60 and above were likely to seek help for their mental illness compared to 26% of middle aged adults.[1] Furthermore, only 1% of older adults were referred to a mental health specialist by their primary care physician [1]. A majority of the geriatric population is unaware of treatment options available and the efficacy of psychotherapies [1]. Additionally, some of the societal beliefs and myths regarding mental health that the older population has acquired over the years, impacts their ability to identify mental health issues as important enough and to actively seek help. The concept of mental health illnesses and appropriate treatments was conceptualized very differently a few decades ago. This generation of adults grew up in an era in which mental illness was considered a taboo and automatically implied a poor prognosis. Mentally ill patients were isolated from society and were routinely treated in long-term residential mental institutions. Over the years, vast advancements and improvements have been made in acceptance and treatment of mental illness. However, this may not change the preconceived notions the older populations of adults have developed about the mental health issues. As a result, it is likely they may still feel threatened by the notion that their dermatological condition is arising from or is perpetuating psychological issues.

Furthermore, adding to the divide between psychotherapists and the geriatric population was a very traditional practice of medicine. Until recently, a majority of old-age care was delivered exclusively by doctors, nurses, and social workers, as care generally focused on physical ailments and the social issues arising from the change in life circumstances with aging. Psychotherapists were not included in traditional care of geriatric patients until the last

* Corresponding author: Ruqiya Shama Tareen. E-mail: shama.tareen@med.wmich.edu

couple of decades. It was a common belief that older adults were not good candidates for psychotherapy due to their advance age and were considered cognitively inflexible.

Although psychotherapy in geriatric patients has been successfully reported in literature for a over eight decades, it is surprising that there remains a limited amount of therapists who are professionally trained to provide psychotherapy to older adults, or who are comfortable doing so [2]. This is due to the fact that the traditional psychology training programs did not provide any in depth gerontology focused psychotherapy training [2]. Despite the initial hesitation, in last few decades psychotherapy with older adults is gaining more acceptance and more psychotherapists are beginning to work with older adults, focusing on the unique aspects of working with these patients.

Special Challenges of Psychotherapy with Older Adults

Although, psychotherapy has proven to be successful in the treatment of older adults, it is not without some challenges. Sensory decline especially hearing deficit, vision decline, and physical limitations in mobility are the most commonly encountered challenges in practice. The therapist may have to accommodate to the physical and sensory challenges of their older adult clients in their office setting. For instance, an office should be handicapped friendly, well lit, and should not have loose rugs or other objects crowding the hallways or walking area to avoid any risk of falls. Furthermore, efficient therapy may require a therapist to sit more closer to the patient, face them directly so they can observe the lip movements, speak clearly while emphasizing consonants, and speak in a low pitch voice [3]. Additionally, cognitive decline related with aging, may cause difficulties in therapy unless therapists help patients develop some techniques to remember and recall the information they are working on. They may have to mutually develop some ways to counter the cognitive problems by using techniques of memory cueing; use of mnemonics, or some other homework assignments to ensure progress [3].

Another challenge in treating older adults with psychotherapy may arise from complications in scheduling. Older adults may deal with physical frailty and medical issues that may surface from time to time, impacting scheduling because of unexpected cancellations. Also older patients may be dependent on others to come to appointments due to inability to drive. Psychotherapists must be aware of these challenges and be willing to accommodate patients when needed and to provide psychotherapy in an optimal way despite these challenges. On the other hand, psychotherapy can be utilized effectively to enhance compliance in older adults with major health issues including psychodermatological issues of chronic nature requiring strict and multiple regimen of biologic treatments. Psychotherapeutic alliance and support can motivate older adults to adhere to the proposed treatment plan, help them adapt to change in level of functioning, and to move them forward psychologically to accept the consequences of nonadherence with treatment. Lack of mobility remains a challenge in treating older adults with psychotherapy.

Patients may be housebound or even immobilized to the extent that they are confined to their room or bed [3] This can be very relevant in a patient with illness like severe psoriatic arthropathy. This should not preclude them from engaging in psychotherapy and in fact may be the only outlet they have to engage in a therapeutic alliance beside the visits from nurses and related health care workers. The interactions they have with nurses are generally limited to focus on the task at hand and do not engage or stimulate the patient psychologically. Medicare covers at-home therapy, and if such service is available psychotherapist should take advantage and strive to engage patients in such therapeutic alliance [3].

Transference and countertransference can be much more pronounced in working with older adults in comparision to other populations. The older adults are usually not comfortable with the idea of being considered as in need of receiving mental health treatment especially psychotherapy and they may consider it as a sign of weakness, being labeled in certain way or fear of being called "crazy" craeating transference issues. While on the other hand therapist specially if they are not used to working with older adults may have difficulties with countertransference because of unique aspects of treating older adults like concerns about their frality and physical difficulties, social issues like transportation,insurance issues etc causing difficulties in engaging and keeping them in treatment. Younger therapist may have countertransfernece issue to identifying older patient with their parents, grandparents or teachers which they had diffuclties with while growing up [3]

Supportive Psychotherapy (ST)

Supportive psychotherapy (ST) is a psychotherapeutic approach at the beginning of the spectrum of psychotherapy. However, it can be argued that all forms of psychotherapy involve some extent of supportive Psychotheraputic work. ST can be employed with relative ease in acute care settings or with patients facing acute changes in their life circumstances affecting their emotional wellbeing. The aim of this therapy is to strengthen a patient's ego by providing them support about their current stressors and to enable patients to adapt well to challenges. ST was conceptualized to identify and enhance the inherent abilities of the patient, in hopes to help them cope with their stressors, help them realize their own potential by motivating them to recognize their own role in coping with what ever the stressors they are facing. ST can involve use of some explorative and interpretative techniques if needed [4]. Older adults often face changes in living environment like moving to a nursing home, medical and physical issues affecting function, loss of loved ones, and disability associated with cognitive deficits. All of these life changes can affect emotional balance, and ST treatment is an ideal treatment option. ST can be especially helpful in the early stages of engaging older patients dealing with psychodermatological diseases as its non-exploratory and non-judgmental approach may put patients at ease and help patient accept the therapy. ST focuses on conscious issues apparent to the patient, what symptoms they are dealing with, and how it is affecting their life. However, if transference issues surface, especially negative transferences, therapist should deal it early on as it will significantly impede the progress of therapy. On the other hand, positive transferences can be utilized and not analyzed to motivate patient in a certain positive direction. ST can be much more flexible and adaptive to the patients and settings requirement then other therapies. Sessions can be timed according to need, and can be brief. The ultimate goal of ST is to create a sense of responsibility in a patient who may feel frozen due to the current stressors to recognize their own responsibility in this situation and to motivate patients to move forward. Additionally, ST strengthens a sense of individuality and helps integrate and enhance positive traits of personality [4, 5]

Psychodynamic Psychotherapy (Insight Oriented Therapy)

Sigmund Freud proposed the psychoanalytic basis of the psychodynamic psychotherapy. He argued that self-directed anger resulted from difficulties experienced during early childhood and affects a person's personality in such a way that it predisposes one to develop depression and melancholia.

Freud later laid down the basic foundation of psychoanalysis and insight oriented therapy utilizing the principles of Id, Ego and Superego. The main techniques utilized are interpreting transference, countertransference, resistance and defense mechanisms.

Psychodynamic psychotherapy is utilized in different therapies essentially focusing on the developmental issues, which have impacted a person's psyche in a profound way affecting their abilities to cope with their current life in a healthy way. It relies heavily on the interplay of therapist – patient relationship. Therapists employ the free association technique while carefully and empathically listening for the emerging themes and patterns. Therapist's ability to interpret the transference, counter transference and resistance phenomenon in expert way and utilizing them in timely manner directs the therapy in the right direction [6]

The empirical evidence to support the efficacy of psychodynamic psychotherapy in late life is not very clear and usually it is not the first choice of therapy for older adults. However, this form of therapy can be utilized very effectively by an expert therapist in older adults to help patients adapt to changes in life, reflect and prepare for what lies ahead, identifying and resolving damaging interpersonal patterns arising from earlier experiences, exploring their fears about the future and present, as well enabling patients to deal with their new reality [3]

Originally, Freud's concept of psychodynamic therapy was thought to be limited in only benefiting younger than 50 years old. However, later work in this field has shown that if carefully selected, older adults can also benefit from this approach in same way as their younger counterparts.

Contrary to common belief, older adults can be good candidates for insight-oriented therapy depending on their cognitive status. Even patients with dementia who have a mild to moderate cognitive impairment can benefit from this therapy. In cases where cognitive status is declined, further involvement of family members is required and therapy can be done both as individual and family therapy [3] It is difficult for older adults to conceptualize the framework of psychodynamic psychotherapy and therefore, this may result in a premature rejection to engage in such therapy. It is imperative for the therapist to explain to the patient in such terms which are easily understandable yet able to establish a clear understanding of the therapeutic process. Helping older adults understand that insight oriented therapy is based on empathic listening while therapist is helping the patient to explore underlying unconscious conflicts and to explore and clarify them with the help of patient to reach a state where they can deal with conflict in healthy ways [3]

Interpersonal Therapy (IPT)

IPT is a time limited structured therapy consisting of 16 weeks of weekly sessions addressing four main areas where interpersonal relations hip can be challenged and can give rise to persisting depression. The first of the four focus areas is grief, which could be related to the death of a loved one or loss in any other meaningful way. This area of focus is often relevant to older adults who are experiencing grief from the loss of spouses, friends, and family members. Older patients may also experience interpersonal conflict as a result of increasing medial and cognitive issues that consequently impact their function and behavior causing interpersonal disputes with others. Furthermore, old age presents a time of role transitions: the third area of focus of IPT. With retirement, change in social structure, decline in physical abilities, and cognitive deficit there are many opportunities for role transition in life which may not be accepted positively, resulting in feeling of worthlessness leading to depression.

All of the above if not dealt well causes interpersonal deficits; the fourth area of IPT [7]. IPT is a manual based treatment, which does not need to be altered much when working with older adults. IPT although not extensively studied in older populations is well suited for this demographic and has shown to be effective in addressing the challenges of interpersonal difficulties older patients experience when depressed. The therapist analyzes the pertinent interpersonal incidents and communication styles in order to help the patient develop an understanding their role in interpersonal difficulties. Once this is identified, the therapist then the works to delineate the interpersonal factors contributing to the depression and anxiety. IPT has shown to be effective when addressing sociality in older adults. By employing IPT to improve interpersonal difficulties, social connectedness, improving sense of self worth and self-esteem, and alleviating despair and dysphoria IPT can reduce the helplessness and hopelessness leading to suicidal thoughts [7]

Interpersonal and Social Rhythm Therapy (IPSRT)

IPSRT is a newer therapy developed by Ellen Frank in 2005 by combining two therapies, interpersonal therapy (IPT) and social rhythm therapy (SRT) for the treatment of major depression and bipolar disorder. IPSRT is a time-limited therapy, consisting of 20-24 sessions of individual therapy delivered over a period of 8 months. IPSRT techniques take into account the fact that most relapses of bipolar disorder occur as a result of major life events causing disruption of interpersonal harmony, non-compliance with treatment and/or interruption of social rhythm [8]. The goals of the IPSRT include: (1) to increase compliance to pharmacotherapy, (2) to develop skills for healthy coping with life-events, and (3) to restore, maintain and monitor of a healthy circadian rhythm.

Most major mood episodes are preceded by major life events. IPT was first developed to address these issues in the four main domains of life events: grief and loss, role transitions, role disputes, and interpersonal sensitivity. IPSRT also addresses an additional domain, "loss of healthy self." A common problem encountered with patients with patients with bipolar disorder is the denial of the disease and not accepting the need for treatment. IPSRT can be employed to help patients develop an acceptance of their diseased-self, with this comes the emergence of the grief about loss of one's healthy-self, and expectation from oneself and recognition of some of the damages to self, social and romantic relations, and possible decline in economic prospects [8, 9]

Affective disorders are associated with disturbances of the basic circadian rhythmslike sleep, appetite, cortisol levels, thermoregulation and activity level. IPSRT emphasizes treatment on establishing social event rhythm like a set time to wake up and go to bed, having a scheduled time for productive activity for school or work, and engaging in meaningful social events and activities. Having a structured social rhythmic activity along with a well-established circadian rhythm promotes stability of mood and prevents relapses of a major mood episode, be it depression, mania or hypomania [8]

Cognitive Behavior Therapy (CBT)

Cognitive therapy (CT) is based on the initial work of Aaron T. Beck conducted in 1963. Beck, the father of cognitive behavioral therapy, was concerned about the lack of empirical evidence regarding psychoanalytical approaches. This led him to search for more structured ways of doing therapy, which can be assessed for efficacy in a meaningful way. He developed CT based on information processing theory, which required a more active role from therapist as well as the patient, by utilizing structured tools and assignments to assess and monitor progress. Beck realized that the difficulties encountered in early development causes cognitive distortions or automatic thoughts, and hence affect the formation of personality. He believed that distorted or negative cognitive schema about self, the future, and the personal world impacts a person's ability to perceive things positively. This in turn impacts a person's feelings negatively and results in faulty behaviors [10].

Behavioral therapy (BT) has been effective especially in older adults with cognitive impairment such as dementia. Behavioral therapy is based on the premise that the stressors create the formation of maladaptive coping mechanisms resulting in negative behavior that leads to decreased response and diminished contingent positive reinforcement. The deficit of positive activities leading to relaxation and pleasure in life while the person employ more faulty coping mechanism gives rise to dysphoria and anxiety. This negative feedback loop results in self-criticism as well as faulty perceptions and behaviors. BT has shown to be effective in older adults especially those living in long term care facilities. The goal of BT in this population is to increase the pleasant experiences and to reduce unpleasant experiences by keeping logs of these events. Training the staff of long term facilities to utilize operant methods and making appropriate changes in milieu while utilizing the logs to document pleasant versus unpleasant events can improve late life depression outcome in older patients even with mild to moderate level of dementia [11]

The combination of cognitive and behavioral therapy is called cognitive behavioral therapy (CBT). In CBT the therapist start with helping patients identify the automatic thoughts and link it to the negative feelings it creates which ultimately results in dysfunctional behaviors. The task for the patient is to learn to make a conscious effort to identify the negative thoughts linking it to unpleasant feeling resulting in maladaptive behaviors. Mastery of linking these together and by practicing how to recognize the automatic negative thoughts early on and attempt to replace it with a positive thoughts, eventually leads to better functional outcomes [10, 11]

The efficacy of CBT in geriatric population has been well established. CBT can be employed with little changes in older adults. There may be some more challenges when the older adults also have physical and cognitive frailty. This may require adjustments in logistics of providing CBT, such as the patient's ability to come for the session and how often and for how long therapy is going to be conducted. Also therapist must also take into account what type of homework assignments can realistically be expected to be completed and in what time frame [10, 11]

Problem Solving Therapy (PST)

An offshoot of cognitive behavioral therapy, PST focuses on training in constructive problem-solving attitudes and skills [12] PST aims to help reduce the symptoms of psychological distress while also addressing behaviors that are counterproductive and may cause relapse of psychiatric issues while trying to improve and maintain quality of life [12] Since its inception in early 1970s, PST has evolved from a simple framework of cognitive mediation to facilitate self control to achieve better behavior outcomes, and has become a more sophisticated concept which can be employed as a stand alone treatment, part of other treatment modalities like group therapy, as an acute treatment, or as a maintenance or prevention program in all age groups including older adults [12]. The initial treatment consists of time limited PST weekly sessions that aim to teach patients a five step problem solving (PS) model. The first five weeks are devoted to learn the PS model and the remaining sessions are devoted to master it by learning and refining problem solving skills [13]. Active participation of patients is required to set the goals and objective of treatment, realist self evaluation about their ability to reach those goals, and alternate ways to achieve goals if initial plan does not work out. The last two sessions focus on devising a plan to prevent relapse and to deal with problems as they arise after treatment [5, 13].

Reminiscence or Life Review Therapy

Reminiscence or life review therapy is a relatively new form of therapy, which was developed especially for the older patients to facilitate and enhance the normal aging process and psychological growth. The elderly population deals with a very unique challenge, not only there is loss of vitality, physical and cognitive abilities, shrinking of social network due to the loss of friends and family members, but also there is a definite sense of loss of relevance to the present world. Reminiscence is a normal process of old age where one reflects back on his or her life and takes an inventory of what was done or not done, and how to reorganize life in a way to accommodate the lessons learned to move forward in life. According to the Erikson's stages of life they stand on the path of "integrity versus despair " and if reminiscence is not dealt in a positive and productive manner they may end up in deep valley of despair as they will be focusing on what was not done right or cannot be done any more [14, 15].

To employ reminiscence as an active tool in therapy, therapist must do so in a structured way in individual or group settings. One of the commonly used techniques is to ask patients to write, the assignments can range from writing letters to loved ones to writing a biographical sketch. Other methods include asking them to make scrapbook or to review old photo albums from certain stages of their life. Life review also promotes discovering the long lost social connections by attending reunions, and revisiting places, which hold special significance in their life. This stage in life also represents a time in which older adults may be interested to rediscover self in light of his or her ethnic or cultural identity. Therapist can encourage this form of life review by assigning tasks like constructing genealogy trees, and actively learning about one's cultural and ethnic background. One drawback associated with life review therapy is that if a patient has negative schema of life to begin with or if they are already chronically or severely depressed, life review techniques may cause negative rumination and obsessive tendencies to linger on the bad memories. In these cases, it will be difficult for the patient to make a shift to the positive side. The life review process tends to bring out for them mostly the negatives in life and they tend to overlook the positive things in life. Such situations may require a more active role from the therapist in order to help the patient process the negative aspects of their life in a way, which leads to a better outcome. Patients with positive egos and higher education are able to move forward despite dealing with significant depression [16, 14, 15].

Group Therapy (GT)

Group therapy has been used in acute and long term care settings for the elderly to provide peer interaction and ability to engage in cognitively stimulating activities. Groups can be purely psychoeducational addressing the issues at hand like how to cope with aging, certain disease, etc. Groups can also be more of psychosocial nature promoting a sense of community, or social connectedness. Another variation in GT arises from organization based on certain therapeutic philosophy like insight oriented psychodynamic model, interpersonal, or cognitive behavioral therapy. Older adults in general tend to enjoy being in groups and are able to establish therapeutic alliances with group leaders and the other participants. Group therapy also encourages the role of a group leader who can guide the discussion in a meaningful way and keep the group focused on the task at hand [17]

Life review therapy groups can be very helpful in patients living in community living establishments such as assisted living or nursing homes. Many older adults living in these settings face difficulties adapting to a totally unfamiliar place where nothing is relevant to them, it is likely that this will impact their emotional equilibrium significantly. Life review therapy employs techniques from various modes of stimulating discussions about the events of the past that are relevant to the geriatric population. The group leader and co-leader use photos, music, TV programs, videos, newspaper articles, magazine articles, and other objects to reminiscence the past years to engage participants in a stimulating discussion by sharing their personal experiences and memories. This form of GT encourages participants to engage with each other on a more personal level, enhancing the sense of attachment, and promoting more social interactions outside the group. Participants also build a strong sense of community in a place where they previously did not feel a sense of belonging. This newly developed sense of community and belongingness prevents depression. Therefore, the GT helps decrease the depression and anxiety which is usually encountered in elders living in such settings where they do not feel socially attached or have a sense of identity and self worth [18]

Music Therapy

Music therapy is known to stimulate the brain by releasing corticotropic hormone and norepinephrine. It has shown to improve general sense of well being, ability of daily functioning, vitality, social functioning, and emotional well being and depressive and anxiety symptoms [19] Music therapy has also shown effectiveness in reducing behavioral deregulation and anxiety in moderate to severe patients with Alzheimer's dementia [20]. As a result of the success seen in the treatment of older patients diagnosed with Alzheimer's, music therapy should be explored in the treatment of older patients with other mental illness es.

Animal/Pet Therapy for Older Adults

Humans have a natural affinity to connect emotionally with pet animals and find it fulfilling. Relatedness with animals can be carried over in human relationships and this was therapeutically utilized for the first time in 18th century when a hospital allowed psychiatrically ill patients in residential treatment to keep and care for small animals to help promote some sense of responsibility, self control, and the ability to develop and sustain relationships [21] Many hospitals and other places of care provisions for elderly employ animal therapy in some form and has been found be of good value. With aging comes loss of relationships, diminished responsibilities, lack of independence, and at times lack of connectedness from others. Having a pet or being in pet therapy on a regular basis promotes the elderly to reconnect in a meaningful way. Furthermore, pet therapy has been shown to increase verbal responses and decrease in latency of verbal responses in elderly patients [21].

Efficacy of Psychotherapy in Older Adults

Thompson et al. compared the efficacy of brief psychodynamic psychotherapy, behavioral therapy, and cognitive behavioral therapy in older adults, in the treatment of major depressive disorder. The study concluded that while there was no post treatment difference, all three treatment groups indicated a significant improvement in depressive symptoms as well as on the measures of improvement in function in older adults. Overall, 70% of older adults who received any of the three types of psychotherapy for six weeks either achieved remission from depression or showed significant improvements in their depression [22].

Interpersonal psychotherapy has also shown significant reduction in overall depressive symptoms, greater sense of wellbeing, and minimized suicidal ideation [7]. These improvements were carried on in some patients at a 6 months follow up [7]. Reminiscence therapies of various kinds including, music, dance, group, art, and movement therapies have gained a central role in residential facilities and nursing homesproviding care to the elderly patients. Reminiscence therapies are shown to improve some of cognitive function by utilizing reality orientation care methods while improvement in physical functioning and behavior in patients with severe dementia was not significantly improved with these techniques [15] Moreover, group reminiscence intervention has been shown to improve depressive symptoms and behavioral disturbances in patients with dementia [18].

Various studies have shown that psychotherapies are effective in treating late life depression. A meta-analysis was conducted to quantify the efficacy of different types of psychotherapies including brief dynamic therapy, cognitive behavioral therapy, cognitive therapy, behavioral therapy, problem-solving therapy, bibliotherapy, interpersonal therapy, interpersonal counseling, reminiscence therapy, and home based problem adaptation therapy. The study analyzed standardized mean difference (SMD) in the score of depression evaluated by the validated depression scales. The authors determined that although psychotherapies are effective in treating late life depression, the size of SMD was dependent on the type of control group used to measure the difference from the baseline. The control groups used in the trials ranged from placebo, waitlist group, attention group, treatment as usual (pharmacotherapy or no treatment at all), and supportive therapy.

The most significant SMD was noted when the comparison was done with the least effect size noted to be when supportive psychotherapy was used as the comparison group. While patients in treatment as usual or waitlist showed greatest difference with psychotherapy. This meta analysis did not find any difference between the efficacy of different therapies however the comparison may not be fair as some therapies examined and compared were fewer in number and/or were conducted with small numbers of participants [23]. CT, BT and CBT have been proven to be effective in decreasing depression in geriatric patients. Overall over 50% older patients have achieved remission in depression and the remissions sustained in over 80% of patients at one year follow up. Over 75% of patients continued to do better at two year follow up [24].

Cuijpers et al. compared 44 studies with older adult subjects comparing efficacy of different psychotherapies to control groupsand other therapies including pharmacotherapy. They included studies of older adults who received psychotherapies including brief psychodynamic, IPT, PST, CBT, internet based CBT (iCBT), self guided help, and dialectical behavioral therapy (DBT). They concluded that receiving psychotherapy irrespective of the type of therapy caused a moderate to high degree of effect on depressive symptomatology in older adults and this effect was sustained at 6 month follow ups. They also confirmed the CBT is most effective treatment, however they also found that life review and PST are also very effective in this population [25]

Conclusion

Psychotherapy is an important and effective tool that has shown efficacy in geriatric population. The earlier notion that elderly patients were unfit candidates for certain types of psychotherapies has limited the use of psychotherapy in this population, however research is proving to negate that notion. Older adults even with some cognitive difficulties continue to retain the abilities to engage, establish therapeutic relationship, ability for reflection and introspection, and to utilize the skills learned to improve their psychological and emotional wellbeing all of which are required to be an active participant in therapy.

References

[1] Klap R, Unroe KT, Unutzer J. Caring for mental illness in the United States: A focus on older adults. *Am. J. Geriatr Psychiatry*. 2013 Oct; 11(5):517-24.

[2] Knight BG. Gerontology with Psychotherapist. In: *Psychotherapy with Older Adults* 3rd ed. California: Sage Publications; 2004.

[3] Morgan AC. Psychodynamic psychotherapy with older adults. *Psychiatric Services*. 2013; 54(12):1592-94.

[4] Dewald PA. Principles of supportive psychotherapy. *Am. J. Psychotherapy*. 1994; 48(4):505-18.

[5] Alexopoulos GS, Raue PJ, Kiosses DN, Mackin RS, Kanellopoulos D, McCulloch C, Areán PA. Problem solving therapy and supportive therapy in older adults with major depression and executive dysfunction: effect on disability. *Arch. Gen. Psychiatry*. 2011 Jan; 68(1): 33–41.

[6] Stein DJ, Kupfer DJ, Schatzber AF, editors. Psychoanalytic and psychodynamic psychotherapy for depression and dysthymia. In: *The American Psychiatric Publishing Textbook of Mood Disorders*. American Psychiatric Pub; 2007.

[7] Heisel MJ, Talbot NL, King DA, Tu XM. Adapting interpersonal psychotherapy for older adults at risk for suicide. *Am. J. Geriatr. Psychiatry*. 2009; 40(2):156-64.

[8] Frank E, Kupfer DJ, Thase ME, Mallinger AG. Two-year outcomes for interpersonal and social rhythm therapy in individuals with bipolar I disorder. *Arch. Gen. Psychiatry*. 2005 Sep;62(9):996-1004.

[9] Bouwkamp CG, de Kruiff ME, van Troost TM, Snippe D, Blom MJ, de Winter RF, Judith Haffmans PM. Interpersonal and social rhythm group therapy for patients with bipolar disorder. *Am. J. Psychiatry*. 2010 Nov; 167(11):1391-8.

[10] Karel MJ, Hinrichsen G. Treatment of depression in late life: psychotheraputic interventions. Clin Psychol Rev. 2000 Aug; 20(6):707-29.

[11] Francis JL, Kumar A. Psychological treatment of late-life depression. *Psychiatr. Clin. North Am*. 2013 Dec;36(4):561-75.

[12] Dobson KS, editor. Problem- solving therapy. In: *Handbook of Cognitive-Behavioral Therapies*. 3rd edi. New York, NY: Guilford Press; 2010.

[13] Areán PA, Raue P, Mackin RS, Kanellopoulos D, McCulloch C, Alexopoulos GS. Problem-solving therapy and supportive therapy in older adults with major depression and executive dysfunction. *Am. J. Psychiatry*. 2010; 167(11):1391–98.

[14] Meléndez-Moral JC. Charco-Ruiz L, VIayordomo-Rodríguez T, Sales-Galán A. Effects of a reminiscence program among institutionalized elderly adults. *Psicothema* 2013; 25(3):319-23.

[15] Wang JJ, Yena M, OuYang WC. Group reminiscence intervention in Taiwanese elders with dementia. *Archives of Gerontology and Geriatrics*. 2009; 49(2):227-32.

[16] Fry PS. Structured and unstructured reminiscence training and depression among the elderly. *Clinical Gerontologist*. 1983; 1:15–37.

[17] Myers WA, editor. Group therapy in later life. In: *Techniques in the Psychotherapy of Older Patients*. Washington, D.C: American Psychiatric Pressl 1991.

[18] Hsu YC, Wang JJ. Physical, affective, and behavioral effects of group reminiscence on depressed institutionalized elders in Taiwan. *Nursing Research*. 2009; 58(4):294-99.

[19] Lee YY, Chan MF, Mok E. Effectiveness of music intervention on the quality of life of older people. *Journal of Advanced Nursing*. 2010; 66(12):2677–87.

[20] Svansdottir HB, Snaedal J. Music therapy in moderate and severe dementia of Alzheimer's type: a case–control study. *International Psychogeriatrics*. 2006 Dec; 18(4):613-21.

[21] Brickel CM. A review of the roles of pet animals in psychotherapy and with the elderly. *Int'l J Aging and Human Development.* 1980; 12(2):119-28.

[22] Thomson LW, Gallagher D, Breckenridge JS. Comparative effectiveness of psychotherapies for depressed elders. *Journal of Consulting and Clinical Psychology* 1987; 55(3):385-90.

[23] Huang AX, Delucchi K, Dunn LB, Nelson CJ. A systematic review and meta-analysis of psychotherapy for late-life depression. *Am. J. Geriatr. Psychiatry. Forthcoming* 2014 Apr.

[24] Gallagher-Thompson D, Hanley-Peterson P, Thompson LW. Maintenance of gains versus relapse following brief psychotherapy for depression. *Journal of Consulting and Clinical Psychology*. 1990; 58(3):371-74.

[25] Cuijpers P, Karyotaki E, Pot AM, Park M, Reynolds CF 3rd. Managing depression in older age: psychological interventions. *Marturitas. Forthcoming* 2014 Jun.

Part II. Psychiatric Disorders with Dermatologic Symptoms

In: Geriatric Psychodermatology
Editors: Mohammad Jafferany and Katlein França
ISBN: 978-1-63463-853-1

Chapter 5

Body Dysmorphic Disorder in the Elderly

Lucia Tomas-Aragones, Ph.D.
and Servando Marron, M.D.

Introduction

The brain forms internal maps of the external world and each person holds within the brain a mental representation of the body and its parts as it moves through space. People do not notice they have a body schema until they lose it or feel it is permanently altered, as for example in Body Dysmorphic Disorder, where a normal part of the body is perceived as distorted.

Mental Health in the Elderly

The world population has never been as mature as now and this figure is increasing rapidly. People aged 60 can now expect to survive an additional 18.5 to 21.6 years. Soon the world will have a higher number of older adults than children.

According to the World Health Organization [1], approximately 15% of adults aged 60 and over suffer from a mental disorder yet mental health problems are under-identified by healthcare professionals and older people themselves. The stigma surrounding mental illness makes people reluctant to seek help, however, mental health has an impact on psychical health and vice versa, thus the importance of prompt recognition and treatment.

Dementia and depression are the mental disordersmost widely studied in the elderly. Other mental disorders, such as Body Dysmorphic Disorder (BDD), have received less attention in this age group and few results have been published. This lack of information is

* Corresponding author: Lucia Tomas-Aragones. Email: luciatomas@cop.es

perhaps due to the fact that many studies have used an > 65 year old exclusion criteria, and in the case of BDD there seems to be a decrease with age. However, the aging of the gobal population and a significant increase in the proportion of older adults in the population are making research into aging issues a priority.

Additionally, the aging process may cause a major adjustment disorder in some people. In fact, the incidence of some psychiatric emergencies such as suicide increases with age. [2]

The epidemiology of mental disorderschanges across age groups. According to the literature, mood, cognitive disorders (e.g., dementias), and secondary disorders (i.e., "organic") appear to predominate in later life. However, most studies have used mixed age samples with a mean age under 45 years or have specifically excluded persons over age 60 or 65 years. Lyness et al. (1999) [3] found that mental disorders are common in older primary care patients; 31.7% of patients had at least one active psychiatric condition at the time of the interview. [3]

As mentioned above, suicide ratesincrease with age – the highest suicide rates being among persons older than 65 years. Psychiatric illness is a major contributing factor and more than 90% of individuals who take their lives suffer from such an illness. [4]

Multimorbidity is also a common problem in the elderly and its occurrence rises with age. In the age group of 65 - 69, 32% of the population suffers three or more chronic conditions. In the age group 80-84 the prevalence of multimorbidity increases to 52%. Multimorbidity is associated with higher mortality, increased disability, a decline of functional status and lower quality of life. [5]

Aging and Ageism

In the process of aging, we begin to lose strength, agility, speed, health, wit and beauty. Large doses of adaptation and acceptance are required to assimilate these changes, and coming to terms with a changed body image can be rather traumatic for some individuals.

Older men seem to be less concerned about their appearances than younger men and women their age, but are more sensitive about the physical decline and disfiguring and disabling conditions, as well as masculinity image loss. [6] On the contrary, older women seem to be as concerned and dissatisfied about their bodily appearance as younger ones [7], although the concern focus shifts from appearance to functionality. [8] However, others say that women of these ages are less concerned about their image due to the fact that they are less exposed to social pressures. [9]

The media promotes athletic skinny bodies wearing fashionable clothes. This helps to promote the idea that being old is "bad". It has been suggested that elderly people reject a stereotyped image in which they do not recognize themselves and their peers, even more so than accepting their age. Consequently, avoidance of this aging image seems reasonable in order to elude the consequent prejudice [10], and a possible reaction to face an old image is to try to conceal it by means of masquerade; creating a façade to try to obscure physical and social manifestations of old age. [11]

The social and cultural meanings of growing old are constantly changing in time, and being old nowadays has negative connotations. Old age is viewed as a medical and social problem that needs to be addressed. There is a high value placed by society on the maintenance of a youthful appearance and even the reversal of some of the aging-related bodily changes. [2]

Society tends to equate both beauty and productivity to youth, especially in women.

The aging of the appearance can elicit certain reactions from others, which can affect the individual's quality of life and psychological well-being.

Aging lies within the spectrum of normal human experience, however aging of the appearance can adversely affect the quality of life. Some of the psychosocial factors associated with aging skin include the effect of an aging appearance upon interpersonal interactions, which can lead to social anxiety, and social isolation. Excessive concerns about an aging appearance may be associated with body image disorders. [2]

Ageism is socially constructed and reproduced at all levels of the society. Ageist practices harm everyone, not just elders. Currently, women of all ages receive anti-aging messages just by turning the pages of fashion magazines. These messages fuel a fear of natural processes of aging, damage female self-esteem, and compel women to hide their true self behind extensive beauty work or engage in unhealthy dietary practices. [12]

Body Image and Self-Esteem

Body image is defined as "a multidimensional construct encompassing self perceptions and attitudes regarding one's physical appearance". It is important for understanding fundamental issues of aging and identity.

Body-image concerns are significant to self-esteem in older adulthood, but vary by age and gender. Women appear to develop various strategies to counter the effects of aging and men seem to be more negatively affected, particularly in relation to body functioning.

Women's discontent with their bodies is relatively stable across the lifespan.

Of all the personal attributes that influence the development of body image, self-esteem may be the most important. Despite indications that self-esteem and body image contribute significantly to one's general wellbeing, neither the development of self-esteem in old age nor the relationship between body image and self-esteem among older adults have received much attention. Self-esteem is an essential component of mental health. Self-esteem rises gradually until the age of 65 years and then declines sharply after the age of 70. [13]

The Skin

The skin is the largest organ of the body and serves an important function in communicating with the world: attachment in the first years of life, self-image and self-esteem as we grow into adolescents and accepting its aging process as we get older. All these functions are highly influenced by emotional, social and psychological issues.

The skin is metaphorically a door to physical and psychological problems and processes, and in order to understand the psychological consequences of cutaneous illness and to treat these effectively, there is a need to view the patient holistically, and to address the reciprocity between body and mind. [14]

The appearance of the face plays an important role in human transactions, and youthful skin contributes significantly to an individual's physical attractiveness.

A youthful appearance has been associated with both increased self-esteem and improved social relations. An attractive appearance has a positive influence upon social functioning. [2]

Many years ago, diseases of the skin were believed to be contagious. Nowadays, skin conditions tend to be depreciated by the medical community because they are not life threatening. Quality of life measurements have helped to understand the impact and burden of some chronic skin diseases. For patients with visible skin diseases, the experience of being "different" is frightening, causing embarrassment, shame and feelings of stigmatization. Disease in any organ affects the sense of personal integrity, but the skin is visible to others and can affect our self-image too. [15]

Aging of the skin is associated with wrinkling, pigmemtary changes, and laxity.

The skin is an external indicator of the overall aging of the body. The skin is also a powerful organ of communication. We are forced to adapt to the aging process and some people find this difficult. [2]

Body Dysmorphic Disorder

Body Dysmorphic Disorder is characterized by excessive concern and preoccupation with an imagined or a slight defect in bodily appearance that is not better accounted for by another mental disorder. The skin and the hair are common body areas of concern. The preoccupations caused by the appearance are intrusive, unwanted, time-consuming and difficult to resist or control. Time-consuming rituals include mirror gazing and constant comparing of their imagined ugliness with others. These patients often seek unnecessary dermatologic treatment and cosmetic surgery.

The newly published DSM-V [16] classifies Body Dysmorphic Disorder (BDD) in the Obsessive-Compulsive and Related Disorders (OCRDs) category. BDD has been included in this category d ue to similarities with OCD, including repetitive behaviours, although BDD is characterized by poorer insight than OCD.

Table 1. DSM-V Diagnostic Criteria [16]

Body Dysmorphic Disorder

Diagnostic Criteria **300.7** (F45.22)

A. Preoccupation with one or more perceived defects or flaws in physical appearance that are not observable or appear slight to others.

B. At some point during the course of the disorder, the individual has performed repetitive behaviors (e.g., mirror checking, excessive grooming, skin picking, reassurance seeking) or mental acts (e.g., comparing his or her appearance with that of others) in response to the appearance concerns.

C. The preoccupation causes clinically significant distress or impairment in social, occupational, or other important areas of functioning.

D. The appearance preoccupation is not better explained by concerns with body fat or weight in an individual whose symptoms meet diagnostic criteria for an eating disorder.

Insight, considered the degree of an individual's conviction in his or her disorder - relevant belief, is an important dimension of psychopathology across many mental health disorders. Patients with BDD typically describe themselves as looking ugly, abnormal, deformed, or disfigured. Those with a delusional form of BDD are completely convinced that their view of their appearance is accurate, and the ones with a nondelusional type may recognize that their perceived deformities may not be accurate. [16]

The diagnosis of body dysmorphic disorder (BDD) is relatively easy to make but is often overlooked because few professionals ask a simple screening question on appearance. The key criterion is a preoccupation with an imagined defect or minor physical anomaly, and the preoccupation must be sufficient to cause significant distress or handicap. [17]

Most people dislike some aspects of their appearance, but individuals with BDD over focus on these details, exaggerating perceived appearance "defects". They may also have maladaptive beliefs about the importance of attractiveness (e.g., "If I am not attractive, I won't be able to be happy"). As appearance is believed to be very important, people with BDD perceive themselves as unattractive and they evaluate themselves negatively and have low self-esteem. These negative beliefs about their appearance often lead them to anxiety, shame and sadness, which in turn lead to maladaptive coping strategies, such as excessive mirror gazing and/or avoidance behaviours. Sufferers of BDD often perceive themselves as vain when admitting how much importance they place on physical appearance and the feeling of shame keeps them from talking about their worries. [18]

Cognitive-behavioural models of BDD suggest that maladaptive beliefs about appearance and self-worth set a person up to get caught in a vicious pattern of unrealistic appearance expectations, followed by increasing distress that one cannot meet the expectations, and repeated attempts to 'fix' one's appearance or give up and avoid situations that elicit appearance concerns [18].

Changes in physical appearance due to aging skin can make some patients, especially women, feel unattractive and this may trigger symptoms of BDD as they initiate a quest for the fountain of youth through repeated cosmetic procedures. [19]

Epidemiology of BDD

BDD is relatively common in both nonclinical and clinical settings, but it is often under diagnosed. It is estimated that BDD occurs in 0.7% to 2.4% of community samples, and in 9% -12% of patients seen by dermatologists. [20]

Etiology of BDD

The etiology of BDD is multifactorial, and these include biological, psychological, and sociocultural factors. The psychological theory of self-discrepancy suggests that BDD patients show a discrepancy between their ideal self and their real self. The importance attached to one's own appearance and the evaluation of one's body image, are important concepts in this disorder. [20]

Several cognitive-behavioural models have been developed to explain BDD. Buhlmann et al. [21] examined facial and object discrimination in BDD patients, but their findings did not support the hypothesis that BDD is characterized by enhanced facial and object discrimination ability.

These authors did however find a response bias to detect facial changes in stimuli that are not changed. These findings would be in accordance with the preoccupation with an imagined or slight appearance flaw that is not shared by other people.

Age of Onset of BDD

Age at onset is an important clinical feature in all disorders. In general, early age at onset has been associated with greater severity of illness, although there are exceptions. Bhornsson et al. [22] looked into age at onset of BDD and clinical correlates of early-onset illness. They conclude that BDD is usually a disorder of child or adolescent onset. No participant in their samples had onset of the illness after their 40s, even though the later decades of life arguably represent a time when appearance concerns become more legitimate. Early onset was significantly associated with a history of suicide attempts.

The authors conclude that BDD is primarily a disorder of childhood or adolescence onset, and that subclinical BDD symptoms begin, on average, several years before individuals experience the full-fledged disorder.

Screening for BDD in a Dermatology Setting

Preliminary Considerations

Most people have some concerns about how they look. However, some individuals experience very high levels of distress about their appearance and their ability to function in daily life becomes impaired.

Generally speaking, there is a low level of awareness about BDD among health care professionals, and BDD is, thus, often overlooked. Direct questioning about appearance satisfaction is needed for the diagnosis, as these patients are often too ashamed to reveal the true nature of their problem.

When they do seek help, they either consult a dermatologist or a cosmetic surgeon, and if they visit a doctor or a mental health care professional, they usually consult for other symptoms, such as depression or social phobia. [23]

Table 2. Question to help diagnose body dysmorphic disorder

- Some people worry a lot about their appearance. Do you worry a lot about the way you look and wish you could think about it less?
- What specific concerns do you have about your appearance? Do you think about them a lot and is it hard to stop thinking about them?
- On a typical day, how many hours a day is your appearance on your mind? (More than one hour is considered excessive)
- What effect does it have on your life?
- Does it make it hard on your social activities?

We need to bear in mind that people with BDD are often ashamed and embarrassed by their condition and may find it very difficult to discuss their symptoms. Therefore, health care professionals should be especially sensitive when exploring the hidden distress and disability commonly associated with this disorder. [23]

Clinicians should ask appearance-specific questions in order to identify patients who are suffering from BDD symptoms and to be able to offer information about their difficulties as well as treatment options. Table 2 offers some screening questions to help diagnose BDD.

Management of BDD

Little research has been performed on the outcome of dermatologic treatment in patients with BDD. The dermatology literature informs that these patients can be difficult to treat and are often dissatisfied with and have a poor response to dermatologic treatment. In addition, these patients consult numerous physicians and pressure dermatologists to prescribe unsuitable and ineffective treatments. [24]

One approach to treating patients with BDD is to change their appearance. However, this is not recommended as the altered appearance may fall short of patient expectations and fail to relieve the underlying problem. Consequently, the most important management is to help these patients to avoid surgical "corrections". [25]

In general, a physician who is empathetic and non-judgmental should not encounter difficulties in fostering a relationship with BDD patients. It is important to remember that skin problems are a means of seeking medical attention without coming to terms with what could be a severe psychological problem. Some recommendations are offered on Table 3.

Table 3. Management of patients with BDD

1. Do not immediately bring up the possibility of psychiatric problems and the need to be seen by a mental health professional.
2. Listen non-critically to the patient's story and perform a thorough dermatological exam.
3. The physician may have to spend several visits dealing with the patient on completely somatic terms before discussing any possibility of a mental health problem.
4. Once the issue of treatment is raised, the dermatologist must assure the patient that the goal of the treatment is to help relief the symptoms.
5. Preparing a patient for psychiatric referral may take several visits.

A stepped-care approach is recommended in the treatment of BDD. This means that the least intrusive intervention, such as education or self-help, should be used first, and only if this proves to be insufficiently effective should we move on to more intense therapy.

With regards to psychological treatment, cognitive behavioural strategies have demonstrated efficacy. Wilhelm et al. [26] have recently published a modular cognitive-behavioural treatment manual specifically for Body Dysmorphic Disorder.

Other Issues of Interest for Clinical Management in Psychodermatology

The Clinical Interview

Dermatologists commonly see patients with underlying psychiatric problems and should therefore be prepared to skillfully manage and treat them.

Interviewing is not simply the task of taking a history. It is the process of determining which illness the patient has and understanding how he or she has been affected by it. To be effective, the clinician must gain an understanding of the patient's perspective on his or her illness. Patient concerns can be wide ranging. Patient values, cultures and preferences need to be explored. Gender is another element that needs to be taken into consideration. The clinician should be careful not to be judgmental because this may rapidly close down communication. Sometimes the patient gains therapeutic benefit just from venting concerns in a safe environment with a caring clinician. [27]

Data gathering for diagnosis and treatment almost exclusively consists of information concerning possible disease symptoms, biomedical history, and diagnostic tests. However, to full y account for health or disease, the social and psychological dimensions of human existence have to be considered along with biomedical data. This requires not only gathering personal or psychosocial data from patients but also competency in interviewing techniques that elicit this information as well as relationship-building skills that nurture confidence and human understanding. The application of these skills in practice is called patient-centered interviewing. [28]

The use of the genogram is useful to gather the patient's family history to be able to draw a family tree. Patients construct their lives by talking about the family members, their relationships, and their life events such as deaths, births, health problems, etc. A wealth of significant information can be gathered through this technique. [29]

In Table 4 some important issues to bear in mind with psychodermatology patients are highlighted. [30]

Table 4. Recommendations for clinical management in psychodermatology [30]

1. Take a psychomatically-oriented history. Elicit patient's explanations and beliefs about the disease and ask about subjective experience helping to express the emotions associated with the illness.
2. The doctor's role is to accept the patient's story and this implies both the somatic and non-somatic problems. Show understanding for the patient's suffering whether it be exaggerated or without foundation.
3. It is necessary to diagnose the dermatological the medical and the underlying mental health condition in these patients.
4. Provide the patient with a biopsychosocial model of disease giving information about the disease and the influence of the psychosocial factors. Promote coping and self-management strategies where possible.

Considerations on the Use of Psychological Measuring Instruments

Use instruments wisely. Explain why you are using them to the patients. You may use some on a regular basis, such as Quality of Life questionnaires or short screening scales for anxiety and depression symptoms. If you want to include a patient in a study, you must inform and get written consent.

Make sure that the instruments you use have adequate psychometric properties, such as reliability and validity. All questionnaires and scales used should be translated, adapted culturally, and standardized in your country. When choosing an instrument to use with your patients, it should be short, easy to complete and it should provide useful information. The instruction guide should be read with attention and if unsure of how to interpretation the test an expert should be consulted. [31]

Always give feedback on the testing undertaken and comment results. Care must be taken not to use diagnoses pejoratively. Overuse of diagnostic terms to label difficult behaviours in patients erodes what may be a useful concept. Adopt an optimistic approach towards the patient, explaining the difficulties but also highlighting the positive aspects you have seen.

Referral of Patients

A relationship of trust and confidence must be established before the dermatologist can transfer a patient to a mental health professional. However, when this happens, it is important for the dermatologist to stay in contact with the patient and to offer further appointments so that the patient does not feel abandoned. During these visits the patient can talk about the experience with the mental health appointments and the dermatologist can offer support with the process. [32]

Patients may resent and even refuse a referral. Some will either abandon the treatment or try "doctor shopping". Some may fear the social stigma associated with having psychiatric care. Others may not be able to afford it. For patients who refuse to be referred to a psychiatrist, a pharmacological approach may be most feasible in a dermatological setting. [2]

Focusing on the distress and disability caused by their concerns, rather than on how they actually look, may be helpful in persuading patients to accept psychiatric referral. [24]

Final Considerations

Body Dysmorphic Disorder in the elderly is not frequent. Patients over 65 years of age may present with body dysmorphic symptoms or concerns but these could be due to an adjustment disorder caused by the aging process.

Gupta and Gupta (2013) [33] refer to Cutaneous Body Image (CBI) to describe an individual's mental perception of the appearance of his or her integumentary system. CBI dissatisfaction can contribute to significant morbidity in dermatologic disorders and is often the primary consideration in deciding whether to proceed with some cosmetic procedures. Assessment of CBI has important clinical implications because it can significantly affect the patient's quality of life. CBI dissatisfaction can increase the overall morbidity in dermatologic disease and has been associated with intentional self-injury, such as self-induced dermatoses and suicide. Poor CBI has been show to be an important factor in adherence to treatment in chronic disorders. [33]

The skin is an important organ of communication throughout the life span. The skin, especially facial skin, is one of the most visible indicators of chronologic age. In the last decades, old age has started to acquire negative connotations. Normal intrinsic aging is often viewed as a medical and social problem that needs to be addressed by health care professionals. Even in later life, the patient may be highly invested in his or her CBI. [33]

Finally, we should remember to assess the risk of self-harm and suicide in patients with BDD, Body Image, or Cutaneous Body Image symptoms or concerns.

References

[1] World Health Organization. (2013). *Mental health and older adults.* (Fact sheet No. 381). Retrieved from http://www.who.int/mediacentre/factsheets/fs381/en/

[2] Gupta M. A., Gupta A. K. Psychological Imapct of Aging and the Skin.Koo, J. Y. M. & Lee C. S. (Eds.) Psychocutaneous Medicine (pp. 365 -382). New York, NY: Marcel Dekker, Inc. 2003.

[3] Lyness J. M., Caine E. D., King D. A., Cox C., & Yoediono Z. Psychiatric Disorders in Older Primary Care Patients. *J. Gen. Intern. Med.* 1999; Apr; 14(4): 249-254. Picardi, A., Lega, I., & Tarolla, E. Suicide risk in skin disorders. *Clinics in Dermatology*, 2013; 31(1), 47–56.

[4] Schäfer, I., von Leitner, E.-C., Schön, G., Koller, D., Hansen, H., Kolonko, T., van den Bussche, H. Multimorbidity Patterns in the Elderly: A New Approach of Disease Clustering Identifies Complex Interrelations between Chronic Conditions. *PLoS ONE*, 2010; *5*(12), e15941. Clarke, L. H., & Korotchenko, A. Aging and the Body: A Review. *Canadian Journal on Aging / La Revue Canadienne Du Vieillissement*, 2011; *30*(03), 495–510.

[5] Webster, Jessica, & Tiggermann, Marika. The relationship Between Women's Body Satisfaction and Self-Image Across the Life Span: The Role of Cognitive Control. *The Journal of Genetic Psychology*, 2003; 164(2), 241-252.

[6] Hurd, L. C. Older women's body image and embodied experience: an exploration. *Journal of Women & Aging*, 2000; *12*(3-4), 77-97.

[7] Baker, L., & Gringart, E. Body image and self-esteem in older adulthood. *Ageing and Society*, 2009; *29*(06), 977-995.

[8] Ginn, J., & Arber, S. Aging and cultural stereotypes of older women. In J. Johnson & R. Slater (Eds.), *Aging and later life* (pp. 60-67). London: Sage. 1993.

[9] Biggs, S. Choosing not to be old? Masks, bodies and identity management in later life. *Ageing and Society*, 1997; *17*(5), 553–570.

[10] Lewis, D. C., Medvedev, K., & Seponski, D. M. Awakening to the desires of older women: Deconstructing ageism within fashion magazines. *Journal of Aging Studies*, 2011; *25*(2), 101–109. Baker, L., & Gringart, E. Body image and self-esteem in older adulthood. *Ageing and Society*, 2009; *29*(06), 977-995. doi:10.1017/ S0144686X09008721

[11] Papadopoulos L, Bor R. Psychological approaches to dermatology. Leicester: The British Psychological Society; 1999.

[12] Koblenzer, C. S. The Emotional Impact of Chronic and Disabling Skin Disease: A Psychoanalytic Perspective. *Dermatologic Clinics*, 2005; *23*(4), 619 – 627. doi:http://dx.doi.org/10.1016/j.det.2005.05.013

[13] American Psychiatric Association. *Diagnostic and statistical manual of mental disorders* (5th ed.). 2013; Arlington, VA: American Psychiatric Publishing.

[14] Veale, D. & Neziroglu, F. *Body Dysmorphic Disorder: A Treatment Manual.* Chichester: Wiley-Blackwell 2010.

[15] Buhlmann, U., Teachman, B. A., Naumann, E., Fehlinger, T., & Rief, W. The meaning of beauty: Implicit and explicit self-esteem and attractiveness beliefs in body dysmorphic disorder. *Journal of Anxiety Disorders*, 2009; *23*(5), 694–702.

[16] Koblenzer, C. S. Psychodermatology of women. *Clinics in Dermatology*, 1997; *15*(1), 127 – 141.

[17] Mufaddel, A., Osman, O. T., Almugaddam, F., & Jafferany, M. A review of body dysmorphic disorder and its presentation in different clinical settings. *The Primary Care Companion to CNS Disorders*, 2013; *15*(4).

[18] Buhlmann, U., Rupf, L., Gleiss, M. J. L., Zschenderlein, K., & Kathmann, N. Seeing "changes" that aren't there: Facial and object discrimination in body dysmorphic disorder. *Comprehensive Psychiatry*, 2014; *55*(3), 468–474.

[19] Bjornsson, A. S., Didie, E. R., Grant, J. E., Menard, W., Stalker, E., & Phillips, K. A. Age at onset and clinical correlates in body dysmorphic disorder. *Comprehensive Psychiatry*, 2013; *54*(7), 893–903. Tomas-Aragones, L. & Marron, S. E. Body dysmorphic disorder in adolescents. In R. S. Tareen, D. E. Greydanus, M. Jafferany, D. R. Patel & J. Merrick. Pediatric *Psychodermatology: A Clinical Manual of Child and Adolescent Psychocutaneous Disorders* (pp. 201-215). Berlin; Boston: De Gruyter. 2013.

[20] Castle, D. J., Phillips, K. A., & Dufresne, R. G. Body dysmorphic disorder and cosmetic dermatology: more than skin deep. *Journal of Cosmetic Dermatology*, 2004; *3*(2), 99–103.

[21] Hunt, T. J., Thienhaus, O., & Ellwood, A. The mirror lies: body dysmorphic disorder. *American Family Physician*, 2008; *78*(2), 217–222.

[22] Wilhelm, S., Phillips, K. A., Didie, E., Buhlmann, U., Greenberg, J. L., Fama, J. M., … Steketee, G. Modular Cognitive-Behavioral Therapy for Body Dysmorphic Disorder: A Randomized Controlled Trial. *Behavior Therapy*, 2014; *45*(3), 314–327.

[23] Teutsch C. Patient-doctor communication. Med Clin North Am. 2002; Sep;87(5):1115-45.

[24] Lyles JS, Dwamena FC, Lein C, Smith RC. Evidence-based patient-centered interviewing. JCOM. 2001; 8(7):29-34.

[25] Poot F, Sampogna F, Onnis L. Basic knowledge in Psychodermatology. JEADV 2007; 21:227-234.

[26] Harth W, Gieler U, Kusnir D, Tausk FA. Clinical management in Psychodermatology. Berlin: Springer-Verlag; 2009.

[27] Tomas-Aragones L, Castillo-Amores AB, Marron SE. Sistemas de medida. Evaluación psicométrica. [Systems of measurement. Psychometric evaluation]. In: Rodriguez-

Cerdeira C. Fundamentos básicos en psicodermatología [Basic principles of psychodermatology]. La Coruña: TresCetres Edit; 2010.
[28] Poot F. What a dermatologist needs to know to transfer dermatological patients to the psychiatrist or psychologist. Dermatol Psychosom 2002; 3:34-37.
[29] Gupta, M. A., & Gupta, A. K. Evaluation of cutaneous body image dissatisfaction in the dermatology patient. *Clinics in Dermatology*, 21013; *31*(1), 72–79.

In: Geriatric Psychodermatology
Editors: Mohammad Jafferany and Katlein França
ISBN: 978-1-63463-853-1

Chapter 6

Hair Disorders and Elderly Populations

Anna Skrok, M.D., Lidia Rudnicka, M.D., Ph.D. *
and Malgorzata Olszewska, M.D.

Introduction

As life expectancy is growing along with longer professional and social activity, the esthetic appearance is gaining increasing importance. The quality of hair seems to be significant to the self-esteem, self-confidence and often to the mental attitude of elderly individuals. Hair changes and hair loss can lead to psychological problems and influence the quality of life. The most common hair-related problems in the elderly patients are hair graying and hair loss.

Hair Graying

On an average, Caucasians begin to gray in their mid-30s, Asians in their late 30s, and Africans, in their mid-40s [1]. Gray hair develops as a result of loss of melanin production and deposition within the hair shafts. Hair shafts appear gray when they start losing melanin in the process of aging (Figure 1 and 2). However, the perception of individuals having gray hair may also result from simultaneous occurrence of non-pigmented (white) and pigmented (dark) scalp hairs [1, 2].

The mechanism of graying is not fully understood. A small number of melanocytes is capable of producing a 1.5 m long pigmented hair shaft [3]. This capability of melanocytes is stable in the first hair cycles and decreases with time. The cyclic melanogenesis and production of pigmented hair shafts occurs in scalp hair folliclesusually during the first 7 to 15 hair cycles, i.e. until approximately the age of 35 - 40 years [4].

* Corresponding author: Lidia Rudnicka. E-mail: lidia.rudnicka@dermatolodzy.com.pl.

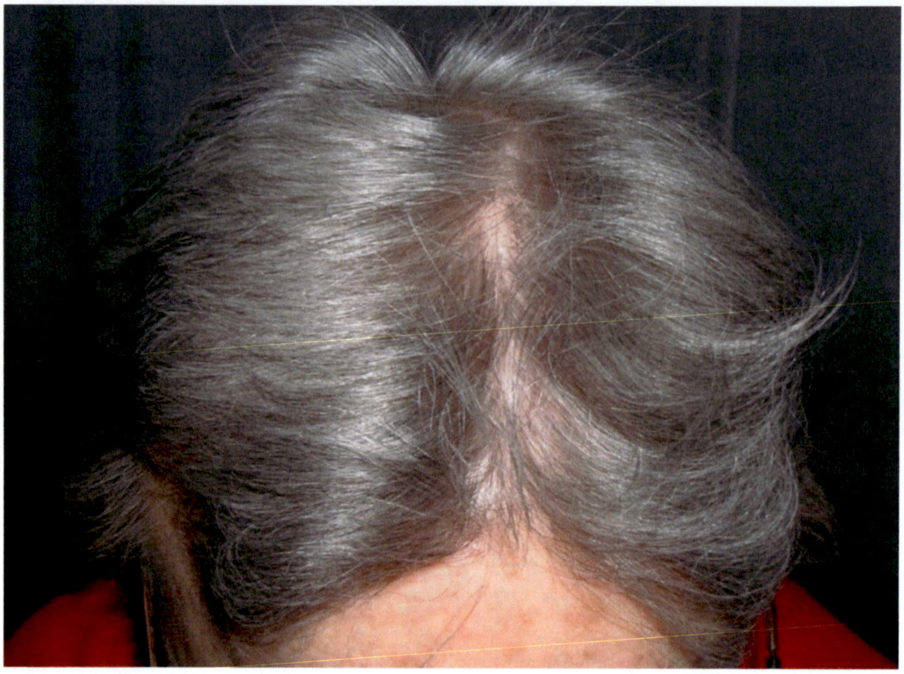

Figure 1. Hair graying. A coexistence of pigmented hair shafts and non-pigmented (white) hair shafts may give the optical impression of "gray hair".

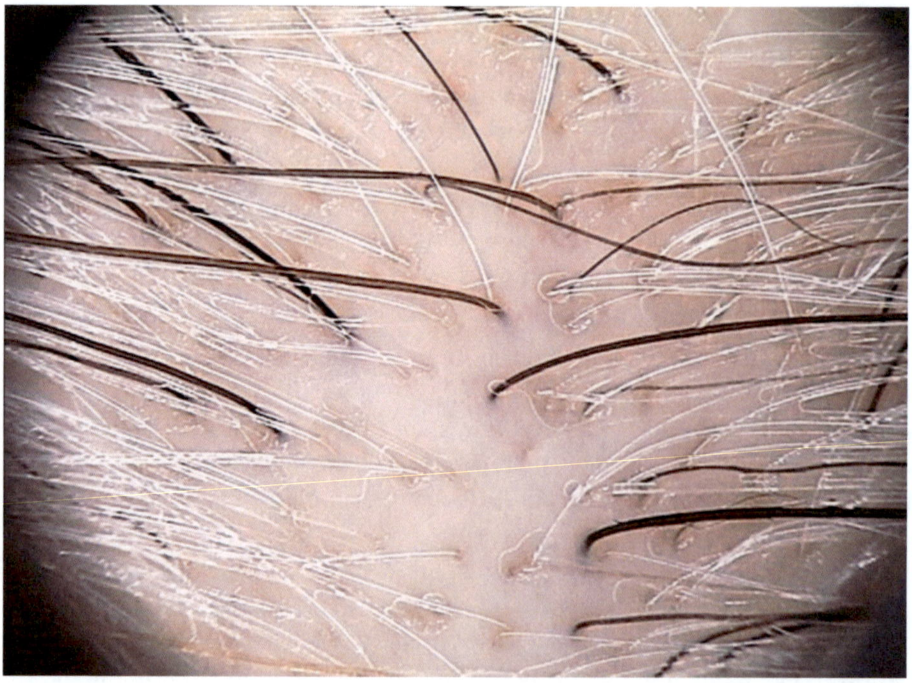

Figure 2. Trichoscopy (hair and scalp dermoscopy) allows for a non-invasive differential diagnosis of various causes of air loss. Performing trichoscopy in elderly patients may be difficult, because the visualization of hypopigmented hairs is more problematic, compared to pigmented hairs. The image shows trichoscopy in a healthy elderly person.

After these hair cycles, there is a partial loss of active melanogenesis with each consecutive cycle. Diluted pigment content results in truly gray hairs, while total lack of melanin results in appearance of white hair shafts (commonly also referred to as "gray hairs") [5]. It has to be noted that follicular melanogenesis is not persistent as in the epidermis, but cyclic, parallel to the cyclic metabolic activity of the hair follicle [6]. It is remarkable that a form of transient loss of pigment, "graying" occurs during each hair cycle. At the end of the anagen phase melanocytes in the hair bulb retract their dendrities and decrease or stop melanogenesis [6]. Cessation of melanogenesis occurs few days before inhibition of keratinocyte proliferation what results in the pigment-free proximal ends of shed telogen hairs.

Multiple mechanisms have been suggested to be responsible for the decrease in melanogenesis with age. The cessation of melanogenesis correlates with a reduction in tyrosinase activity of hair bulbar melanocytes, decrease in interactions between melanocytes and cortical keratinocytes, and disruption of the migration of melanocytes within a pigment hair unit [2]. Also, down-regulation of melanocyte activity in hair follicleshas been associated with decrease in alpha-MSH expression, changes in innervation and neuropeptide stimulation and oxidative stress [7, 8]. It has been observed in few cases that the hair graying may be retarded in patients after sympathectomy, indicating a possible neurogenic effect on hair graying [9].

Several intrinsic and extrinsic factors may lead to premature hair graying. The intrinsic factors include medical conditions such as thyroid insufficiency, Werner syndrome, Williams syndrome or pernicious anemia [1]. Extrinsic factors include smoking, ultraviolet radiation, toxins and nutritional deficiencies [1, 10, 11].

Research data indicate that the age of onset of hair graying is not associated with biological ageing or predicted life span [11]. The age of onset of hair graying is similar in women and men [11]. The temporal and occipital area are significantly more involved in men than in women whereas in women the frontal and parietal areas are affected more frequently. The average time from onset of hair graying to total or near-total involvement of all scalp hairs is above 25 years [11].

The effect of hair graying on quality of life has not been investigated in detail. The common desire to reverse this process indicates that the hair color is a significant factor contributing to self-esteem and psychological wellbeing.

Currently, hair dyeing is the only available option for individuals who wish to "reverse" graying and change their hair color. Permanent, semi-permanent and plant-based dyes are most popular. Several health safety concerns have been raised. For this reason the products containing hair dyes are highly regulated by international and national regulatory agencies. A recent study indicates that over 40% of individuals who have a tendency to develop gray hair use hair dyes to change their hair appearance [12]. Women dye their hair significantly more often than men and individuals below the age of 70 more often than older persons [12]. Individuals who felt that graying has advanced by more than 20% of the overall hair were more likely to dye their hair than those with less advanced graying of hair.

Prevention or genuine reversal of hair graying appears to be within an easy reach of dermatological research. In vitro research, animal studies and reports in humans have documented that various types of treatment may (temporarily) reverse hair graying [13, 14]. Some authors indicate that melanocyte stem cells may serve as potential future solution in hair graying [15]. It seems probable that the upcoming years will be devoted to developing a high safety profile product that prevents or reverses hair graying.

Age-Related Hair Loss

A slow, but steady, decrease in hair density is associated with ageing [16]. The average hair density is above 300 hair shafts per cm at the age of 20 and it decreases by over 50% by the age of 70 [16]. This process affects predominantly the frontal area, and to a lesser extent the occipital area. It remains unclear whether this process is associated solely with age or with other factors, such as subclinical androgenetic alopecia, general health or environmental factors. Research data indicate that the percentage of anagen hairs is decreasing after the age of 45 [16]. This may explain the decrease in hair density with age. It has been shown that post-menopausal women have a lower hair density compared to pre-menopausal women [16], what may indicate that hormonal factors may contribute to the decrease in hair density with age. Also, the average hair thickness decreases with age from over 80 micrometers at the age of 20 to slightly over 60 micrometers at the age of 80 [16].

Androgenetic Alopecia

The most frequent cause of hair loss in the elderly population is androgenetic alopecia (AGA) (Figure 3 and 4). Androgenetic alopecia is an androgen -related condition, which develops in genetically predisposed individuals [17]. The disease affects up to 80% Caucasian men and 40% women. The prevalence of androgenetic alopecia is lower in Asian and African-American men and women [18]. The prevalence of the disease increases with age [17]. Androgenetic alopecia (male pattern hair loss) and female androgenetic alopecia (female pattern hair loss) share the same histopathological feature of hair follicle miniaturization and a similar pathogenic pathway. In susceptible hair follicles, dihydrotestosterone binds to the androgen receptor, and the hormone-receptor complex activates the genes responsible for the gradual transformation of large terminal follicles to miniaturized follicles [17]. In both men and women there is no correlation between serum androgen concentrations and the severity or activity of the disease.

In androgenetic alopecia the duration of the anagen phase gradually decreases. As the anagen phase shortens, the new anagen hairs become shorter and thinner. This process of miniaturization may eventually lead to clinically apparent balding [17]. The diagnosis of androgenetic alopecia is based on clinical evaluation and trichoscopy [19]. Histopathology may be useful in doubtful cases [20].

The clinical presentation and severity of disease is estimated according to the modified Norwood-Hamilton classification in men and the Ludwig scale in women [20]. The basic and specific classification (BASP) has been introduced a few years ago, but it has not gained significant interest in clinical practice because of its high complexity [21].

In women, typically three patterns are observed: a diffuse thinning of the crown area with preservation of the frontal hair line, thinning and widening of the central part of the scalp with breach of the frontal hair line, and thinning associated with bitemporal recession [22].

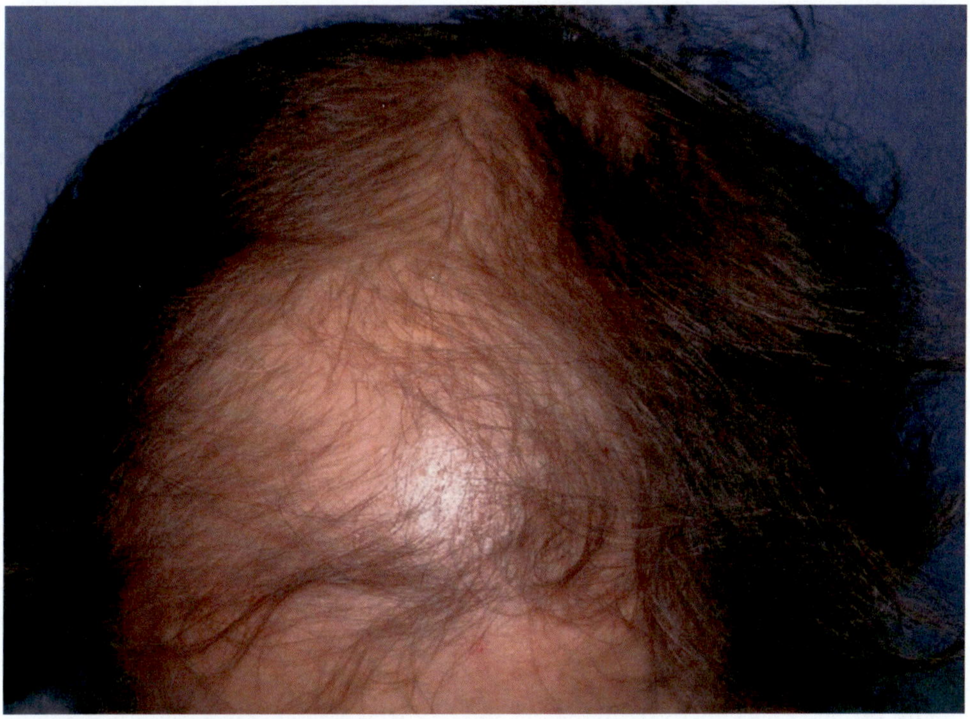

Figure 3. Female androgenetic alopecia.

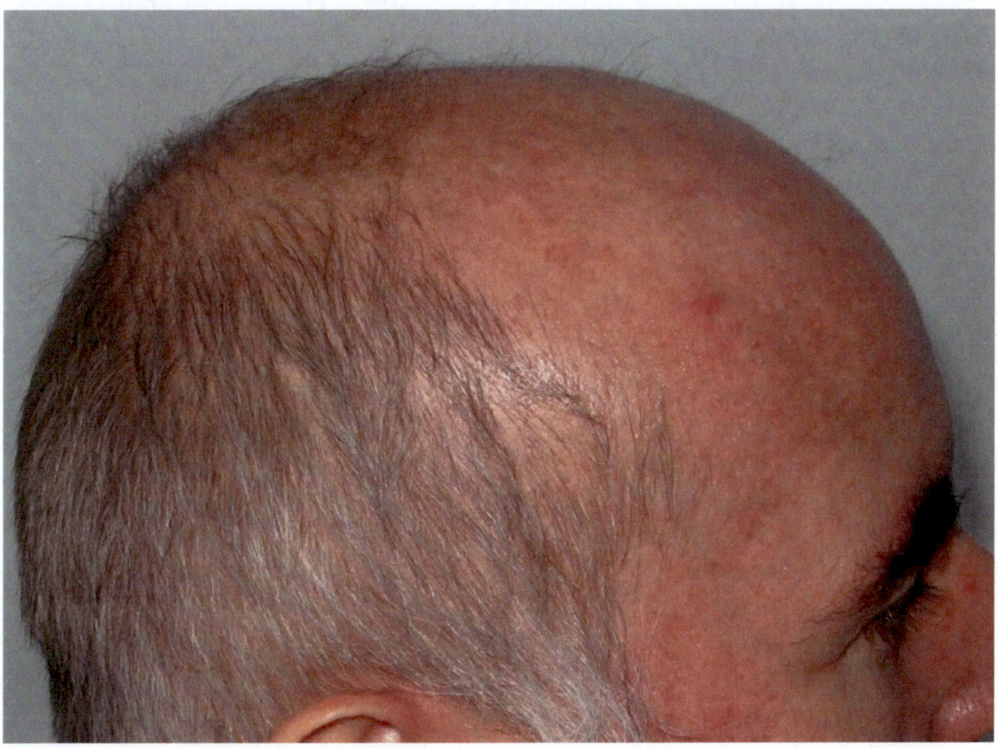

Figure 4. Androgenetic alopecia in a man.

During the European Hair Research Society Meeting in 2013 prof. Vera H. Price has suggested to differentiate the spectrum of female androgenetic alopecia according to age: puberty to age 40 (androgenetic alopecia), approx. 45 - 55 years (female pattern hair loss) and after age 60 (senescent alopecia). We consider this classification very controversial from the biological and diagnostic point of view. However, our experience shows that indeed anti-dihydrotestosterone therapy is the most efficient in young and middle-aged women, indicating that the role of androgens in elderly patients is less prominent.

A relevant recent finding is that androgenetic alopecia in women and men is associated with higher body mass index, higher risk of coronary artery disease and diabetes mellitus [23].

Male androgenetic alopecia and female androgenetic alopecia share similar trichoscopy features, such as: hair shaft thickness heterogeneity, thin hairs, yellow dots, perifollicular discoloration (peripilar sign), an increased proportion of vellus hairs and high number of follicular units with only one emerging hair shaft [19, 24]. Thin, wavy hair shafts and honeycomb hyperpigmentation often coexist as additional, non-specific features [25, 26]. Trichoscopy criteria for the diagnosis of androgenetic alopecia have been developed by Rakowska et al. [27]. They are currently being revised by the authors to better fit the needs of everyday clinical practice.

Androgenetic alopecia has a significant impact on the quality of life. Zhuang et al. [28] investigated 125 first-visit patients with female androgenetic alopecia and found that the average DLQI score was 9.62±5.92, which is close to 10 (very large impact on patient's life). The impact of the disease on quality of life is somewhat less relevant in men. Yamazaki et al. [29] reported that the average DLQI in men with androgenetic alopecia is 5.74±6.14 (small to moderate impact). However, for many men loss of hair is associated with a significant psychological distress. There is a correlation between the severity of balding and the impact of disease on the quality of life. Interestingly, in patients with the late onset androgenetic alopecia there is a tendency of higher effect of the disease on quality of life compared to patients with an early onset AGA [28]. Women and men with long-lasting androgenetic alopecia develop some coping mechanisms, such as avoiding negative emotions from their surroundings by reducing their outdoor activities or by wearing hats or wigs to prevent discomfort [28].

The goal of current treatment in androgenetic alopecia is rather to decelerate ongoing hair loss than to achieve full hair regrowth. The latter appears not possible in advanced cases at the current level of dermatological knowledge. Topical 2% and 5% minoxidil solution is the first choice method recommended by majority of authors [30]. In many countries the 5% solution is used in women off-label. The improvement is usually seen after few months, however telogen effluvium may be observed during the first 8 weeks of therapy [30]. Oral 5-alpha reductase inhibitors have an established position in treatment of androgenetic alopecia. Finasteride for men, applied at a dose of 1 mg per day is the only officially approved treatment. However, finasteride and dutasteride have been used with success in both women and men in reported studies [30-32]. Whereas 1 mg/day of finasteride appears to be sufficient for the therapy of androgenetic alopecia in men, many authors indicate that a higher dose should be used in women. Finasteride at a dose of 5 mg/day was found effective and safe for the treatment of female androgenetic alopecia in postmenopausal women in the absence of clinical or laboratory signs of hyperandrogenism [31]. The efficacy of topical finasteride remains controversial [33]. Other types of antiandrogenetic therapies include cyproterone acetate and spironolactone [34]. Spironolactone has to be used with special caution in the elderly patients as it may lead to hyperkalemia. The efficacy of other suggested therapies, such as platelet-rich plasma or Ginseng extracts has not been sufficiently confirmed. However, we have some relatively good experience with both, platelet-rich plasma and the use of Ginseng extracts as diet supplements in women with androgenetic alopecia. Hair transplantation may be used to rapidly improve the patient's appearance, but the procedure does not replace pharmacological therapy. Hairpieces and wigs may be an alternative to medical therapy.

Only two types of therapy, topical minoxidil and oral finasteride have been shown to significantly improve the quality of life of patients with androgenetic alopecia [28, 29]. Interestingly, the improvement of quality of life was observed in both, responders and non-responders [28].

Taken into consideration that the disease has a significant impact on the quality of life and that the treatment results may be disappointing, dermatologists should devote sufficient time to consultation at the first visit to discuss the planned treatment timetable, the therapeutic options and patient's expectations. Due to the 'placebo effect', some patients may be satisfied with the treatment even if they are poor responders, implying that dermatologists should take the psychological aspects of therapy into account throughout the therapeutic process. Psychological counseling may be required in certain patients in parallel to pharmacological management of hair loss [35].

Senescent Alopecia

The controversial concept of senescent alopecia (senile alopecia, Figure 5) has evolved from the observation that diffuse hair thinning may develop after the age of 50 years in patients, who have otherwise no features of androgenetic alopecia and no family history of balding [16]. Senescent alopecia was believed to be a non-androgen -dependent cause of hair follicle miniaturization. However studies of senescent alopecia are complicated by the commonly coexisting (subclinical) androgenetic alopecia. It was suggested that following features are most characteristic of senescent alopecia: 1) onset after 60 years of age, 2) diffuse hair thinning over the whole scalp, 3) reduced hair density, 4) reduced hair diameter, 5) hair follicle miniaturization often present, 6) usually minor inflammatory changes, 7) potential response to minoxidil and finasteride [16]. Despite many years of research the concept of senescent alopecia remains controversial. A microarray analysis may indicate that androgenetic and senescent alopecia show distinct gene expression profiles [36]. However, a major drawback of this study is that the age at onset of disease was chosen as the major feature to distinguish the two entities.

The results of a histopathology study, performed by Whiting [37] leads to the conclusion that most cases of significant hair loss in the elderly patients are androgen driven. Our trichoscopy experience [38] shows that senescent alopecia shares with androgenetic alopecia the predominance of follicular units with only one hair, increased percentage of thin hairs and decreased hair shaft density with honeycomb pattern pigmentation of the affected scalp. The tendency to form brown perifollicular discoloration (peripilar sign) is less common compared to typical androgenetic alopecia. We hypothesize that senescent alopecia is a subtype of androgenetic alopecia in the elderly population that shows less dynamics and poorer response to therapy.

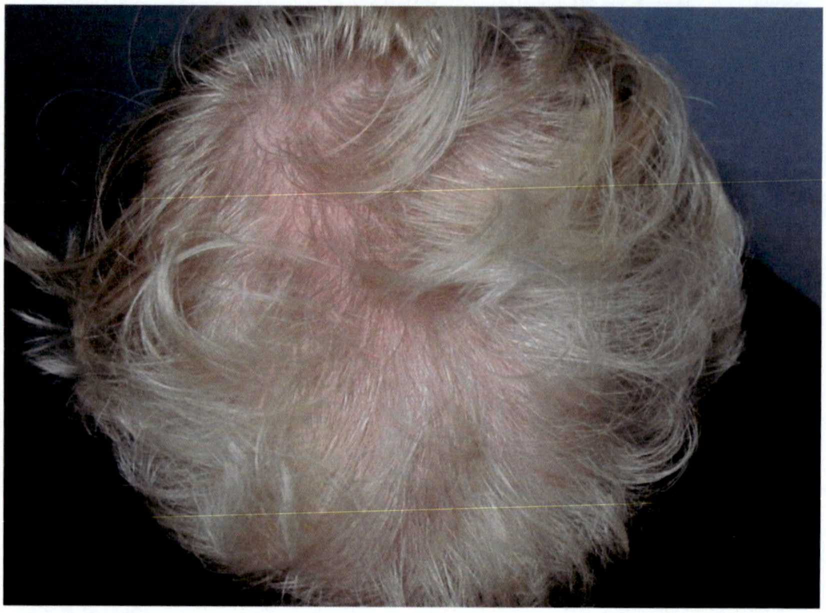

Figure 5. Senescent alopecia. The concept of this diagnosis remains controversial.

Taken this into consideration, we believe that all psychodermatology considerations in senescent alopecia should be analogous to androgenetic alopecia.

Fibrosing Alopecia in Pattern Distribution

Fibrosing alopecia in pattern distribution (Figure 6) develops in patients with underlying androgenetic alopecia [16]. Women are more commonly affected than men. The disorder shares features of androgenetic alopecia (miniaturization of hair follicle s) with features of lichen planopilaris (perifollicular lymphohistiocytic infiltrates and fibrosis, loss of sebaceous glands) [39]. Published case reports show that progression of hair loss may be halted with anti-androgen therapy [40].

Frontal Fibrosing Alopecia

Frontal fibrosing alopecia (FFA, Figure 7 and 8), called previously also "postmenopausal frontal fibrosing alopecia", is a primary lymphocytic cicatricial alopecia within the spectrum of lichen planopilaris [41]. It usually, but not exclusively, affects postmenopausal women. According to a literature review by Chew et al. [42], only 7.6% of all reported patients with FFA were premenopausal women and 1.9% were men. The disease is characterized clinically by slowly progressing symmetric hair line recession in the frontotemporal and/or frontoparietal region. The usual rate of hairline recession is 0.3 to 1.7 mm per month [43].

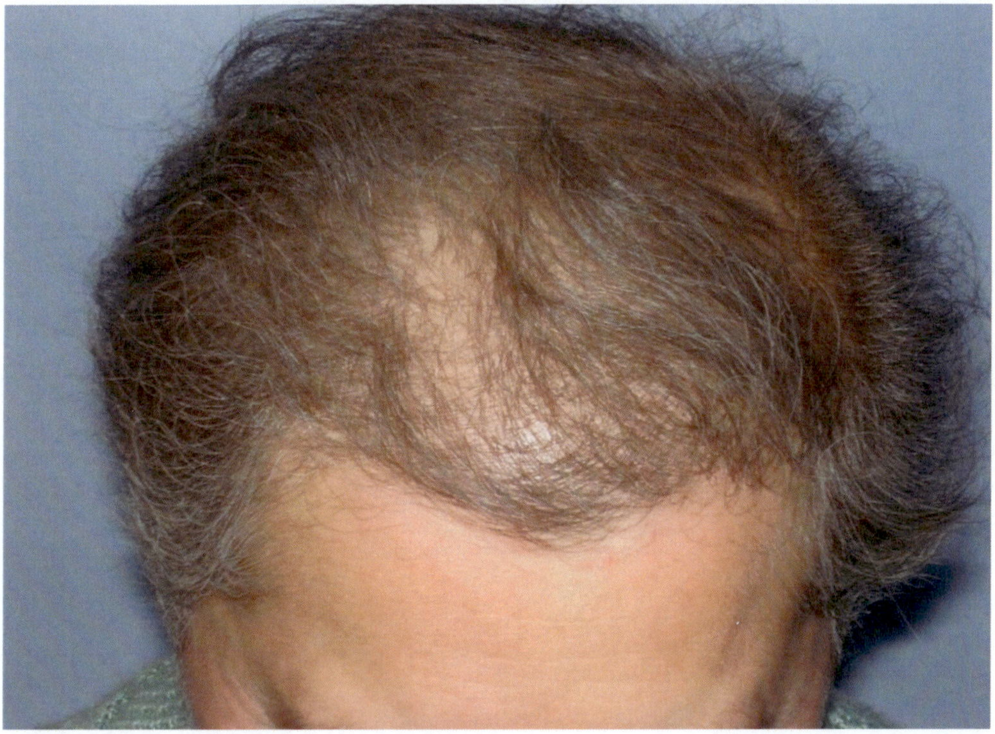

Figure 6. Fibrosing alopecia in pattern distribution.

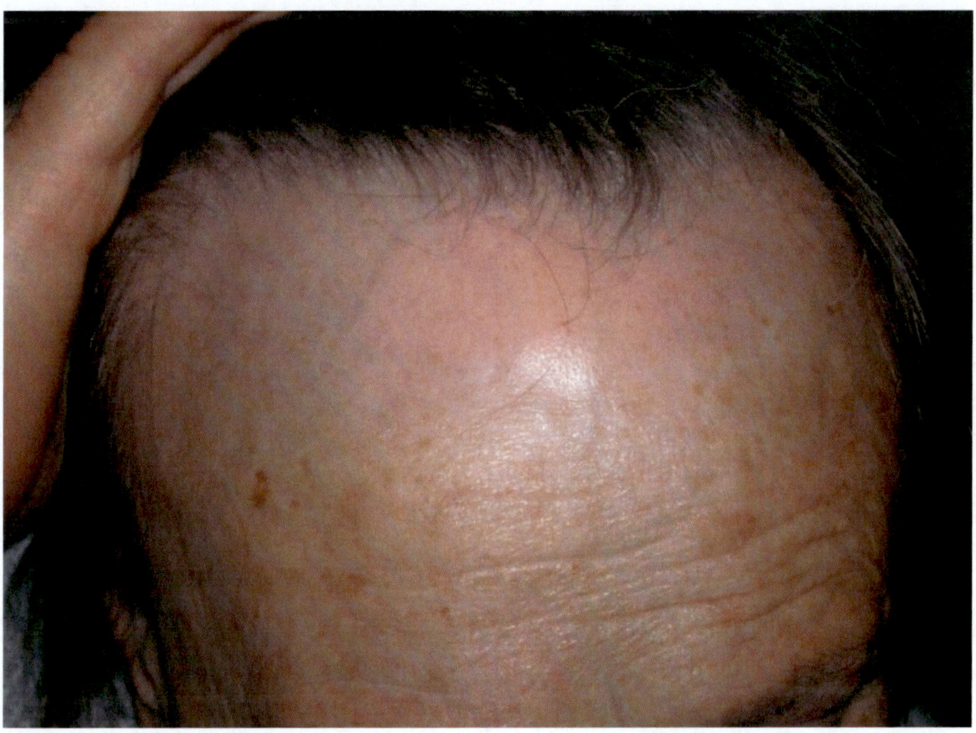

Figure 7. Frontal fibrosing alopecia.

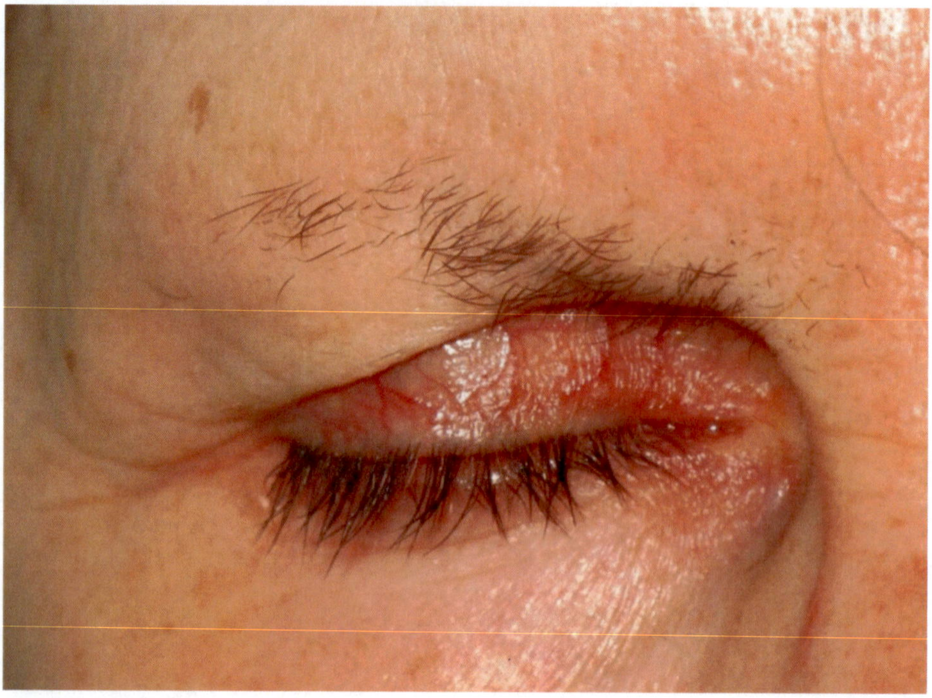

Figure 8. Madarosis (loss of eyebrows) is a common finding in patients with frontal fibrosing alopecia.

Eyebrow loss is observed in 50% to 83% of patients. Characteristically, eyebrow loss begins at the lateral third of the brow and uncommonly progresses to total eyebrow loss. Body hair loss may be associated with FFA in 27% to 77% of patients and usually affects the axilla, pubic area, and occasionally the upper or lower limbs [42, 44]. The diagnosis is based on characteristic clinical appearance. Histopathology and trichoscopy may aid in the differential diagnosis [45, 46]. Intralesional or oral corticosteroids, hydroxychloroquine, tetracyclines or 5-alpha reductase inhibitors (finasteride, dutasteride) have been applied with some benefit in halting the hair loss process and decreasing itching [47, 48]. As in all cicatricial alopecias hair regrowth is not possible in the hair folliclesthat have been replaced by fibrotic tissue. The permanent hair loss is associated with significant impact on psychological status, quality of life, and social interactions [49]. A recent study in 105 patients with frontal fibrosing alopecia and lichen planus showed that patients perceive their condition as a chronic disease with significant personal consequences and emotional impact. A significant level of psychological distress was observed as evaluated with means of the Hospital Anxiety and Depression Scale (mean total score was 11.3 ± 8.1). The level of psychological distress correlated with the activity of the disease [50].

Hair Loss Secondary to General Health Problems

Hair loss associated with general health problems in the elderly population is most commonly telogen effluvium that may be induced by drugs, psychological stress, severe infectious diseases or surgery in general anesthesia [51, 52]. The hair loss never leads to balding and in most cases (partial) spontaneous hair regrowth is observed within few months.

The most psychologically distressing type of hair loss in the elderly population is chemotherapy -induced alopecia. In such cases hair loss occurs when the metabolic and mitotic activity of the follicles is rapidly suppressed by a cytotoxic drug [53]. The incidence and severity of chemotherapy-induced alopecia varies depending on the chemotherapy protocol, but general prevalence of alopecia is estimated to range from 65 to 85% of patients receiving chemotherapy [53, 54]. Alkylating agents (cyclophosphamide, ifosfamide), cytotoxic drugs (doxorubicin, daunorubicin), antimicrotubule agents (docetaxel, paclitaxel), and topoisomerase inhibitors (etoposide) cause hair loss most frequently. Fluorouracil, hydroxycarbamide, and methotrexate induce alopecia much less commonly, and the effects are usually less severe [53, 54].

Almost 50% of women feel that hair loss is the most traumatic aspect of chemotherapy, and 8% declare that would consider declining chemotherapy because of fear of hair loss [54]. There are no significant differences between women and men with regard to lack of psychological well-being associated with chemotherapy-induced alopecia [55]. A Chemotherapy-induced Alopecia Distress Scale (CADS) was recently developed as a tool for measuring distress from chemotherapy-induced alopecia [56]. The need is being raised for developing specific interventions to minimize distress due to alopecia associated with chemotherapy.

Conclusion

Hair loss can be associated with serious psychological consequences, particularly anxiety, depression and an impairment in the quality of life. Taken into consideration that the treatment efficacy of hair loss in the elderly population is very limited, it is important for the consulting physician to devote sufficient time for consultation. The patient's expectations and the therapeutic options should be discussed in detail. It is important not to underestimate the psychological importance of hair appearance, also in elderly patients who may have other coexisting medical conditions, seemin to the physician more "serious".

References

[1] Pandhi D., Khanna D. Premature graying of hair. *Indian J. Dermatol. Venereol. Leprol.*, 2013 Sep.-Oct.; 79(5):641-53.

[2] Tobin D. J., Paus R. Graying: gerontobiology of the hair follicle pigmentary unit. *Exp. Gerontol.*, 2001 Jan.; 36(1):29-54.

[3] Van Neste D., Tobin D. J. Hair cycle and hair pigmentation: dynamic interactions and changes associated with aging. *Micron,* 2004; 35(3):193-200.

[4] Keogh E. V., Walsh R. J. Rate of greying of human hair. *Nature,* 1965 Aug. 21; 207 (999):877-8.

[5] Seiberg M. Age-induced hair greying - the multiple effects of oxidative stress. *Int. J. Cosmet. Sci.,* 2013 Dec.; 35(6):532-8.

[6] Slominski A., Paus R. Melanogenesis is coupled to murine anagen: toward new concepts for the role of melanocytes and the regulation of melanogenesis in hair growth. *J. Invest. Dermatol.,* 1993 Jul.; 101(1 Suppl.):90S-7S.

[7] Peters E. M., Imfeld D., Graub R. Graying of the human hair follicle. *J. Cosmet. Sci.,* 2011 Mar.-Apr.; 62(2):121-5.

[8] Shi Y., Luo L. F., Liu X. M., Zhou Q., Xu S. Z., Lei T. C. Premature graying as a consequence of compromised antioxidant activity in hair bulb melanocytes and their precursors. *PLoS One,* 2014; 9(4):e93589.

[9] Ortonne J. P., Thivolet J., Guillet R. Graying of hair with age and sympathectomy. *Arch. Dermatol.,* 1982 Nov.; 118(11):876-7.

[10] Zayed A. A., Shahait A. D., Ayoub M. N., Yousef A. M. Smokers' hair: Does smoking cause premature hair graying? *Indian Dermatol. Online J.*, 2013 Apr.; 4(2):90-2.

[11] Jo S. J., Paik S. H., Choi J. W., Lee J. H., Cho S., Kim K. H., et al. Hair graying pattern depends on gender, onset age and smoking habits. *Acta. Derm. Venereol.,* 2012 Mar.; 92(2):160-1.

[12] Jo S. J., Shin H., Paik S. H., Choi J. W., Lee J. H., Cho S., et al. The pattern of hair dyeing in koreans with gray hair. *Ann. Dermatol.,* 2013 Nov.; 25(4):401-4.

[13] Endou M., Aoki H., Kobayashi T., Kunisada T. Prevention of hair graying by factors that promote the growth and differentiation of melanocytes. *J. Dermatol.,* 2014 Aug.; 41(8):716-23.

[14] Park W. S., Kwon O., Yoon T. J., Chung J. H. Anti-graying effect of the extract of Pueraria thunbergiana via upregulation of cAMP/MITF-M signaling pathway. *J. Dermatol. Sci.*, 2014 Aug.; 75(2):153-5.

[15] Lee J. H., Fisher D. E. Melanocyte stem cells as potential therapeutics in skin disorders. *Expert Opin. Biol. Ther.,* 2014 Aug. 8:1-11.

[16] Trüeb R. M., Tobin D. J. Aging hair. Heidelberg: Springer; 2010.

[17] Otberg N., Finner A. M., Shapiro J. Androgenetic alopecia. Endocrinol. Metab. *Clin. North Am.,* 2007 Jun.; 36(2):379-98.

[18] Wang T. L., Zhou C., Shen Y. W., Wang X. Y., Ding X. L., Tian S., et al. Prevalence of androgenetic alopecia in China: a community -based study in six cities. *Br. J. Dermatol.,* 2010 Apr.; 162(4):843-7.

[19] Mubki T., Rudnicka L., Olszewska M., Shapiro J. Evaluation and diagnosis of the hair loss patient: Part II. Trichoscopic and laboratory evaluations. *J. Am. Acad. Dermatol.,* 2014 Sep.; 71(3):431 e1- e11.

[20] Mubki T., Rudnicka L., Olszewska M., Shapiro J. Evaluation and diagnosis of the hair loss patient: Part I. History and clinical examination. *J. Am. Acad. Dermatol.,* 2014 Sep.; 71(3):415 e1- e15.

[21] Lee W. S., Oh Y., Ji J. H., Park J. K., Kim do W., Sim W. Y., et al. Analysis of familial factors using the basic and specific (BASP) classification in Korean patients with androgenetic alopecia. *J. Am. Acad. Dermatol*., 2011 Jul.; 65(1):40-7.

[22] Blume-Peytavi U., Blumeyer A., Tosti A., Finner A., Marmol V., Trakatelli M., et al. S1 guideline for diagnostic evaluation in androgenetic alopecia in men, women and adolescents. *Br. J. Dermatol.*, 2011 Jan.; 164(1):5-15.

[23] Sharma K. H., Jindal A. Association between androgenetic alopecia and coronary artery disease in young male patients. *Int. J. Trichology,* 2014 Jan.; 6(1):5-7.

[24] Rudnicka L., Olszewska M., Rakowska A., Kowalska-Oledzka E., Slowinska M. Trichoscopy: a new method for diagnosing hair loss. *J. Drugs Dermatol.*, 2008 Jul.; 7(7):651-4.

[25] Ross E. K., Vincenzi C., Tosti A. Videodermoscopy in the evaluation of hair and scalp disorders. *J. Am. Acad. Dermatol.,* 2006 Nov.; 55(5):799-806.

[26] Rudnicka L., Olszewska M., A. R., Slowinska M. Trichoscopy update 2011. *J. Dermatol. Case Rep.,* 2011; 5(4):82-8.

[27] Rakowska A., Slowinska M., Kowalska-Oledzka E., Olszewska M., Rudnicka L. Dermoscopy in female androgenic alopecia: method standardization and diagnostic criteria. *Int. J. Trichology,* 2009 Jul.; 1(2):123-30.

[28] Zhuang X. S., Zheng Y. Y., Xu J. J., Fan W. X. Quality of life in women with female pattern hair loss and the impact of topical minoxidil treatment on quality of life in these patients. *Exp. Ther. Med.*, 2013 Aug.; 6(2):542-6.

[29] Yamazaki M., Miyakura T., Uchiyama M., Hobo A., Irisawa R., Tsuboi R. Oral finasteride improved the quality of life of androgenetic alopecia patients. *J. Dermatol.,* 2011 Aug.; 38(8):773-7.

[30] Varothai S., Bergfeld W. F. Androgenetic alopecia: an evidence -based treatment update. *Am. J. Clin. Dermatol.*, 2014 Jul.; 15(3):217-30.

[31] Oliveira-Soares R., J. M. E. S., Correia M. P., Andre M. C. Finasteride 5 mg/day Treatment of Patterned Hair Loss in Normo-androgenetic Postmenopausal Women. *Int. J. Trichology,* 2013 Jan.; 5(1):22-5.

[32] Olszewska M., Rudnicka L. Effective treatment of female androgenic alopecia with dutasteride. *J. Drugs Dermatol.*, 2005 Sep.-Oct.; 4(5):637-40.

[33] Caserini M., Radicioni M., Leuratti C., Annoni O., Palmieri R. A novel finasteride 0.25% topical solution for androgenetic alopecia: pharmacokinetics and effects on plasma androgen levels in healthy male volunteers. *Int. J. Clin. Pharmacol. Ther.,* 2014 Jul. 30.

[34] Olsen E. A., Messenger A. G., Shapiro J., Bergfeld W. F., Hordinsky M. K., Roberts J. L., et al. Evaluation and treatment of male and female pattern hair loss. *J. Am. Acad. Dermatol.*, 2005 Feb.; 52(2):301-11.

[35] Stough D., Stenn K., Haber R., Parsley W. M., Vogel J. E., Whiting D. A., et al. Psychological effect, pathophysiology, and management of androgenetic alopecia in men. *Mayo. Clin. Proc.*, 2005 Oct.; 80(10):1316-22.

[36] Karnik P., Shah S., Dvorkin-Wininger Y., Oshtory S., Mirmirani P. Microarray analysis of androgenetic and senescent alopecia: comparison of gene expression shows two distinct profiles. *J. Dermatol. Sci.*, 2013 Nov.; 72(2):183-6.

[37] Whiting D. A. How real is senescent alopecia? A histopathologic approach. *Clin. Dermatol.*, 2011 Jan.-Feb.; 29(1):49-53.

[38] Atlas of trichoscopy: dermoscopy in hair and scalp disease. New York: Springer; 2012.

[39] Olsen E. A. Female pattern hair loss and its relationship to permanent/cicatricial alopecia: a new perspective. *J. Investig. Dermatol. Symp. Proc.,* 2005 Dec.; 10(3): 217-21.

[40] Zinkernagel M. S., Trueb R. M. Fibrosing alopecia in a pattern distribution: patterned lichen planopilaris or androgenetic alopecia with a lichenoid tissue reaction pattern? *Arch. Dermatol.*, 2000 Feb.; 136(2):205-11.

[41] Filbrandt R., Rufaut N., Jones L., Sinclair R. Primary cicatricial alopecia: diagnosis and treatment. *CMAJ,* 2013 Dec. 10; 185(18):1579-85.

[42] Chew A. L., Bashir S. J., Wain E. M., Fenton D. A., Stefanato C. M. Expanding the spectrum of frontal fibrosing alopecia: a unifying concept. *J. Am. Acad. Dermatol.,* 2010 Oct.; 63(4):653-60.

[43] Tan K. T., Messenger A. G. Frontal fibrosing alopecia: clinical presentationsand prognosis. *Br. J. Dermatol.,* 2009 Jan.; 160(1):75-9.

[44] Vano-Galvan S., Molina-Ruiz A. M., Serrano-Falcon C., Arias-Santiago S., Rodrigues-Barata A. R., Garnacho-Saucedo G., et al. Frontal fibrosing alopecia: a multicenter review of 355 patients. *J. Am. Acad. Dermatol.*, 2014 Apr.; 70(4):670-8.

[45] Rakowska A., Slowinska M., Kowalska-Oledzka E., Warszawik O., Czuwara J., Olszewska M., et al. Trichoscopy of cicatricial alopecia. *J. Drugs Dermatol.,* 2012 Jun.; 11(6):753-8.

[46] Otberg N. Primary cicatricial alopecias. *Dermatol. Clin.,* 2013 Jan.; 31(1):155-66.

[47] Banka N., Mubki T., Bunagan M. J., McElwee K., Shapiro J. Frontal fibrosing alopecia: a retrospective clinical review of 62 patients with treatment outcome and long-term follow-up. *Int. J. Dermatol.*, 2014 Apr. 16.

[48] Harries M. J., Messenger A. Treatment of frontal fibrosing alopecia and lichen planopilaris. *J. Eur. Acad. Dermatol. Venereol.,* 2014 Jan. 20.

[49] Pradhan P., D'Souza M., Bade B. A., Thappa D. M., Chandrashekar L. Psychosocial impact of cicatricial alopecias. *Indian J. Dermatol.,* 2011 Nov.; 56(6):684-8.

[50] Y Z. C., Bundy C., CE M. G., Paus R., M J. H. The role of beliefs: Lessons from a pilot study on illness perception, psychological distress, and quality of life in patients with primary cicatricial alopecia. *Br. J. Dermatol.,* 2014 Jul. 12.

[51] Patel M., Harrison S., Sinclair R. Drugs and hair loss. *Dermatol. Clin.,* 2013 Jan.; 31 (1):67-73.

[52] Rebora A. Telogen effluvium revisited. *G. Ital. Dermatol. Venereol.*, 2014 Feb.;149(1): 47-54.

[53] Shin H., Jo S. J., Kim D. H., Kwon O., Myung S. K. Efficacy of interventions for prevention of chemotherapy -induced alopecia: A systematic review and meta-analysis. *Int. J. Cancer,* 2014 Aug. 1.

[54] Trueb R. M. Chemotherapy-induced alopecia. *Curr. Opin. Support Palliat. Care,* 2010 Dec.; 4(4):281-4.

[55] Can G., Demir M., Erol O., Aydiner A. A comparison of men and women's experiences of chemotherapy -induced alopecia. *Eur. J. Oncol. Nurs.,* 2013 Jun.; 17(3):255-60.

[56] Cho J., Choi E. K., Kim I. R., Im Y. H., Park Y. H., Lee S., et al. Development and validation of Chemotherapy-induced Alopecia Distress Scale (CADS) for breast cancer patients. *Ann. Oncol.*, 2014 Feb.; 25(2):346-51.

In: Geriatric Psychodermatology
Editors: Mohammad Jafferany and Katlein França
ISBN: 978-1-63463-853-1

Chapter 7

Nail Disorders in Geriatric Population

Adam Reich, M.D.* and Jacek C. Szepietowski, M.D.

Introduction

Nails are important organs of human body; however, their significance is often neglected unless their appearance and/or structure are disturbed. Nails fulfil a number of relevant functions: they protect tips of fingers and toes from mechanical injuries, fingernails enhance fine touching and tactile sensitivity as well as aid fine manipulation and picking up small objects. Nails are also used during scratching to relieve itch and in some occasions they may be even used as a defensive weapon. Last but not least, healthy looking nails are part of own body image, playing an important role in interpersonal relations hips [1]. Remarkably, as shown by Kim et al. [2] all elderly people have at least one kind of a foot problem and the most prevalent ones are nail abnormalities, and this phenomenon cannot be overlooked by healthcare professional.

It is generally known that elderly people often suffer from numerous internal diseases, like arterial hypertension, diabetes, ischemic heart disease s, chronic kidney insufficiency, etc., which results from the natural process of aging, previous lifestyle and lifelong cumulative exposure to various environmental hazards. If left untreated, they are potentially life-threatening and may lead to significant morbidity and life shortening. Therefore, physicians, nurses and other health care providers are usually focused on these "important" diseases while treating elderly people, often forgetting about "milder" health problems like nail abnormalities, or considering them as irrelevant. However, at least for some elderly persons abnormal nails may be a very significant problem, e.g., thickened toenails may prevent from matching shoes and cause pain while walking. Damaged toenails, e.g., due to onychomycosis, may facilitate invasion of other pathogens resulting in bacterial cellulitis or erysipelas of the lower leg [3]. On rare occasions, pathogens found in the nails may even disseminate via blood resulting in sepsis and patient's death [3, 4].

* Corresponding author: Adam Reich. E-mail: adam.reich@umed.wroc.pl.

To maintain the proper function of nails they should be correctly look after. Remarkably, proper care of toenails in elderly people is significantly altered due to movement and bending difficulties and frequent visual disturbances further facilitating development of nail abnormalities or even dystrophy. Thus, the proper care of nails in elderly people often requires participation of third parties to be done correctly. Unfortunately, for many elderly persons such help is, for different reasons, unavailable.

Onychomycosis

Onychomycosis is the most frequent nail disease and it is also the best studied nail condition with regard to health related quality of life (HRQoL) [1, 5]. The prevalence of onychomycosis in the general population is estimated between 2 to 8% [6-11], however, it is much more prevalent in elderly people [6, 8-10]. In our study including 198 patients older than 65 years onychomycosis was observed in 17.2% of subjects [12]. The frequency can be even higher, if predisposing factors are present, e.g., Papini et al. [13] found that more than a half of patients with diabetic foot suffered concomitantly from toenail onychomycosis.

Onychomycosis in elderly people is not only more prevalent, but is also more severe. Comparing with younger people, we have found that older subjects have significantly more toenails involved (patients with toenail onychomycosis >60 years old had on average 5.1±2.8 toenails involved, while patients younger than 30 years had only 3.3±2.1 toenails with onychomycosis and subjects between 30 and 60 years had 4.3±2.6 toenails involved; $p<0.001$), more frequently suffered from bilateral toenail onychomycosis (84% of patients >60 years old compared to 64.1% and 74.3% in the other age groups, respectively, $p<0.001$) and also suffered from toenail onychomycosis significantly longer than the other patients (mean disease duration: 25.2±25.0 months vs. 10.0±9.7 months and 16.6±18.1 months, respectively, $p<0.001$) [14]. Even more importantly, toenail onychomycosis in elderly people was accompanied more commonly by tinea pedis (38.6%) than it was observed in other age groups (patients <30 years old: 30.1%, patients between 30 and 60 years old: 32.6%, $p=0.01$) [15].

Onychomycosis is not a life-threatening disease, however, it cannot be considered as a cosmetic problem. Due to its chronic course, significant difficulties in achieving complete and durable clinical and mycological cure, common relapses and visibility for other people, onychomycosis has significant influence on HRQoL [1]. The disease is usually long lasting, even if appropriate antifungal therapy is introduced, it causes pain and significant problems of wearing shoes [16-18].

Assessment of HRQoL in onychomycosis patients was an objective of many scientific projects which used numerous generic or disease-specific instruments [15-26]. However, none of these studies were specifically dedicated elderly people, albeit in all studies persons older than 60 (or 65) years constituted significant portion of studied populations. Therefore, results of these studies may be, at least partially and with some caution, extrapolated to elderly population. As showed by Drake et al. [17] about 70% of toenail onychomycosis patients considered their nail disease to be at least a moderate problem for them. Other studies showed that subjects with onychomycosis had significantly poorer ratings of general health perception, bodily pain, mental health, social functioning, physical appearance and functional limitations, when compared to gender- and age -matched healthy controls [20, 21]. Patients with onychomycosis frequently experience reduced self-esteem, embarrassment and are less willing to participate in social and leisure activities [5]. Pain within toes was present in 41-60% of studied subjects and nearly one fifth of patients avoided various social activities due to onychomycosis [17]. Other sensations related to onychomycosis included tin gling, burning, numbness, pressure, or discomfort [17]. According to the Achilles Foot-Screening Project, 51% of patients with onychomycosis suffered from discomfort in walking, 33% had foot pain, 28% were embarrassed by the nail condition, and 13% were limited in work or other activities because of the affection of toenails [27].

As mentioned above, older patients suffer from onychomycosis significantly longer and had usually more nails involved than the younger counterparts. Elewski [16] observed, that patients suffering from onychomycosis for 10 years or longer had more psychosocially impaired HRQoL and subjects with five or more toenails involved experienced more psychosocial effects than those with four or fewer toenails infected. Similarly, Drake et al. [22] reported that long duration of toenail onychomycosis and involvement of 5 or more toenails significantly impaired emotional and physical domains of HRQoL. Coexisting fingernail involvement was another important co-factor significantly reducing HRQoL comparing with subjects having only toenail onychomycosis [28]. Significant numbers of patients feel to be unattractive and stigmatized by onychomycosis, indicating that other people stare at the changed nails and consider their disease as contagious [29]. Majority of toenail onychomycosis patients express the feeling that other people found it unpleasant to look at infected nails and had problems in wearing shoes, difficulties of cutting their nails as well as complained that they had to spent significant amount of money to treat their nail disease [16-18]. Nevertheless, Drake et al. [17] found, that more than 95% of onychomycosis subjects would be willing to pay for an anti-fungal therapy with an 80% cure rate, even if their insurance would not cover the cost and even more importantly, anti-mycotic therapy resulted in significant reduction of stigmatization caused by onychomycosis [29].

There are, however, some differences in disease perception between elderly patients and younger counterparts. Older patients usually experience more symptoms due to onychomycosis, while younger people are more emotionally affected by the fungal disease [18, 20, 22]. As shown in Table 1, elderly people had been found to be less severely affected by onychomycosis than younger people: significantly more elderly subjects only demonstrated small effect on HRQoL, while in younger subjects the disease usually had at least moderate effect. Such dimensions like leisure activities, school and work activities and personal relations hipswere significantly less affected by onychomycosis in older people than in younger individuals, however, problems with symptoms and feelings, daily activities and treatment were similarly expressed by both groups.

Nail Psoriasis

Nail psoriasis is another nail condition which might be responsible for significant disfigurement and emotional stress in elderly patients.

Nail psoriasis affects about half of all psoriatic individuals [30-33]. Taking into account, that the prevalence of psoriasis in general population is estimated to be 1-3%, it could be assumed, that the prevalence of nail psoriasis is around 0.5-1.5%. Nail psoriasis is believed to be an indicator of more advanced disease, both in respect to skin manifestation as well as to severity of joint symptoms [32, 34-36]. Nail involvement in psoriasis may manifest as nail pitting (tiny depressions of the nail plate), nail bed discoloration ("salmon spots", "oil drops"), splinter haemorrhages, red spots within the lunula, subungual hyperkeratosis, nail plate thickening or crumbling, onycholysis, and in the most severe cases even as a complete dystrophy of the nail plate [32, 37, 38]. Similarly to onychomycosis, there is no study analyzing particularly the relevance of nail psoriasis with respect to well-being of elderly people.

Table 1. Comparison of HRQoL in onychomycosis between elderly patients defined as persons ≥65 years old and younger counterparts (DLQI – Dermatology Life Quality Index, scale scoring ranges from 0 to 30 points, higher scoring indicating greater impairment of HRQoL)

	Patients ≥65 years old	**Patients <65 years old**	**p**
N	86	685	-
DLQI total scoring (range 0 – 30)	4.5±3.7	7.5±5.4	<0.001
DLQI dimensions			
Symptoms and feelings (range 0 – 6)	2.0±1.3	2.2±1.3	0.11
Daily activities (range 0 – 6)	1.3±1.3	1.5±1.4	0.11
Leisure (range 0 – 6)	0.5±1.0	1.3±1.4	<0.001
Work and School (range 0 – 3)	0.01±0.1	0.3±0.6	<0.001
Personal relationships (0 – 6)	0.3±0.6	1.6±1.6	<0.001
Treatment (0 – 3)	0.4±0.6	0.5±0.7	0.28
DLQI categories			
No effect on HRQoL	20.9%	13.1%	<0.001
Small effect on HRQoL	44.2%	28.2%	
Moderate effect on HRQoL	32.6%	40.3%	
Very large effect on HRQoL	2.3%	17.5%	
Extremely large effect on HRQoL	0%	0.9%	

However, taking into consideration visibility of nail lesions (especially within fingernails), limited treatment options showing frequently unsatisfactory efficacy as well as long-lasting nail disfigurements, it seems, that the negative influence of nail lesions in psoriasis on patients should be at least as big as that caused by onychomycosis.

Nail problems were mentioned among the most bothersome symptoms of psoriasis by 36.4% psoriatic individuals [39]. Only pruritus (63.6%), extensive skin scaling (56.4%), redness of the skin (52.7%), skin burning (41.8%), and prominent scaling within scalp (38.2%) were more frequently indicated as the most disturbing psoriasis symptoms [39]. However, the proper assessment of the influence of nail lesions on HRQoL in psoriasis is difficult, as frequently these patients demonstrate simultaneously extensive skin lesions and/or joint involvement. Furthermore, as shown by Augustin et al. [40], patients with nail involvement had higher disease severity (mean Psoriasis Area and Severity Index 12.7 points vs. 9.3 points), higher frequency of psoriatic arthritis (26.0% vs. 12.7%), and a 2.5-fold higher rate of inpatient treatments compared to psoriatic patients without nail lesions. Subjects with nail psoriasis also showed stronger impairment of HRQoL (mean DLQI 8.9 points vs. 7.3

points), but this difference cannot simply be attributed to the presence of nail lesions, as they also had more severe psoriasis in general.

Nevertheless, it is clearly evident that nail psoriasis leads to significant functional impairment, may cause pain and psychosocial distress and has a negative impact on social activities [37, 38, 41]. Remarkably, more than 90% of patients with nail psoriasis were concerned about the cosmetic appearance of their nails [41]. Based on the NailQoL [25] very important aspects of nail psoriasis were being ashamed of, embarrassed about or frustrated with the appearance of their nails, and high degree of the worry, that the nail condition may get worse [42]. Subjects with nail psoriasis demonstrated also significantly worse satisfaction with their therapy, higher stress, and had to spend more time for the treatment procedures [35]. In general, psoriatics with nail lesions displayed significantly lower HRQoL according to the DLQI (7.2±6.4 points vs. 5.3±5.3 points; $p<0.001$) and poorer health state based on the EQ5-D (EuroQoL) (60.1±21.6 points vs. 67.3±21.0 points; $p<0.001$) [35]. In addition, severe nail disease was found to be associated with functional impairment related to psoriatic arthritis and more severe nail lesions correlated with more depression and anxiety [34]. Higher suffering in psoriatics with nail involvement also resulted in the higher number of medical consultations sought from both dermatologists and orthopedic surgeons/ rheumatologists [35].

Despite the fact, that all the discussed data refers to patients with nail psoriasis in general, we do believe that they are also valid for elderly psoriatic patients with nail involvement as we did not observed hardly any relationship between age and the degree of HRQoL [42], similarly to Ortonne group [43]. The only difference was found regarding symptoms severity, which was more prone in older subjects suggesting that older patients may be even more affected than the younger counterparts [42].

Other Nail Conditions

Onychophagia is defined as a chronic nail biting behavior, while onychotillomania is a form of self-induced nail destruction caused by recurrent picking and manicuring of the nails [44]. Habitual nail biting is a common behavior in children and young adults, but may also be observed in older patients [44]. The prevalence of nail biting among people older than 60 years is estimated to be between 4.5% and 10.7% [45]. Nail biting behavior should be classified among an obsessive-compulsive spectrum disorder. Despite nail biting can be considered in most cases as a cosmetic problem, if uncontrolled, it can cause serious morbidity. The most common complications of nail biting are damage of the cuticles and nails, paronychia and secondary bacterial infection, self-inflicted gingival injuries, and on some occasions, even temporo-mandibular dysfunction and osteomyelitis [46-49]. Nail biting is also often embarrassing and socially undesirable. Treatment of nail biting may be based on behavioral therapy, including self-monitoring and habit reversal. In more severe cases serotonin re-uptake inhibitors, such as clomipramine or sertraline seem to be a good alternative. They are effective in approximately 60–70% of patients with onychophagia [44].

Brittle nail syndrome, defined as an increased fragility of nail plates, is another nail condition that may cause significant cosmetic concerns and decrease of self-esteem [50]. The impact of brittle nails on HRQoL has not been well evaluated so far, however, the vast majority of patients with brittle nails consider them as a significant cosmetic problem and a number of sufferers indicated that these nail abnormalities are painful and impair daily activities [50, 51].

Chemotherapy is another important factor, which may cause nail problems. A number of chemotherapeutics were shown to induce nail abnormalities, taxanes and anthracyclines being the most commonly implicated [52-55]. As elderly people quite commonly suffer from malignancies, nail complications of chemotherapy are probable more prevalent in this age group than in the other people. Nail toxicities can be asymptomatic and limited to cosmetic concerns, but may also be quite severe, causing considerable pain and discomfort, subungual hemorrhages and nail plate avulsion [52-55].

Remarkably, in a study by Winther et al. [54] more than 40% of individuals with docetaxel nail toxicities experienced various degrees of functional problems like difficulties in housekeeping, writing, or sewing, up to 37% had problems finding proper footwear and nearly one third declared difficulties in walking.

Conclusion

Elderly people often suffer from numerous severe medical conditions that must be adequately treated. However, besides this "important" disorders old people may also suffer from other health problems, which although not so severe, but may alter very much the daily functioning. Among them, nail abnormalities seem to be very common. So far, no many studies have been performed to analyze the relevance of nail problems in respect to well-being of elderly population. However, extrapolating available data it could be assumed that nail diseases may be a significant ailment in this patient group. Nail abnormalities cause not only significant cosmetic concerns, but, even more importantly, may cause physical pain and limit daily activity and social functioning. Thus, nail diseases should be considered as an relevant medical problem, and must gain adequate attention from health care providers.

References

[1] Reich A., Szepietowski J. C. Health-related quality of life in patients with nail disorders. *Am. J. Clin. Dermatol.*, 2011; 12:313-320.

[2] Kim S., Ahn J., Choi S., Lee Y. Geriatric foot problems and related factors in two provinces of Korea. *J. Korean Acad. Nurs.*, 2010; 40:161-171.

[3] Reich A., Schwartz R. A., Szepietowski J. C. Complications of superficial mycoses. In: Fratamico P. M., Smith J. L., Brogden K. A. (eds.). Sequelae and long-term consequences of infectious diseases. ASM Press, Washington, DC, 2009;407-413.

[4] Arrese J. E., Piérard-Franchimont C., Piérard G. E. Fatal hyalohyphomycosis following Fusarium onychomycosis in an immunocompromised patient. *Am. J. Dermatopathol.*, 1996; 18:196-198.

[5] Szepietowski J. C., Reich A. Onychomycosis and quality of life. *Eur. Dermatol.*, 2009; 4:85-87.

[6] Roberts D. T. Prevalence of dermatophyte onychomycosis in the United Kingdom: results of an omnibus survey. *Br. J. Dermatol.,* 1992; 126, Suppl 39:23-27.
[7] Heikkilä H., Stubb S. The prevalence of onychomycosis in Finland. *Br. J. Dermatol.,* 1995; 133:699-703.
[8] Sais G., Jucglà A., Peyrí J. Prevalence of dermatophyte onychomycosis in Spain: a cross-sectional study. *Br. J. Dermatol.,* 1995; 132:758-761.
[9] Gupta A. K., Jain H. C., Lynde C. W., Watteel G. N., Summerbell R. C. Prevalence and epidemiology of unsuspected onychomycosis in patients visiting dermatologists' offices in Ontario, Canada – a multicenter survey of 2001 patients. *Int. J. Dermatol.,* 1997; 36:783-787.
[10] Gupta A. K., Jain H. C., Lynde C. W., Macdonald P., Cooper E. A., Summerbell R. C. Prevalence and epidemiology of onychomycosis in patients visiting physicians' offices: a multicenter canadian survey of 15,000 patients. *J. Am. Acad. Dermatol.,* 2000; 43: 244-248.
[11] Ioannidou D. J., Maraki S., Krasagakis S. K., Tosca A., Tselentis Y. The epidemiology of onychomycoses in Crete, Greece, between 1992 and 2001. *J. Eur. Acad. Dermatol. Venereol.,* 2006; 20:170-174.
[12] Reszke R., Pełka D., Walasek A., Machaj Z., Reich A. Skin problems of the elderly patient. *Int. J. Dermatol.* 2014; doi: 10.1111/ijd.12832 [in press].
[13] Papini M., Cicoletti M., Fabrizi V., Landucci P. Skin and nail mycoses in patients with diabetic foot. *G. Ital. Dermatol. Venereol.,* 2013; 148:603-608.
[14] Szepietowski J., Reich A., Garłowska E., Kulig M., Baran E. Predisposing factors to onychomycosis in Polish population. *Mikol. Lek.,* 2005; 12:231-234.
[15] Szepietowski J. C., Reich A., Garłowska E., Kulig M., Baran E. Factors influencing coexistence of toenail onychomycosis with tinea pedis and other dermatomycoses: a survey of 2761 patients. *Arch. Dermatol.,* 2006; 142:1279-1284.
[16] Elewski B. E. The effect of toenail onychomycosis on patient quality of life. *Int. J. Dermatol.,* 1997; 36:754-756.
[17] Drake L. A., Scher R. K., Smith E. B., Faich G. A., Smith S. L., Hong J. J., Stiller M. J. Effect of onychomycosis on quality of life. *J. Am. Acad. Dermatol.,* 1998; 38:702-704.
[18] Szepietowski J. C., Reich A., Pacan P., Garlowska E., Baran E. Evaluation of quality of life in patients with toenail onychomycosis by Polish version of an international onychomycosis-specific questionnaire. *J. Eur. Acad. Dermatol. Venerol.,* 2007; 21:491-496.
[19] Drake L. Quality of life issues with patients with fungal nail infection s. *AIDS Patient Care,* 1995;9,Suppl. 1:S15-17.
[20] Lubeck D. P., Gause D., Schein J. R., Prebil L. E., Potter L. P. A health -related quality of life measure for use in patients with onychomycosis: a validation study. *Qual. Life Res.,* 1999; 8:121-129.
[21] Lubeck D. P., Schein J. R., Gause D., Prebil L. A., Potter L. P. Health-related quality of life in patients with toenail onychomycosis: data from 9-month observational study. *J. Clin. Outcomes Manage.,* 1999; 6:37-42.
[22] Drake L. A., Patrick D. L., Fleckman P., Andr J., Baran R., Haneke E., Sapède C., Tosti A. The impact of onychomycosis on quality of life: development of an international onychomycosis-specific questionnaire to measure patient quality of life. *J. Am. Acad. Dermatol.,* 1999; 41:189-196.

[23] Turner R. R., Testa M. A. Measuring the impact of onychomycosis on patient quality of life. *Qual. Life Res.,* 2000; 9:39-53.

[24] Potter L. P., Mathias S. D., Raut M., Kianifard F., Tavakkol A. The OnyCOE-t questionnaire: responsiveness and clinical meaningfulness of a patient-reported outcomes questionnaire for toenail onychomycosis. *Health Qual. Life Outcomes* 2006; 4:50.

[25] Warshaw E. M., Foster J. K., Cham P. M., Grill J. P., Chen S. C. NailQoL: a quality-of-life instrument for onychomycosis. *Int. J. Dermatol.,* 2007; 46:1279-1286.

[26] Milobratović D., Janković S., Vukičević J., Marinković J., Janković J., Railić Z. Quality of life in patients with toenail onychomycosis. *Mycoses,* 2013; 56:543-551.

[27] Katsambas A., Abeck D., Haneke E., van de Kerkhof P., Burzykowski T., Molenberghs G., Marynissen G. The effects of foot disease on quality of life: results of the Achilles Project. *J. Eur. Acad. Dermatol. Venereol.,* 2005; 19:191-195.

[28] Szepietowski J. C., Reich A., Woźniak M., Baran E. Evaluation of quality of life in patients with onychomycosis using the Polish version of Dermatology Life Quality Index. *Mikol. Lek.,* 2006; 13:193-198.

[29] Szepietowski J. C., Reich A.; for the National Quality of Life in Dermatology Group. Stigmatisation in onychomycosis patients: a population -based study. *Mycoses,* 2008; 52:343-349.

[30] Jiaravuthisan M. M., Sasseville D., Vender R. B., Murphy F., Muhn C. Y. Psoriasis of the nail: anatomy, pathology, clinical presentation, and a review of the literature on therapy. *J. Am. Acad. Dermatol.,* 2007; 57:1-27.

[31] Edwards F., de Berker D. Nail psoriasis: clinical presentation and best practice recommendations. *Drugs,* 2009; 69:2351-2361.

[32] Reich K. Approach to managing patients with nail psoriasis. *J. Eur. Acad. Dermatol. Venereol.,* 2009; 23,Suppl. 1:15-21.

[33] Klaassen K. M., van de Kerkhof P. C., Pasch M. C. Nail psoriasis: a questionnaire - based survey. *Br. J. Dermatol.,* 2013; 169:314-319.

[34] Williamson L., Dalbeth N., Dockerty J. L., et al. Extended report: nail disease in psoriatic arthritis – clinically important, potentially treatable and often overlooked. *Rheumatology,* (Oxford) 2004; 43:790-794.

[35] Radtke M. A., Langenbruch A. K., Schäfer I., Herberger K., Reich K., Augustin M. Nail psoriasis as a severity indicator: results from the PsoReal study. *Patient Relat. Outcome Meas.,* 2011; 2:1-6.

[36] Langenbruch A., Radtke M. A., Krensel M., Jacobi A., Reich K., Augustin M. Nail involvement as a predictor of concomitant psoriatic arthritis in patients with psoriasis. *Br. J. Dermatol.,* 2014; doi: 10.1111/bjd.13272. [Epub ahead of print]

[37] Baran R. The burden of nail psoriasis: an introduction. *Dermatology,* 2010; 221,Suppl. 1:1-5.

[38] Salomon J., Szepietowski J. C., Proniewicz A. Psoriatic nails: a prospective clinical study. *J. Cutan. Med. Surg.,* 2003; 7:317-321.

[39] Reich A., Welz-Kubiak K., Rams Ł. The disease apprehension by patients suffering from psoriasis. *Adv. Dermatol. Allergol.,* 2014; 31:289-293.

[40] Augustin M., Reich K., Blome C., Schäfer I., Laass A., Radtke M. A. Nail psoriasis in Germany: epidemiology and burden of disease. *Br. J. Dermatol.,* 2010; 163:580-585.

[41] de Jong E. M., Seegers B. A., Gulinck M. K., Boezeman J. B., van de Kerkhof P. C. Psoriasis of the nails associated with disability in a large number of patients: results of a recent interview with 1,728 patients. *Dermatology,* 1996; 193:300-303.

[42] Zdrojowy M., Szepietowski J., Zazulak N. Gutfreund K., Lis J., Reich A. Quality of life in nail psoriasis. *Acta. Derm. Venereol.,* 2009; 89:561.

[43] Ortonne J. P., Baran R., Corvest M., Schmitt C., Voisard J. J., Taieb C. Development and validation of nail psoriasis quality of life scale (NPQ10). *J. Eur. Acad. Dermatol. Venereol.,* 2010; 24:22-27.

[44] Pacan P., Grzesiak M., Reich A., Szepietowski J. C. Onychophagia as a spectrum of obsessive-compulsive disorder. *Acta. Derm. Venereol.,* 2009; 89:278-280.

[45] Heaton K. W., Mountford R. A. Nail-biting in the population and its relationship to irritable bowel syndrome. *J. R. Soc. Med.,* 1992; 85:457.

[46] Tosti A., Peluso A. M., Bardazzi F., Morelli R., Bassi F. Phalangeal osteomyelitis due to nail biting. *Acta. Derm. Venereol.,* 1994; 74: 206-207.

[47] Baydas B., Uslu H., Yavuz I., Ceylan I., Dagsuyu I. M. Effect of a chronic nail-biting habit on the oral carriage of *Enterobacteraceae. Oral Microbiol. Immunol.,* 2007; 22: 1-4.

[48] Williams T. I., Rose R., Chisholm S. What is the function of nail biting: an analog assessment study. *Behav. Res. Ther.,* 2006; 45: 989-995.

[49] Lee D. Y. Chronic nail biting and irreversible shortening of the fingernails. *J. Eur. Acad. Dermatol. Venereol.,* 2009; 23:185.

[50] van de Kerkhof P. C., Pasch M. C., Scher R. K., Kerscher M., Gieler U., Haneke E., Fleckman P. Brittle nail syndrome: a pathogenesis -based approach with a proposed grading system. *J. Am. Acad. Dermatol.,* 2005; 53:644-651.

[51] Scher R. K. Brittle nails. *Int. J. Dermatol.,* 1989; 28:515-516.

[52] Gilbar P., Hain A., Peereboom V. M. Nail toxicity induced by cancer chemotherapy. *J. Oncol. Pharm. Pract.,* 2009; 15:143-155.

[53] Hong J., Park S. H., Choi S. J., Lee S. H., Lee K. C., Lee J. I., Kyung S. Y., An C. H., Lee S. P., Park J. W., Jeong S. H., Nam E., Bang S. M., Cho E. K., Shin D. B., Lee J. H. Nail toxicity after treatment with docetaxel: a prospective analysis in patients with advanced non-small cell lung cancer. *Jpn. J. Clin. Oncol.,* 2007; 37:424-428.

[54] Winther D., Saunte D. M., Knap M., Haahr V., Jensen A. B. Nail changes due to Docetaxel – a neglected side effect and nuisance for the patient. *Support Care Cancer,* 2007; 15:1191-1197.

[55] Fenniche S., Hammami H., Badri T., Mokhtar I., Benmously R. Subungueal haemorrhages following docetaxel (taxotere) treatment. *Curr. Drug Saf.,* 2012; 7:247-249.

In: Geriatric Psychodermatology
Editors: Mohammad Jafferany and Katlein França

ISBN: 978-1-63463-853-1

Chapter 8

Obsessive Compulsive Disorder in the Elderly

Thelda Kestenbaum, M.D.*

Introduction

The number of elderly people (65 years of age and older) is increasing in both developed and developing countries. By the year 2030 it is estimated that there will be 71 million elderly in the United States [1] and in 2050 it is projected that there will be 86.7 million elderly in the United States. [2] Twenty years ago, in 1994, 8% of the American population was elderly [3] and in 2050 it has been projected that 21% of the American population will be elderly. [2]

Obsessive compulsive disorder (OCD) afflicts significant numbers of the elderly with cutaneous signs and symptoms of OCD often presenting to dermatologists and primary care physicians. Excoriations, some recalcitrant eczemas (especially hand eczemas), trichotillomania, onychotillomania, and onychophagia are among the most common cutaneous manifestations across all age groups. [4]

In the elderly, excoriations, eczemas (lichen simplex chronicus), prurigo, and onychotillomania are probably more prevalent as cutaneous manifestations of OCD whereas trichotillomania (hair pulling) is less common than in the population overall. [2, 3] Fear of forgetting (especially of names) and of having sinned may be more common in older patients with OCD. [5]

According to Jafferany et al. only 18% of dermatologists have an understanding of psychodermatology but 39% of dermatologists have an interest in increasing their knowledge of psychodermatology. [6] Interestingly, most patients with skin signs of OCD present to their primary care physicians or to dermatologists so it is imperative that these physicians in particular have familiarity with common skin manifestations of obsessive compulsive disorder. About 90% of psychiatrists surveyed were not aware of patient or family resources on manifestations of OCD. [7] Psychiatrists are not much better than dermatologists in their

* Corresponding author: Thelda Kestenbaum. Email: tkestenb@kumc.edu

feeling at ease with psychodermatology. [7] About 21% of psychiatrists in one survey had a clear idea of psychodermatology; 85% expressed interest in obtaining more instruction on this topic. [7]

Prevalence

OCD was previously thought to be rare but it is now known the prevalence is 2% to 3% in the general population. Prevalence is much higher (between 14% to almost 25%)in patients presenting with cutaneous complaints other than those with just skin cancers and this has been shown in multiple surveys and in different ethnicities. [4] DSM-5 cites a 12 month prevalence in the United States as 1.2% with a similar prevalence internationally (1.1%-1.8%). [8] Since OCD is a chronic disorder, it often persists into old age. It may be present in 1.5% of adults over age 65 years of age. [5] Research in late life OCD spectrum disorders is modest. [5]

Definition

The new DSM-5 categorizes obsessive compulsive and related disorders separately from anxiety disorders and include obsessive-compulsive disorder, body dysmorphic disorder, hoarding disorder, trichotillomania, excoriation (skin picking), substance/medication -induced obsessive-compulsive disorder, obsessive-compulsive and related disorder due to another medical condition and other specified and unspecified obsessive-compulsive and related disorders (such as obsessional jealousy). It is stressed that there is close overlap of the related disorders and also a close relationship to anxiety disorders from which now it has a separate category. [8]

Obsessions are defined in DSM-5 as recurrent and persistent thoughts, urges, or images that are experienced as intrusive and unwanted. Compulsions are defined as repetitive behaviorsor mental acts that an individual feels driven to perform in response to an obsession or according to rules that must be applied rigidly. The definition requires that obsessions and compulsions must be time consuming (often taking more than an hour a day).

Onset

The mean age of onset of OCD is 19.5 years and 25% of cases start by 14 years of age. Onset after age 35 years is unusual but can occur. [8] Older people, then, with OCD have had it chronically since youth as opposed to having a new onset of OCD in old age.

Late onset of OCD is said to be fairly uncommon [5] and when it does occur is said to be more frequent in women than in men. Late onset OCD may indicate associated cerebral lesions. Dysregulation in serotonergic pathways of the basal ganglia and orbital frontal cortex may represent an underlying vulnerability. In elderly patients with OCD this may indicate cerebrovascular disease (which in the new DSM-5 might be classified as OCD related to another medical condition). Another vulnerability to late-onset OCD is concern about a decline in cognitive function ing whether the concern is warranted or not. [5]

Skin Signs of OCD

The most common cutaneous signs of OCD in the elderly are excoriations, lichen simplex chronicus, prurigo, and onychotillomaia. [2, 3]

Excoriations (skin picking; psychogenic excoriations; formerly called neurotic excoriations) are defined in DSM-5 as recurrent skin picking resulting in skin lesions; repeated attempts to decrease or stop picking; and skin picking causing significant stress or impairment in social, occupational or other important areas of functioning. One must rule out other causes of excoriation such as substance abuse (for example, cocaine) or infestation (such as scabies) or other skin disorders. One cannot explain the picking behavior by symptoms of another mental disorder such as tactile hallucinations or body dysmorphic disorder or intention to harm oneself in order to place it just as OCD. The face, arms and hands are the most common areas of involvement. Most patients use their fingernails but some rub, squeeze, lance, or tweeze the skin. Lifetime prevalence is said to be 1.4% at least in DSM-5. Other sources have found a prevalence of 2% in dermatology clinics, 5.4% in a community sample and 4.6% in a college student sample. [4] Most admit to the picking and this helps differentiate them from patients with factitial skin disorders.

The elderly are more likely to have dry skin and often that causes itching resulting in excoriations. Not all picking is a sign of OCD. People can pick their skin when they are angry, depressed, have body dysmorphic disorder, borderline personality, delusional states, guilt, habit, narcissism and other organic causes. Patients with Prader-Willi syndrome have a great propensity to excoriations; this would now be classified in DSM-5 as OCD secondary to another condition rather than just OCD.

Most patients with excoriations are women (75%) with the onset in middle age. Typically at least a decade or more has gone by before patients receive the correct diagnosis and the problem is usually chronic. It is important to realize that both depression and anxiety are common co-morbidities. If patients complain of pruritus then oral doxepin may be used. Most patients do not itch. Depending on the location of the excoriations, Unna wraps changed weekly may be helpful. A useful website for patients is StopPicking.com.

Eczemas like lichen simplex chronicus (LSC) (also termed neurodermatitis) may be a manifestation of OCD. Prurigo is really a variant of lichen simplex chronicus and is more of a scaly nodule whereas lichen simplex chronicus is usually a scaly plaque. Both result from chronic scratching. The chronic scratching leads to thickening of the skin; usually the epidermis remains intact (unlike in excoriations).While chronic hand eczemas may result from OCD, most hand eczemas are caused by irritant or atopic dermatitis. One must rule out fungal infection, id reaction to a fungal infection of the feet, psoriasis, contact dermatitis, and dyshidrosis. The elderly are more likely to have fungal infections in general and although they do not develop contact dermatitis as readily as younger people often they are using more topical potentially sensitizing agents such as topical antibiotics because they itch from dry skin or stasis dermatitis. Recalcitrant hand eczema patients of any age should be asked how often they wash their hands and if it seems excessive further queries on why they are washing and with what types of soaps and for how long a time they are washing is helpful.

Favorite sites of LSC are the neck, genitals and lower legs. The areas of involvement have to be accessible to the patient by their hands or other instruments like back scratchers which they employ. It is notable that in the elderly with LSC there may be personality differences in those with LSC including a greater tendency to pain avoidance, [2]and conformity compared to a control group. Also, Dr. Jafferany [2] cites a study suggesting that older patients with LSC on the limbs may suggest damage to the peripheral nervous system such as radiculopathy and neuropathy. Nerve root compression on MRI and radiculopathy in nerve conduction studies are more common in those with LSC than in controls. [2] Neuropathic changes are more common in the elderly with LSC and should be considered.

Onychotillomania is not classified separately in DSM-5 but may well be a skin manifestation of OCD, depression, or fixed hypochondriacal delusion. [9, 10] It is defined as a neurotic picking at a nail until it is permanently altered. Some say it encompasses onychophagia (nail biting), nail picking, hangnail, finger sucking, and habit-tic deformity [9].Others say it is just picking of the nailfolds and would classify it separately from onychophagia. [11] It is seen in 85% of cases of trichotillomania which in many cases is a skin manifestation of OCD. Depression is higher in the elderly so definitely should be excluded. In addition, onychotillomania may be seen in syndromes such as Smith-Magenis or Lesch-Nyan whose presentation would be in children. Certain medications, spinal cord injury and congenital indifference and insensitivity to pain may lead to this self- destructive behavior also. [9] One must diagnose the associated psychiatric illness in order to properly address the treatment. Cognitive behavioral therapy and hypnosis have been used [11] and these may be the safest treatments to try for elderly patients with this problem. Onychotillomania may result in melanonychia striata (longitudinal hyperpigmented streak). [12]

Since OCD tends to be chronic, all the skin manifestations of OCD are seen in the elderly just as in other age groups even though excoriations, lichen simplex chronicus and onychotillomania are more common skin manifestations of it in the elderly.

Trichotillomania (hair pulling) is classified under OCD and spectrum disorders in DSM-5. It is a heterogeneous disorder. The essential feature of trichotillomania according to DSM-5 is recurrent pulling out of one's own hair resulting in hair loss which leads to distress or impairment in social, occupational or other important areas of functioning. One must determine that it is not caused by another medical condition and rule out other mental illness (such as body dysmorphic disorder). Usually the scalp (in 75% of cases) [13] is the most common site involved but eyebrow, eyelash, axillary, facial, genital and perirectal hair may also be involved. The 12 month prevalence for trichotillomania in adults and adolescents is 1%-2%. [14] Lifetime prevalence may be as high as 3.4% of women and 1.5% of men. [13]

There are some interesting variants of hair pulling including trichotemnomania [15] (hair loss caused by cutting or shaving the hair), trichodaganomania [16] (hair loss from compulsive habit of biting one's own hair), and trichoteiromania [17] (hair loss from perpetual rubbing of the scalp with fracturing of the hair shafts resulting in white distal tips of hair).

In addition to the usual treatments of OCD, one might mention oral N-acetylcysteine, which is an amino acid and a glutamate modulator that may restore extracellular glutamate concentration in the nucleus accumbens and prove helpful. In a 12 week study of 50 patients

(45 women and 5 men) treated for trichotillomania with 1200 to 2400 mg daily of N-acetylcysteine, the patients in the treatment group were 3 times more likely to have improvement than those in the placebo group (56% vs 16%). [18] The use of this medication is not a definitively proven treatment [19] but is worth more exploration. The trichotillomania learning center website (www.trich.org) may be helpful as well as the website StopPulling.com.

There are animal models of trichotillomania and it is often worsened in animals under stress such as confinement. Cats can demonstrate wool sucking behavior and psychogenic alopecia. Feather picking in birds may represent a similar phenomenon. [13]

Body dysmorphic disorder (BDD) has been called by many other names in the past including dysmorphophobia, dermatologic non-disease, primary monosymptomatic or hypochondriacal psychosis. As defined in DSM-5, it is a preoccupation with one or more perceived defects or flaws in physical appearance that are not observable or appear slight to others. As some point the patient has performed repetitive behaviors(such as mirror checking, excessive grooming, skin picking, etc.) in response to this concern. The preoccupation causes clinically significant distress or impairment in social, occupational or other important areas of functioning. [8] The median age of onset is 15 years. Little is known about BDD in the elderly. [8] Interestingly there are gender related issues in that males seem to be more likely to have genital pre-occupations and females are more likely to have comorbid eating disorders. In males almost exclusively there is a "muscle dysmorphia" form of BDD in which there is preoccupation with the idea that one's body is too small or insufficiently lean or muscular. Most of these men diet, exercise, and or lift weights excessively. Culture can influence the type of BDD issues. For example, the fear of a deformed body is seen more in Japanese. [8]

The description by Dr. Morselli in 1891 describes BDD well; he coined the term dysmorphophobia. He describes a patient who is miserable and who throughout all daily activities including mealtime is consumed with the doubt of his perceived deformity. [13, 20] Patients with eating disorders have a very high rate of BDD. Overall the prevalence of BDD in a recent survey was 2% in a control group; 6.7% in dermatology patients and 14% in dermatology patients seeking cosmetic treatments. [21] In DSM-5 the point prevalence among US adults is 2.4% (2.5% in females and 2.2% in males). It is important to recognize these patients since not only are they dissatisfied with their appearance but they tend to be dissatisfied with treatment of their perceived cosmetic defect. Older patients may be seeking cosmetic treatments and it behooves physicians to recognize patients with BDD because these patients tend to be dissatisfied with whatever is done for them and tend to seek more and more unnecessary cosmetic procedures. There is significant association of BDD with a decrease in quality of life in that about a third stay at home for at least a week; 80% have suicidal ideation and 25% have attempted suicide. [20]

Excessive tanning is often a cutaneous identifier of patients with BDD and of OCD. Sometimes the tanning is a way that the patient has of hiding their BDD. Asking patients to stop tanning so as to avoid developing skin cancers will usually not be incorporated into the behavior any more than telling an anorexic, cachectic patient to eat. [20, 22-24]

Another potential behavior in addition to tanning that may be an identifier of OCD is rhinotillexomania (nose picking). Certainly people who pick their nose excessively are more likely to have other behaviors such as onychotillomania, skin picking, and trichotillomania. This was established in an interesting article establishing that in a sample of people randomly selected to answer questions about their habit of nose picking, 3.5% of the responders had excessive nose picking which took more than one hour per day, interfered with their activities, and even caused nasal septal perforation (2 patients out of 254). [25] Even more severe injury has been described with this behavior. [26]

Etiology of OCD

Brain abnormalities, both structural and neurochemical, have been etiologically implicated. Abnormalities in serotonin, dopamine and glutamate pathways seem to be important in etiology. Drugs affecting these latter three pathways offer therapeutic options. PET scan of patients with OCD are abnormal and then return to more normal patterns after successful treatment whether the treatment is through drug therapy or behavioral therapy. [4, 13]

Ventromedial caudate dysfunction is associated with the obsessions and compulsions of OCD and putamen dysfunction is associated with Tourette's. [13] Functional neuroimaging studies suggest that cortico-striatal-thalamo-cortical circuit dysfunction is the core pathophysiologic feature of OCD [27] Differences in the white matter in OCD; [28-30] differences in the hippocampal neurochemistry and shape in OCD may be most pertinent in etiology. [31, 32]

Certainly the improvements in OCD with use of selective serotonin reuptake inhibitors(SSRIs) group of medications support serotonin being involved. The use of antipsychotics in therapy would lend some thought that dopamine may play a role. Glutamate concentrations in the caudate and anterior cingulate cortex of patients with OCD are altered. [33, 34] Some mice models with glutamate signaling dysfunction have abnormal compulsive, OCD-like, grooming behavior. Treatment with compounds that decrease glutamate activity such as riluzole and memantine may be helpful for treatment [33, 34] D-cycloserine which is a partial N-methyl-D-aspartate (NMDA) agonist has been shown to increase the effectiveness of exposure therapy in patients with OCD [35] by some but its efficacy is still debatable. [36] This drug has been used for treatment of tuberculosis for more than twenty years and is fairly safe.

It is intriguing to speculate that perhaps infection, in certain predisposed individuals, can precipitate OCD or OCD-like behavior. There may be a subset of OCD pediatric patients in whom Group A streptococcal infection precipitates OCD behavior suddenly. This has been termed pediatric autoimmune neuropsychiatric disorder associated with streptococcal infections (PANDAS) [8]. Because this category is under debate, the current DSM-5 states it might be better to give the more expanded entity of pediatric acute -onset neuropsychiatric syndrome (PANS) or idiopathic childhood acute neuropsychiatric symptoms (CANS) and this area deserves further study it goes on to state. In any case, in DSM-5, this group would be placed under OCD and related disorder due to another medical condition (as opposed to just plain OCD).

Genetics of OCD

The observance that OCD seemed to be clustered in certain families date back to the 1930's and concordance rates of 50% in fraternal twins and 80%-87% in identical twins supports this. [13, 37] Glutamate transporter genes may well be involved in OCD; relatives of patients with OCD are four times more likely to develop OCD than the population at large. [38]

Treatment of OCD

Proper diagnosis is imperative. In older patients with OCD remember that underlying cerebrovascular disease is more likely to be responsible in the late onset group as well as in the chronic group with early onset. Physical disability which is more common in older people may be a source of fear for the patient which may lead to behavior such as repeated checking in someone with decreased vision or repeatedly asking instructions over and over in someone with decreased hearing which can be misconstrued as obsessive compulsive behavior when in fact it is a method of coping with a physical ailment. [5] Social taboos in the elderly for example in sexual or religious matters may make assessment of obsessions more difficult to evaluate since they may be more reluctant to admit to any sexual taboo topics or blasphemous topics. Parameters for assessing OCD have not been well worked out for the elderly. The standard Yale-Brown Obsessive Compulsive Scale is used by clinicians to assess OCD symptom severity and monitor improvements with treatment but its psychometric properties has not been evaluated in elderly OCD patients. The Brief Symptom Inventory which is a self-report questionnaire of OCD symptoms is the only measure that has published norms for the elderly. [5]

Treatment for OCD is primarily behavioral therapy and pharmacotherapy. There are some novel therapies some of which are adjunctive. Certainly focusing first on behavioral therapy for elderly patients with OCD is prudent and should be used first in patients of all ages. Elderly patients are more likely to have other medical issues and be on multiple medications that make behavioral therapy a safer choice of treatment. [5]

Cognitive behavioral therapy [39] has been shown to be effective looking at 16 randomized controlled trials involving 756 patients with OCD total compared to controls. Interestingly, older patients may not show as great effect of the treatment but it is effective overall. There are no controlled studies in older adults to examine exact effectiveness of exposure and response prevention therapy. [5] Exposure and response therapy involves gradually and repeatedly bringing the patient into contact with the feared object for as long as possible (exposure). The patient is then asked to try and refrain from the compulsive behavior for as long as possible (such as hand washing or checking). Older patients may not be able to do this sometimes because of decrease in senses such as hearing and it may appear to be less effective when in actuality physical disability interfered. Also, in older patients one must be cognizant that they are more likely to feel a stigmatization for psychiatric disease. Only 10% of older patients with OCD obtain treatment. [5] There may be cognitive limitations as well as intermittent medical conditions that interrupt therapy. [5] Stress can exacerbate OCD behavior and certainly in elderly people there are stresses from medical illnesses, death of a spouse, fear of injury such as falling because of unstable gait that can make good outcomes more difficult to achieve.

Pharmacotherapy for OCD is primarily selective serotonin inhibitors (SSRIs) and the one tricyclic antidepressant (TCA), clomipramine. [40] In recalcitrant cases some of the newer antipsychotics may be added but these are less studied than SSRIs and clomipramine.

Clomipramine (Anafranil) was the first drug approved by the FDA for treatment of OCD in 1989.It is a highly serotonergic tricyclic antidepressant; perhaps that is why it seems to be the most efficacious of its class of drugs for treatment of OCD. SSRIs or clomipramine should be started at low doses with the intent of raising the dosage to the effective one. It may be necessary to go to the highest recommended dosages for at least 3 months to ascertain success. It takes a higher dosage of these medications for treatment of OCD and a longer treatment trial (of at least 3 months) than it does for treatment of depression.

Pharmacological Treatment of OCD

SELECTIVE SEROTONIN RE- UPTAKE INHIBITORS		
Brand (Generic)	Initial starting daily dose	Target daily dose
Prozac (fluoxetine)	20 mg	60-80 mg
Luvox (fluvoxamine)	50 mg	300 mg
Zoloft (sertraline)	50 mg	200 mg
Paxil (paroxetine)	20 mg	60 mg
Celexa (citalopram)	20 mg	20 -60 mg?*
Lexapro (escitalopram)	10 mg	20-30 mg?**
TRICYCLIC ANTIDEPRESSANT		
Anafranil (clomipramine)	25-50 mg	250 mg

Dosages of two of the SSRI drugs, citalopram (Celexa) [41, 42] and escitalopram (Lexapro), perhaps should not be raised to the highest dosages in older patients. In 2011 the FDA raised concern for drug safety with citalopram* because of abnormal heart rhythms with high doses of citalopram; in 2012 recommendations were that those over 60 years of age not use more than 20 mg per day. A large study of more than 600,000 patients on citalopram for depression was looked at by Zivin [42] and this admonition could not be substantiated. In fact, a higher dose of citalopram was associated with less cardiac arrhythmiasthan was a lower dose!* It might be fair to say there is debate on whether or not cardio-toxicity is a valid concern for citalopram.*

Escitalopram (Lexapro) is closely related to citalopram and so one might worry about similar side effects. It is a therapeutic active S- enantiomer of the race mic citalopram. [43] Escitalopram has been used in more than 240 million patients since it was approved in 2001. It seems to be more efficacious than citalopram and has a fast onset of action in treating depression. It seems to have more prolonged serotonin reuptake inhibition than the other drugs in the SSRI group of drugs. Interestingly, when the cardio safety of escitalopram was looked at in over 17 studies involving more than 3000 patients it was found to be safe.**Two of the 17 studies included older patients. No meaningful effect on EKG or blood pressure was noted. The drug seems almost never, even in over-dosage, to cause significant cardio-toxicity. [44] Escitalopram at 30 mg may be better than at 20 mg [45] for treatment of OCD.**

Of the SSRIs for treatment of OCD, there are no absolute guidelines for "the best". Overall of the SSRIs, escitalopram (Lexapro) and sertraline (Zoloft) seem to have less drug interactionswith other medications and this may be of particular importance when treating older patients who are frequently on more medications than younger people. If a family member of the patient had success with a specific SSRI drug, one may want to consider choosing that particular drug.

SSRI drugs are used more commonly than TCA drugs because it is believed they are safer. Once symptoms of OCD are controlled by the medication usually patients have to be on them long term for at least a year. Side effects of all the SSRI drugs include nausea, diarrhea, headaches, insomnia, jitteriness, fatigue and sexual dysfunction. Some patients do better with one SSRI than another.

Do not suddenly stop an SSRI because you could precipitate the discontinuation syndrome. These symptoms include agitation, anxiety, anorexia, confusion, impaired coordination, diarrhea, headache, insomnia, sensory disturbances, sweating, tremor, vomiting, shock -like sensations and flu-like illness. Tapering the patient off an SSRI, rather than abrupt cessation, should be done. Fluoxetine (Prozac), because of its long half-life, is less likely to cause this discontinuation syndrome and paroxetine (Paxil) is more likely to cause a severe discontinuation syndrome unless it is slowly tapered.

For recalcitrant cases of OCD if one has tried several different SSRIs and then clomipramine you could consider adding (but very cautiously if at all) newer atypical antipsychotics. Probably safer choices of an adjunct like odansetron (see novel therapies) might be chosen. Atypical antipsychotic drugs have been used off-label for adjunctive treatment of OCD but in the elderly one should be very leery and some authors feel the dangers (not just weight gain and sedation but increased mortality in the elderly) outweigh the benefit. Having said all that, of the atypical antipsychotics, resperidone (Resperdol) may have some benefit in treating OCD. [46]

Novel treatments for OCD include in addition to N-acetylcysteine [18] and D-cycloserine (mentioned under etiology), the additional glutamate modulating drugs memantine and riluzole. [34, 47] Also, naltrexone, [48, 49] ondansetron (Zofran), [50] exercise, and hypnosis may be beneficial. Even some of the anti-epileptic medications like topiramate and lamotrigine may deserve further exploration. Naltrexone seems to be helpful in some cases of trichotillomania but not necessarily in other types of OCD but perhaps that is because trichotillomania in some cases is a type of addiction and we know that naltrexone is approved by the FDA for both alcohol and opioid addiction. [49]

It is more recently being appreciated from both animal models and clinical research that the glutamatergic system is a promising potential target for pharmacotherapy; glutamate is the most ubiquitous CNS excitatory neurotransmitter with several receptors. [51, 52] This is leading to more close examination of drugs like memantine, riluzole, amantadine, ketamine and certain anti-convulsants. Memantine is a N-methyl-D-aspartate (NMDA) receptor antagonist approved for treatment of Alzheimer's dementia. There is an open label study of its help in OCD. [53] Riluzole is a calcium and sodium -channel blocker, which inhibits synaptic glutamate release and enhances glutamate uptake by astrocytes. [54, 55] It is approved for the treatment of amyotrophic lateral sclerosis (ALS) [56] only in the United States.

Development of this drug was in France as an anti-epileptic drug. In a small study of thirteen patients it was added at a dosage of 50 mg po bid to standard psychotropic medications in treatment resistant OCD patients with significant improvement. One half of patients treated with this medication develop transient elevation in their liver function tests so these tests have to be monitored very regularly.

Odansetron (Zofran) at 0.25 mg bid for two weeks and then raised to 0.5 mg bid for another ten weeks was found to be a very good adjunct to SSRI therapy and when it was discontinued relapse occureed. [50] Odansetron may prove not only slightly more efficacious than added atypical antipsychotics but seems safer. [50] Usually it is used as an antiemetic agent in doses such as 4 mg IV at the end of a surgical procedure to prevent post op nausea and vomiting. [57]

It has been used in pregnancy complicated by nausea and vomiting. Odansetron is thought to modulate dopamine turnover in the nucleus accumbens and the net result is reduction in dopamine induced repetitive behavior. It binds to a serotonin receptor (5-HT3) as well. It can, however prolong QT interval on EKG so do not use it in patients with QT prolongation, but overall it is a safe drug. Dosages used for adjunctive treatment for OCD are much less than dosages for prevention of emesis.

Exercise has been shown promising for treatment of OCD. [58, 59] Moderate intensity exercise sessions weekly for just between 20 and 40 minutes for 12 weeks with participants doing two or three sessions per week on their own in addition led to improvement in OCD symptoms as well as improvement in concurrent depression and anxiety. Hypnotherapy is also a treatment that has shown promise. [60, 61, 11]

Hypnosis was helpful in a pregnant patient with acne excoriée (a variant of excoriations) [61]. A good website for more information on hypnosis and qualified hypnotherapists is www.asch.net. Both exercise and hypnotherapy may be safer than medications if behavioral therapy is not effective alone; they may prove to be effective as an adjunct to behavioral or drug therapy.

Treatment of OCD has come a long way from exorcism [13, 60] and as we understand more about the underlying chemical pathways that may be involved hopefully more efficacious treatments are forthcoming. Recognition of the disorder by dermatologists and primary care physicians in a more timely manner may increase the abysmal figures that overall less than 20% of all patients with OCD are in treatment and many have waited up to 17 years for appropriate therapy to be done. [13] Only 10% of the elderly with OCD seek treatment [5].

Overall more than half of the patients benefit from just behavioral therapy and more than half benefit from just drug therapy. Combining behavioral therapy with drug therapy is often necessary.

Some of the adjuncts such as exercise, hypnotherapy, odansetron, naltrexone, N-acetylcysteine and D-cycloserine may improve outcomes further. The obsessive-compulsive foundation (www.ocfoundation.org) is a helpful website for physicians and patients providing educational information and support group information. A warm accepting attitude from the physician is very important and will increase the chances that physicians can recognize and help their patients with OCD improve their quality of life.

References

[1] Yaar M, A. GB. Aging of Skin. In: Goldsmith L, Katz S, Gilchrest B, Paller A, Leffell D, Wolff K, editors. *Fitzpatrick's Dermatology in General Medicine*. 8th ed. New York: McGraw-Hill; 2012.

[2] Jafferany M, Huynh TV, Silverman MA, Zaidi Z. Geriatric dermatoses: a clinical review of skin diseases in an aging population. *Int. J. Dermatol*. 2012;51(5):509-22.

[3] Koblenzer CS. Psychologic aspects of aging and the skin. *Clin. Dermatol.* 1996;14(2):171-7.

[4] Kestenbaum T. Obsessive-compulsive disorder in dermatology. *Semin. Cutan. Med. Surg*. 2013;32(2):83-7.

[5] Ayers C, Najmi S. Treatment of obsessive-compulsive spectrum disorders in late life. In: Storch EA, McKay D, editors. *Obsessive-compulsive disorder and its spectrum: A life-span approach.* Washington, DC US: American Psychological Association; 2014. p. 97-116.

[6] Jafferany M, Vander Stoep A, Dumitrescu A, Hornung RL. The knowledge, awareness, and practice patterns of dermatologists toward psychocutaneous disorders: results of a survey study. *Int. J. Dermatol*. 2010;49(7):784-9.

[7] Jafferany M, Stoep AV, Dumitrescu A, Hornung RL. Psychocutaneous disorders: a survey study of psychiatrists ' awareness and treatment patterns. *South Med. J.* 2010;103(12):1199-203.

[8] Diagnostic and statistical manual of mental disorder s: DSM-5. 5th ed. ed. American Psychiatric A, American Psychiatric Association DSMTF, editors. Arlington, VA: American Psychiatric Association; 2013.

[9] Reese JM, Hudacek KD, Rubin AI. Onychotillomania: clinicopathologic correlations. *J. Cutan. Patho*l. 2013;40(4):419-23.

[10] Lin YC, Lin YC. Onychotillomania, major depressive disorder and suicide. *Clin. Exp. Dermatol*. 2006;31(4):597-9.

[11] Shenefelt PD. Biofeedback, cognitive-behavioral methods, and hypnosis in dermatology: is it all in your mind? *Dermatol. Ther*. 2003;16(2):114-22.

[12] Baran R. Nail biting and picking as a possible cause of longitudinal melanonychia. A study of 6 cases. *Dermatologica*. 1990;181(2):126-8.

[13] Jenike MA, Baer, Lee and Minichiello, William O. Obsessive-Compulsive Disorders Practical Management. 3rd ed. St Louis: Mosby; 1998.

[14] Thomsen PH. Obsessive-compulsive disorders. *Eur. Child Adolesc. Psychiatry*. 2013;22 Suppl 1:S23-8.

[15] Happle R. Trichotemnomania: obsessive-compulsive habit of cutting or shaving the hair. *J. Am. Acad. Dermatol*. 2005;52(1):157-9.

[16] Jafferany M, Feng J, Hornung RL. Trichodaganomania: the compulsive habit of biting one's own hair. *J. Am. Acad. Dermatol*. 2009;60(4):689-91.

[17] Reich S, Trueb RM. [Trichoteiromania]. *J. Dtsch. Dermatol. Ges*. 2003;1(1):22-8.

[18] Grant JE, Odlaug BL, Kim SW. N-acetylcysteine, a glutamate modulator, in the treatment of trichotillomania: a double-blind, placebo -controlled study. *Arch. Gen. Psychiatry*. 2009;66(7):756-63.

[19] Bloch MH, Panza KE, Grant JE, Pittenger C, Leckman JF. N-acetylcysteine in the treatment of pediatric trichotillomania: a randomized, double-blind, placebo -controlled add-on trial. *J. Am. Acad. Child Adolesc. Psychiatry*. 2013;52(3):231-40.

[20] Gupta R, Huynh M, Ginsburg IH. Body dysmorphic disorder. *Semin. Cutan. Med. Surg*. 2013;32(2):78-82.

[21] Conrado LA, Hounie AG, Diniz JB, Fossaluza V, Torres AR, Miguel EC, et al. Body dysmorphic disorder among dermatologic patients: Prevalence and clinical features. *J. Am. Acad. Dermatol*. 2010;63(2):235-43.

[22] Hunter -Yates J, Dufresne RG, Jr., Phillips KA. Tanning in body dysmorphic disorder. *J. Am. Acad. Dermatol*. 2007;56(5 Suppl):S107-9.

[23] Ashrafioun L, Bonar EE. Tanning addiction and psychopathology: Further evaluation of anxiety disorders and substance abuse. *J. Am. Acad. Dermatol*. 2014;70(3):473-80.

[24] Phillips KA, Conroy M, Dufresne RG, Menard W, Didie ER, Hunter -Yates J, et al. Tanning in body dysmorphic disorder. *Psychiatr. Q*. 2006;77(2):129-38.

[25] Jefferson JW, Thompson TD. Rhinotillexomania: psychiatric disorder or habit? *J. Clin. Psychiatry*. 1995;56(2):56-9.

[26] Rathore D, Ahmed SK, Ahluwalia HS, Mehta P. Rhinotillexomania: a rare cause of medial orbital wall erosion. *Ophthal. Plast. Reconstr. Surg. 2013*;29(5):e134-5.

[27] Brennan BP, Rauch SL, Jensen JE, Pope HG, Jr. A critical review of magnetic resonance spectroscopy studies of obsessive-compulsive disorder. *Biol. Psychiatry*. 2013;73(1):24-31.

[28] Gruner P, Vo A, Ikuta T, Mahon K, Peters BD, Malhotra AK, et al. White matter abnormalities in pediatric obsessive-compulsive disorder. *Neuropsychopharmacology*. 2012;37(12):2730-9.

[29] Szeszko PR, Ardekani BA, Ashtari M, Malhotra AK, Robinson DG, Bilder RM, et al. White matter abnormalities in obsessive-compulsive disorder: a diffusion tensor imaging study. *Arch. Gen. Psychiatry*. 2005;62(7):782-90.

[30] Weber AM, Soreni N, Stanley JA, Greco A, Mendlowitz S, Szatmari P, et al. Proton magnetic resonance spectroscopy of prefrontal white matter in psychotropic naive children and adolescents with obsessive-compulsive disorder. *Psychiatry Res*. 2014;222(1-2):67-74.

[31] Atmaca M, Yildirim H, Ozdemir H, Koc M, Ozler S, Tezcan E. Neurochemistry of the hippocampus in patients with obsessive-compulsive disorder. *Psychiatry Clin. Neurosci*. 2009;63(4):486-90.

[32] Atmaca M, Yildirim H, Ozdemir H, Ozler S, Kara B, Ozler Z, et al. Hippocampus and amygdalar volumes in patients with refractory obsessive-compulsive disorder. *Prog Neuropsychopharmacol Biol. Psychiatry*. 2008;32(5):1283-6.

[33] Wu K, Hanna GL, Easter P, Kennedy JL, Rosenberg DR, Arnold PD. Glutamate system genes and brain volume alterations in pediatric obsessive-compulsive disorder: a preliminary study. *Psychiatry Res*. 2013;211(3):214-20.

[34] Wu K, Hanna GL, Rosenberg DR, Arnold PD. The role of glutamate signaling in the pathogenesis and treatment of obsessive-compulsive disorder. *Pharmacol. Biochem. Behav*. 2012;100(4):726-35.

[35] Rothbaum BO. Critical parameters for D-cycloserine enhancement of cognitive-behaviorial therapy for obsessive-compulsive disorder. *Am. J. Psychiatry*. 2008;165(3):293-6.

[36] Storch EA, Merlo LJ, Bengtson M, Murphy TK, Lewis MH, Yang MC, et al. D-cycloserine does not enhance exposure -response prevention therapy in obsessive-compulsive disorder. *Int. Clin. Psychopharmacol*. 2007;22(4):230-7.
[37] Taylor S. Molecular genetics of obsessive-compulsive disorder: a comprehensive meta-analysis of genetic association studies. *Mol. Psychiatry*. 2013;18(7):799-805.
[38] Bloch MH, Pittenger C. The Genetics of Obsessive-Compulsive Disorder. *Curr. Psychiatry Rev*. 2010;6(2):91-103.
[39] Olatunji BO, Davis ML, Powers MB, Smits JA. Cognitive-behavioral therapy for obsessive-compulsive disorder: a meta-analysis of treatment outcome and moderators. *J. Psychiatr. Res*. 2013;47(1):33-41.
[40] Fineberg NA, Reghunandanan S, Brown A, Pampaloni I. Pharmacotherapy of obsessive-compulsive disorder: evidence -base d treatment and beyond. *Aust. N. Z. J. Psychiatry*. 2013;47(2):121-41.
[41] Bird ST, Crentsil V, Temple R, Pinheiro S, Demczar D, Stone M. Cardiac safety concerns remain for citalopram at dosages above 40 mg/day. *Am. J. Psychiatry*. 2014;171(1):17-9.
[42] Zivin K, Pfeiffer PN, Bohnert AS, Ganoczy D, Blow FC, Nallamothu BK, et al. Evaluation of the FDA warning against prescribing citalopram at doses exceeding 40 mg. *Am. J. Psychiatry*. 2013;170(6):642-50.
[43] Zhong H, Haddjeri N, Sanchez C. Escitalopram, an antidepressant with an allosteric effect at the serotonin transporter--a review of current understanding of its mechanism of action. *Psychopharmacology* (Berl). 2012;219(1):1-13.
[44] Thase ME, Larsen KG, Reines E, Kennedy SH. The cardiovascular safety profile of escitalopram. *Eur. Neuropsychopharmacol*. 2013;23(11):1391-400.
[45] Dougherty DD, Jameson M, Deckersbach T, Loh R, Thompson-Hollands J, Jenike M, et al. Open-label study of high (30 mg) and moderate (20 mg) dose escitalopram for the treatment of obsessive-compulsive disorder. *Int. Clin. Psychopharmacol*. 2009;24(6):306-11.
[46] Maher AR, Theodore G. Summary of the comparative effectiveness review on off-label use of atypical antipsychotics. *J. Manag. Care Pharm*. 2012;18(5 Suppl B):S1-20.
[47] Sani G, Serra G, Kotzalidis GD, Romano S, Tamorri SM, Manfredi G, et al. The role of memantine in the treatment of psychiatric disorders other than the dementias: a review of current preclinical and clinical evidence. *CNS Drugs*. 2012;26(8):663-90.
[48] De Sousa A. An open-label pilot study of naltrexone in childhood -onset trichotillomania. *J. Child Adolesc. Psychopharmacol*. 2008;18(1):30-3.
[49] Grant JE, Odlaug BL, Potenza MN. Addicted to hair pulling? How an alternate model of trichotillomania may improve treatment outcome. *Harv. Rev. Psychiatry*. 2007;15(2):80-5.
[50] Pallanti S, Bernardi S, Antonini S, Singh N, Hollander E. Ondansetron augmentation in patients with obsessive-compulsive disorder who are inadequate responders to serotonin reuptake inhibitors: improvement with treatment and worsening following discontinuation. *Eur. Neuropsychopharmacol*. 2014;24(3):375-80.
[51] Kariuki-Nyuthe C, Gomez-Mancilla B, Stein DJ. Obsessive compulsive disorder and the glutamatergic system. *Curr. Opin. Psychiatry*. 2014;27(1):32-7.

[52] Grados MA, Specht MW, Sung HM, Fortune D. Glutamate drugs and pharmacogenetics of OCD: a pathway-based exploratory approach. *Expert. Opin. Drug* Discov. 2013;8(12):1515-27.

[53] Aboujaoude E, Barry JJ, Gamel N. Memantine augmentation in treatment -resistant obsessive-compulsive disorder: an open-label trial. *J. Clin. Psychopharmacol.* 2009;29(1):51-5.

[54] Grant P, Song JY, Swedo SE. Review of the use of the glutamate antagonist riluzole in psychiatric disorders and a description of recent use in childhood obsessive-compulsive disorder. *J. Child Adolesc.Psychopharmacol.* 2010;20(4):309-15.

[55] Coric V, Taskiran S, Pittenger C, Wasylink S, Mathalon DH, Valentine G, et al. Riluzole augmentation in treatment -resistant obsessive-compulsive disorder: an open-label trial. *Biol. Psychiatry*. 2005;58(5):424-8.

[56] Bellingham MC. A review of the neural mechanisms of action and clinical efficiency of riluzole in treating amyotrophic lateral sclerosis: what have we learned in the last decade? *CNS Neurosci. Ther*. 2011;17(1):4-31.

[57] Christofaki M, Papaioannou A. Ondansetron: a review of pharmacokinetics and clinical experience in postoperative nausea and vomiting. *Expert Opin Drug Metab Toxicol.* 2014;10(3):437-44.

[58] Brown RA, Abrantes AM, Strong DR, Mancebo MC, Menard J, Rasmussen SA, et al. A pilot study of moderate-intensity aerobic exercise for obsessive compulsive disorder. *J. Nerv. Ment. Dis*. 2007;195(6):514-20.

[59] Abrantes AM, Strong DR, Cohn A, Cameron AY, Greenberg BD, Mancebo MC, et al. Acute changes in obsessions and compulsions following moderate-intensity aerobic exercise among patients with obsessive-compulsive disorder. *J. Anxiety Disord.* 2009;23(7):923-7.

[60] Frederick C. Hypnotically facilitated treatment of obsessive-compulsive disorder: can it be evidence -based? *Int. J. Clin. Exp. Hypn*. 2007;55(2):189-206.

[61] Shenefelt PD. Using hypnosis to facilitate resolution of psychogenic excoriations in acne excoriee. *Am. J. Clin. Hypn*. 2004;46(3):239-45.

Part III. Psychophysiological Disorders

In: Geriatric Psychodermatology
Editors: Mohammad Jafferany and Katlein França
ISBN: 978-1-63463-853-1

Chapter 9

Vitiligo

Tania Nely Rocha, M.D. ***and Rafael Henrique Rocha, M.D.***

Introduction

Vitiligo is an acquired depigmentation disorder characterized by completely amelanotic achromatic spots and hypopigmented patches with a few active melanocytes. It affects 0.5% to 2% of the world's population. People of different ethnicities, skin types and gender can be affected. The onset of this condition is most commonly observed from 10 to 30 years old, with the average age of onset being 20 years. [1]

According to Roberto Azambuja, one of the most important precursors of Psychodermatology in Brazil, the pathogenesis of vitiligo is unknown, as only unproven theories exist. [2]

According to Taieb & Picardo, the initial appearance of vitiligo is often focal and can progress to affect larger areas. The pathogenesis is multifactorial and not clearly elucidated; it may include mechanisms involving autoimmunity, intrinsic defects of melanocytes, and oxidative stress. [3]

In some cultures, patients with vitiligo are sometimes blamed for having the disease. In Iran, women with vitiligo reported that the disease is perceived as a "punishment from God " for sins or any moral and spiritual impurities. In India, vitiligo has been considered "Sweta Kustha" which simply means white leprosy. In the bible, vitiligo was sometimes confused with leprosy, which led to prejudice concerning certain individuals. [1]

Several therapeutic modalities lead to good improvement depending on the patient. Factors influencing improvement include whether or not treatment was initiated in its early stages, the appearance of the lesions, and the location. It is known that the achromatic spots on the face are more responsive to treatment [4, 5]

* Corresponding author: Tania Nely Rocha. Email: tanianely@hotmail.com

Characteristics

In September 2011, during the Global Consensus of Vitiligo in Bordeaux, a classification for vitiligo was defined. The classification presented here is the final one; after the creation of this consensus, all research should follow the new classification. [2]

Localized Vitiligo: Includes focal, segmental and mucosal forms.

- *Focal vitiligo:* characterized by one or a few small vitiligo lesions confined to a specific area of the skin with a non-dermatomal distribution (a dermatome is an area innervated by a particular nerve).
- *Mucosal vitiligo:* involvement of areas with mucous membranes (such as lips and genital area).
- *Segmental vitiligo:* vitiligo lesions occur in a dermatomal distribution or almost dermatomal, involving one or more dermatomes. There is also a rare form called bilateral segmental which can be difficult to diagnose because of its similarity to vitiligo vulgaris. The bilateral segmental form is limited (and remains fixed without evolution of the lesion size) and localized, which differs from vitiligo vulgaris.

Generalized Vitiligo: Includes acrofacial, common and universal forms.

- *Acrofacial Vitiligo:* Depigmented lesions in the distal part of the fingers, on periorificial areas of the face (around the mouth and eyes, for example).
- *Common Vitiligo (vulgaris):* vitiligo lesions that appear beyond the areas already affected by the acrofacial form such as: the chest, abdomen, thighs, groin, legs, buttocks, arms, neck and armpits.
- *Universal Vitiligo:* the affected individuals have few (or no) areas of normal skin pigmentation.

Mixed Vitiligo: this group consists of patients with concomitant segmental vitiligo and the type acrofacial or common.

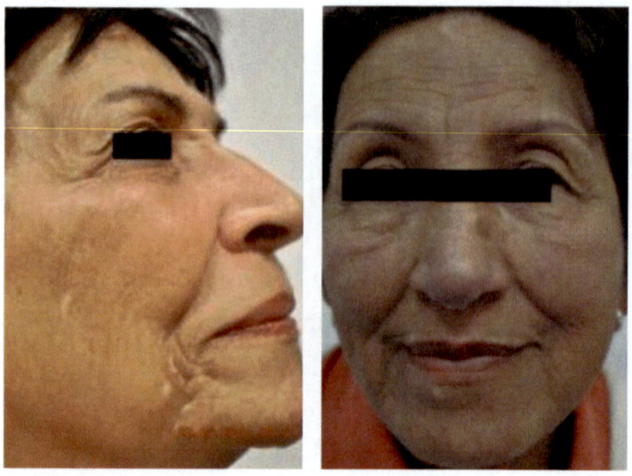

Figure 1. Female patients with facial vitiligo.

Differential Diagnosis

Elderly patients present many skin changes caused by sun exposure during life. This prolonged exposure may cause various skin lesions that result in the appearance of white spots.

There are various diseases that cause white spots. Dermatologists should watch for the differential diagnosis of vitiligo. [6]

1. Chemically induced leucoderma (often occupational)
   - Arsenic
   - Phenols and other derivatives, catechols.
2. Infections
   - Leishmaniasis
   - Leprosy
   - Onchocerciasis
   - Secondary syphilis
   - Pityriasis versicolor
   - Treponematosis
3. Genetic syndromes
   - Chediac-Higashi syndrome
   - Hypomelanosis of Ito
   - Oculocutaneous albinism
   - Piebaldism
   - Tuberous Sclerosis
   - Vogt-Koyanagi-Harada Syndrome
   - Waardenburg syndrome
4. Inflammatory post Hypopigmentation
   - Atopic dermatitis /contact dermatitis
   - Nummular dermatitis
   - Hypopigmentation induced by Phototherapy or radiotherapy
   - Pityriasis Alba
   - Post traumatic hypopigmentation
   - Psoriasis
   - Sarcoidosis
   - Systemic Lupus Erythematosus
   - Depigmentation induced by topical or systemic medications
5. Neoplastic
   - Amelanotic melanoma
   - Halo nevi
   - Melanoma associated to leucodermas
   - Mycosis fungoid
6. Idiopathic
   - Hypomelanosis idiopathic guttate
   - Lichen sclerosus et atrophicus

- Striated lichen
- Scleroderma (morphea)
- Melasma (residual stains, contrast between dark skin and light skin)
- Progressive macular hypomelanosis or acquired progressive hypomelanosis

7. Malformation
    - Anemic nevi
    - Non pigmented nevus / hypopigmented
8. Nutritionals
9. Kwashiorkor
10. Selenium Deficiency

Possible Causes

Although advances in the treatment of vitiligo have been recorded, especially in recent years, its pathogenesis is not yet fully known. Recent studies reveal important associations of the immune system and the melanocyte system itself.

Vitiligo and Evidence That Suggests It to Be a Disease Caused by Autoimmunity

The cause of vitiligo is not yet fully understood and several theories have been proposed to explain the origin of disease. Of these, the autoimmune hypothesis is still the most widely accepted among experts. Autoimmunity is explained by the attack of the defense cells of the patients, who do not recognize their own body's cells (in the case of vitiligo, the melanocytes). This leads to the destruction of the melanocytes. Due to this, the melanin production stops, causing the affected skin to become an intense white. The idea that vitiligo cases have autoimmune cause was initially based on the frequency of other autoimmune diseases in patients affected by vitiligo and positive response to treatment with immunosuppressive drugs (which reduce the autoimmune defense). These treatments would include photochemotherapy with UVA (ultraviolet A) and topical corticosteroids, both locally and orally.

The last part of important data related to the autoimmune vitiligo was the discovery that vitiligo patients have a decrease in the cell type known as Treg (regulatory T cell lymphocytes). With the decrease of these regulatory cells of the immune response, people with vitiligo would be subject to frequent autoimmune attacks (especially under stress), causing new areas of depigmentation. [2]

It was reported in Brazil that a case of segmental vitiligo appeared after the use of infliximade for rheumatoid arthritis (in this case the patient was 46 years old, female, who was using infliximab for 8 months). This same article also reinforces the idea that the pathogenesis is related to autoimmunity, occurring association with thyroid diseases, diabetes mellitus, and alopecia areata, as well as with HDLAs DR4, DW7, DR1, CW6, DR53, A19 and DR52. The use of inhibitors has frequently been associated whit skin diseases and also autoimmune manifestations, since laboratory abnormalities of asymptomatic nature until systemic diseases include the finding of autoantibodies such as ANA and anti-DNA. [7]

Comorbidities Associated to Vitiligo

Other autoimmune diseases can be found in patients with vitiligo; in other words, the patient may genetically inherit vitiligo as well as other autoimmune diseases. To prove this theory, two large epidemiological studies found different prevalence of comorbidities in patients with autoimmune vitiligo, especially thyroid disease. Even so, there are important differences in the prevalence of this association. For example, in Chinese subjects this association occurs in 7.7% of patients, contrasting with a higher prevalence in Caucasians where it occurs in 20%. Considering this, thyroid exams should always be requested in patients with vitiligo. Furthermore, patients should be informed that the thyroid treatment will not improve vitiligo, and vice versa. Other autoimmune diseases found concomitantly in patients with vitiligo include: psoriasis (3%), alopecia areata, halo nevus, diabetes mellitus, scleroderma, lupus erythematosus, rheumatoid arthritis, etc. [7]

Because of these associations, dermatologists should request further tests to investigate other comorbidities when diagnosing vitiligo.

Medical Exam

Some precautions are essential when treating the elderly. Waiting rooms should be prepared within the guidelines of health monitoring of each country. The waiting room and the toilet must be prepared to receive the elderly. The examination room should have a special chair for examining elderly patients.

During the consultation, it is advisable for dermatologists to ask elderly patients or their companions the following questions:

- Do you mind undressing completely to be examined?
- Do you need extra help to undress, put clothes on, take off shoes, or untie your hair?
- Do you want to see yourself in the mirror?
- Do you care if your companion helps you to undress?
- Do you mind if someone notices the white spots on your body?

To resolve these issues, the dermatologist should ask the patient what he or she wants:

- How would you feel more comfortable during your exam?
- Did you notice the white spots, or did someone in the family notice?
- When did you first see the white spots?
- How many spots appeared initially?
- Where did the spots appear initially?
- Do these spots bother you a lot or a little?

- Do the patches have any symptoms? Did you notice the skin itching before the emergence of the spots?

After these procedures, the examination should be continued with the aid of a Wood's lamp, in which the achromatic spots flourish in a characteristic manner. Only after this examination is it possible to conclude the diagnosis and report the result to the patient and their family. [8] A biopsy is rarely necessary.

If a biopsy should be requested, this should be taken in a white spot and in a contralateral site without a spot, so it will be possible to observe and compare the amount of viable melanocytes in the different tissues. The issues of Spirituality, Religion and Faith of the patient can be taken into consideration if the patient addresses these topics. [9, 10, 11]

A practical and valid suggestion in the clinic is to ask the elderly patient to complete the Dermatology Life Quality Index (DLQI) questionnaire. [1] This questionnaire consists of ten items divided into six categories: symptoms and feelings; daily activities; leisure; work / school; interpersonal relations hips; and treatment. The responses generate scores from zero to three, and the final calculation is a simple sum of these scores, with the highest rates indicating worse disease-related quality of life. The psychological impact caused by dermatosis should be carefully assessed and treated individually because it undoubtedly influences the development of a skin disease and the adherence to treatment. There is also a specific DLQI for patients with Vitiligo. [1]

Communicating the Diagnosis

After the correct diagnosis, a specialist in dermatology should develop a strategy to communicate the diagnosis to the patient or the relatives who may accompany the patient to the consultation. It is known that in most cases the diagnosis has significant impact on the patients and their family. Thus it comes to mind: How and when does one tell the patient the diagnosis? Using what words? Do elderly patients who develop vitiligo have the same concerns with self-esteem and body image of a patient who developed the disease during childhood or as a teenager?

It is certain that a cautious approach at this stage of communication of diagnosis, allowing, and creating and strengthening the bond with the patient will enable greater compliance and better outcomes to proposed treatments.

In a medical consultation, much is achieved through conversations between doctor and patient. Based on studies of neurolinguistic programming, it is known that the most relevant communication are not the words themselves, but the tone of words and phrases and the body language used when talking to the other person. The way of talking with the patient, especially with the elderly with Vitiligo, constitutes a major topic for discussion.

It should be emphasized that the problem is not only in the dermatosis (Vitiligo) itself, but also in the patient. While discussing the disease, the focus should be only the patient and his or her perceptions. When the patient or family asks about the diagnosis, the doctor should be well prepared for the emotional reaction to the patient and family may have to have certainty of diagnosis of Vitiligo. There are still many misconceptions regarding this disease.

The physician should have adequate time to the questions that arise after confirmation of the diagnosis.

Vitiligo Treatments

Commonly used treatments include corticosteroids, topical calcineurin inhibitors, phototherapy, laser therapy, and surgical repigmentation therapies [12, 13]. Unlike many other skin diseases, vitiligo lesions are usually asymptomatic (i.e no associated itching, burning or pain). It is important to consider some issues regarding the diagnosis of vitiligo in elderly patients. For example, a patient who lives alone may have limitations concerning the use of topical medications in certain regions of the body like the back.

Another case to be considered refers to an elderly patient who developed vitiligo but has no concern for this particular injury to the skin. The patient does not want to treat the white spots, but the family wants the patient to treat the condition.

Another disease of the elderly that deserves special consideration is Alzheimer's disease. Doctor's should be aware of how to prescribe dermatologic drugs for these patients, taking into consideration that many patients will hardly remember taking or applying medication unless someone else assumes these responsibilities.

Many medications commonly used by elderly patients can worsen the disease such as: Chloroquine, hydroquinone, alpha interferon, Levodopa, beta-blockers, and lansoprazole, among others. [10]. There are some foods and spices that also should be avoided by patients with vitiligo such as mango, pepper, cranberry, goji berry, acai, pistachios, curry or turmeric from India. There is evidence that certain foods can improve vitiligo such as: apple, onion, milk, red meat (source of vitamin B1 2) and food containing omega three. [14]

Dermatological Treatments

The development of an effective treatment for patients with Vitiligo depends on the maximum understanding of the mechanisms of depigmentation and repigmentation of the skin and the excellence and effectiveness of the doctor- patient relationship.

The quality of the individual's thoughts influences their skin, including the melanin unit. Thoughts are processed in the limbic-hypothalamic system and transmitted to the skin and other organs through the nerves and blood stream via "chemical messengers." These "messengers" connect the central nervous system to the skin, thus establishing the concept of "dermatological-psiconeuroimunoendocrino" system.

It is proven that the calcitonin gene related peptide (CGRP) has modulatory effects on Langerhans cells, which are in constant contact with epidermal nerves that secrete the peptide. The alpha-MSH is also a potent immunomodulator, inhibitor of the production of IL-1 and 2 and IFN -gamma. Under the action of stress, CGRP inhibits antigen presentation of Langerhans cell and alpha- MSH acts as an immunosuppressant. Due to its photoprotective effect, the substance has been approved in Europe for use in patients with erythropoietic protoporphyria only. To be indicated in the treatment of patients with Vitiligo, more studies still need to be performed.

Developed at the University of Arizona and at the Arizona Cancer Center, the melanotan I and melanotan II, both afamelanotide, are the two synthetic versions of a melanocyte-stimulating hormone. Melanotan I is a 13 amino acid molecule in a linear pattern, and melanotan II is the abbreviated version, circular of the melanotan I. Both stimulate skin pigmentation without exposure to the sun. The melanotan II also presented side effects such as increased libido and spontaneous erections. Considering this, it is now being studied as a drug for sexual and erectile dysfunction.

Phototherapy with narrowband UVB and phototherapy with the excimer laser and excimer lamp 308 nm has been commonly used [1]. An oral drug, considered an oral sunscreen, contains a chemical substance from the genus of fern called Polypodium Leucotomos [15]. It is also used as an immunomodulator, antioxidant and oral photoprotective in the treatment of Vitiligo. The drugs, which are effective in the treatment of vitiligo, that are considered "natural" may have contraindications. For example, Polypodium Leucotomos can lead patients with irritable bowel to have more intense diarrhea and patients with diabetes to have elevated glycaemia. Every day there is more proof that "natural" medications can also have side effects.

There are published articles on the use of kellin (topical and oral), which is based on the extract of the plant Ammi visnaga. A modified pseudocatalase is also being studied for the treatment of patients with Vitiligo. [16]

Autologous melanocyte transplantation is another treatment option that should be discussed with the patient. Autologous melanocyte transplantation associated with the use of excimer laser 308 nm or 308 nm excimer lamp can cause benefits, thus accelerating the process of repigmentation. [13]

Psychological Treatments

Psychotherapy, meditation, hypnosis, and dialogues about spirituality, religion and faith can be used by dermatologists to conduct a therapeutic approach with elderly patients who present the disease during or after emotional stress, or for patients who are not living in a balanced way with the disease. [17]

Homeopathy, anthroposophic medicine, herbal medicine, psychotherapy, speech therapy, aromatherapy, color therapy, crystal therapy, acupuncture, emotional acupuncture without needles, healing code, and prayers may be used for patients who are fans of holistic treatments. [18]

Support Groups

Support groups for patients with skin diseases may help patients who consider dermatosis as disfiguring and patients that have difficulties related to self-esteem or social impairment. The benefits of a support group are mutual: dermatologists and patients who meet both benefit from them. Patients can be taught different techniques to deal with stress and improve their quality of life [19, 20, 21, 22, 23]. Self-help books can be suggested by the dermatologist and discussed during the support groups meetings.

As we all know, medical therapeutic success is closely related to the quality of the doctor-patient relationship, the quality of life of the patients and the shared interest in conducting the necessary and indicated treatment. [20]

Doctor-Patient Relationship

The doctor-patient relationship in dermatology is well discussed by Katlein França in her book. The author emphasizes that the daily work of a dermatologist requires close attention and a relevant concern with the psychological issues of patients. [24] The proper diagnosis and treatment of skin diseases are entirely based on the harmonic interaction between dermatologists and their patients.

In 2001, an article published in the Brazilian Annals of Dermatology suggested different types of approaches to be used with the patient. These would be: [18]

- Physiological: where are the skin lesions?
- Behavioral: what worsens or improves the disease?
- Cognitive: why does the patient have the disease and why at this time of his life?
- Affective: how does the patient feel about having the disease?
- Systemic: what is the meaning of dermatological disease in the body?
- Ecological: What is the meaning of people's reactions to the disease?

Dealing with the Disease

Each patient is unique. We are all unique on this planet! None of us have the same fingerprint. None of us will be a senior like any other. None of us knows how we would react to the diagnosis of a disease until we develop a disease ourselves, or a loved one develops one.

Is it right to tell the patient that the disease has no cure? We think we should keep in mind that the healing process belongs to each patient. Dermatologists should teach the patient the way to treat the disease [21]

What would the message from the body be to the patient with Vitiligo? That is the main question to be asked by the patient himself – a question that the dermatologist, at the right time, can ask his or her elderly patient. The patient expects a lot from the physician – not only as a doctor but as a sensible and caring person. The good results depend on the professional that is guiding the patient and his family!

Conclusion

In the above text the authors presented different aspects of the diagnosis and treatment of elderly patients with vitiligo. The psychological aspects and treatments of the disease were emphasized. A different and more sensible approach is necessary when dealing with elderly patients. Remember that we should always treat the patient and not the disease.

References

[1] Lilly E1, Lu PD, at al.Development and validation of a vitiligo -specific quality-of-life instrument (VitiQoL). *J. Am. Acad. Dermatol.* 2013 Jul;69(1):11-8.

[2] Castro CC, Azambuja RD. *Vitiligo: Manual para pacientes e familiares.* Curitiba: Champagnat, 2013.

[3] Taïeb A Picardo M. Clinical practice. *Vitiligo N. Engl J. Med.* 2009 Jan 8;360(2):160-9.

[4] Rocha, TN, Rocha RH. Excimer laser 308 nm no tratamento do vitiligo. *Surg.Cosmet. Dermatol.* 2010; 2 (2):124-129.

[5] Antônio CB, Antônio JB, Marques AMB.Excimer Laser no tratamento do vitiligo em 123 pacientes: estudo retrospectivo. *Surg. Cosmet. Dermatol.* 2011;3(3):213-8.

[6] B. Lotti T, Salafi A.Vitiligo- questions & Answers- The vitiligo Research Foundation *Handbook for answering the most common questions on Vitiligo.*

[7] Carvalho CLDL, Ortigosa LCM. Vitiligo segmentar após o uso de infliximabe para artrite reumatóide- Relato de caso. Anais Brasileiros de Dermatologia. 2014;89(1):158-60.

[8] Steiner D, Bedin V; Moraes MB; Villas RT; Steiner T *An. Bras. Dermatol.*, 2004, 79(3)335-351.

[9] Pessini L.Espiritualidade e Arte de Cuidar-O sentido da fé para a saúde. São Paulo: Centro Universitário São Camilo e Edições Paulinas, 2010.

[10] Martini A, Martins AA.Teologia e Saúde. São Paulo: Paulinas, 2012.

[11] Frankl VE.A vontade de sentido- Fundamentos e aplicações da logoterapia. São Paulo: Paulus,2011.

[12] Falabella R. Treatment of localized vitiligo by autologous minigrafting. *Arch. Dermatol* 1988;124:1649-55.

[13] Ramos MG, Ramos DG, at al.Transplante de suspensão celular de melanócitos/queratinócitos para o tratamento de vitiligo estável na face: relato de dois casos. *An Bras Dermatol.* 2013; 88(5):815-8.

[14] Lupi, O. *Doutor eu tenho Vitiligo.* São Paulo: Grupo Gen, 2013.

[15] Middelkamp-Hup MA, Bos JD, Rius-Diaz F, Gonzalez S, Westerhof W. Treatment of vitiligo vulgaris with narrow-band UVB and oral Polypodium leucotomos extract: a randomized double-blind placebo -controlled study. *J. Eur Acad Dermatol Venereol.* 2007 Aug;21(7):942-50.

[16] Cestari TF, Dias MCS, Fernandes EI, Correia RB et al. Estudo Comparativo entre 2 psoralenos na fototerapia tópica do Vitiligo. *An Bras Dermatol.* 76(6): 2001 52-56.

[17] Nogueira LSC; Zancanaro PCQ; Roberto D. Azambuja Vitligo e emoções *An. Bras. Dermatol.* 2009 84 (1) 45-47.

[18] Rocha, TN. Uma contextualização sob a ótica integrativa. An. Bras. Dermatol. 2003; 78(5):619-624.

[19] Dogra S, Parsad D, Handa S, Kanwar AJ. Late onset vitiligo: A study of 182 patients International Journal of Dermatology, 2005,44(3), 193–19.

[20] Grossbart TA, ShermanC.Skin Deep- a mind/body program for healthy skin. NY: William Morrow and Company 1986.

[21] Dethlefsen T, Dahlke R - A Doença Como Caminho - Uma visão nova da cura como ponto de mutação em que um mal se deixa transformar em bem - 6ª Edição - São Paulo: Cultrix, 1998.

[22] Anzieu D. O Eu, pele. São Paulo: Casa do psicólogo, 2000.

[23] Dossey L. Reinventing Medicine: Beyond Mind-Body to a New Era of Healing, Sao Francisco: Harper Collins, 1999.

[24] França Katlein., Dermatologia e o Relacionamento Médico-Paciente - *Aspectos Psicossociais e Bioéticos*. São Paulo: Jurua, 2012.

In: Geriatric Psychodermatology
Editors: Mohammad Jafferany and Katlein França
ISBN: 978-1-63463-853-1

Chapter 10

Atopic Dermatitis in the Elderly: A Behavioral Approach

Christopher Bridgett, M.D.* and Peter Noren, M.D.

Introduction

The Combined Approach to atopic dermatitis is a programmed treatment approach that combines optimised topical treatment with the behaviour modification technique *habit reversal* for habitual scratching (Norén, P 1995). The Manual for Practitioners sets out suggested detailed protocols and provides patient handbooks (Bridgett, C. et al., 2009). As a several week programme it has an emphasis on staged treatment interventions with monitored progress and follow-up.

Habit reversal is a simple common-sense method that can be easily understood and taught, without any special training. Although the programme can be offered by practitioners as a clinic-based approach, it is also successful as a self-help treatment (www. atopicskindisease.com).

Atopic dermatitis remains predominately a skin disease of childhood. Most grow out of it by adulthood, but the prevalence of continuing atopic dermatitis in adulthood may be increasing (Falk, S Faergemann, J 2006), including in the elderly, when it can present for the first time (Tanei, R 2009).

The approach has three levels, with three additional dimensions (Box 1). The essentials of the programme for younger children and their parents, and older children and adults (Bridgett, C 2014) are the same, but are modified according to the age of the patient. This chapter gives an account of how the approach can be used in the elderly.

* Corresponding author: Christopher Bridgett: Email: email@ckbridgett.com

BOX 1. The Combined Approach to atopic dermatitis in the elderly

Three levels

- Emollients
- Topical steroids
- Habit reversal

Three dimensions

- Attitudes of the Elderly
- Attitudes to the Elderly
- Stress

For the elderly there are particular issues to account for, both dermatological and psychological. Thus the skin in old age is thinner and more easily damaged by scratching and rubbing compared to the skin in the younger patient, and the healing process of the skin is slower (Farage, MA et al., 2010). Psychologically, the treatment level habit reversal is adapted from that successful for younger patients, and particular attention may need to be paid to the important dimension of attitude to ageing, both in the elderly and in those caring for them, if the treatment approach is to be successful. Moreover, with cognitive impairment, involving others in habit reversal may become necessary, and greater time may be required.

The Treatment Programme

The Combined Approach treatment programme for the elderly with atopic dermatitis is organised in four stages (Box 2). The average program of five to seven weeks for younger adults may require seven to nine weeks for the elderly.

BOX 2. The Treatment Programme

- Assessment
- Treatment
- Trouble-shooting
- Follow-up

1. Assessment

The approach is especially indicated when there is a clinical history of frequently relapsing and remitting acute atopic eczema that does not completely clear-up between exacerbations: areas of long-term lichenification (Figure 1) secondary to habitual scratching and rubbing are characteristic, and resistance to conventional treatment is reported. Such skin is relatively unstable and sensitive, and more easily provoked to acute eczema than healthy skin.

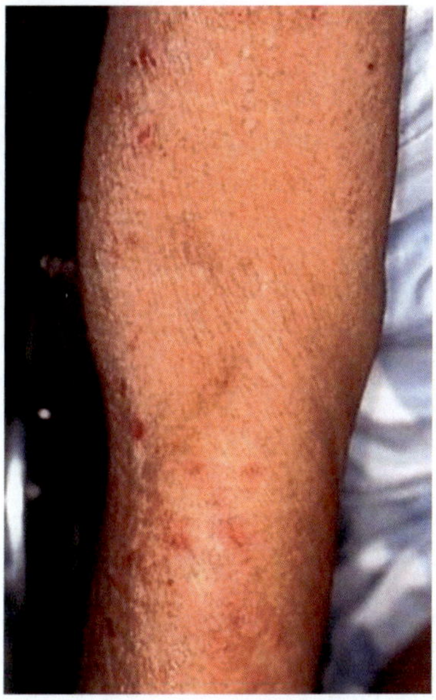

Reproduced with permission of Dr Ryoji Tanei.

Figure 1. Arm. 70 years old, with lichenification and excoriations.

Assessment is partly in clinic and partly home-based, often supported by others. In clinic there is an opportunity to explain the rationale of the programme, especially the link between apparent resistance to topical treatment and lichenification due to habitual scratching. The first week of the programme requires a record of the daily scratching and rubbing frequency to be established by the patient using a hand tally counter. This process makes conscious what has become unconscious, automatic scratching behaviour that is often associated with triggers other than itch. These triggers are also recorded: they may include periods of stress, episodes of boredom and being absentminded, and exposure of the skin as when washing, or when changing clothing.

2. Treatment

The treatment instructions require discussion and instruction in all three levels of treatment - emollients, topical steroids and habit reversal (see below). The advice given is supported by the patient handbook, where the recommended topical treatment is recorded. During treatment it is important that the hand tally counter continues to be used, showing how habit reversal gradually eliminates habitual scratching.

3. Trouble-shooting

After three weeks following all three treatment levels it helpful to review progress and ensure the programme is being adhered to correctly, and to re-enforce all three levels of treatment.

4. Follow-up

After another four weeks of treatment a review of progress will allow decisions to be made about follow-up. If the treatment programme has been successful habit reversal is no longer required. Continuing use of emollients needs to be discussed and the future appropriate intermittent use of topical steroids can be recommended. From now on it is important to ensure that acute relapse is recognised promptly and treated with topical steroids of adequate potency for long enough: while the chronic syndrome requires treatment for several weeks, acute eczema responds to a few days treatment, but this also takes longer to achieve in the elderly. As time passes with this firm regime the skin becomes increasingly resilient and less liable to acute eczema.

The Three Levels of Treatment for the Elderly with Chronic Atopic Dermatitis

I. Emollients

Account needs to be taken of the factors that dry the skin in the elderly. With age the skin thins, and less sebum is secreted. Although trans-epidermal water loss decreases with age in healthy skin, with acute inflammation and damage caused by scratching water loss will increase. Central heating in cold weather and air conditioning in hot weather contribute. Any associated dehydration and malnutrition will also increase drying, as will certain medical conditions, and their treatment.

Generally the elderly prefer lotions and creams to ointments as they are easier to apply. As the aged skin is fragile it is particularly important that application of moisturiser is gentle. To achieve optimal results involving someone else can be important, partly because of increasing joint stiffness and partly to offer distraction and diversion in the twenty minutes after moisturising, when otherwise habitual scratching is likely to occur.

For the elderly the use of an emollient as a soap substitute is especially useful: skin cleaning is best achieved by first applying the emollient, then gently washing it off with warm, rather than hot, water. Washing by hand, and showering, are safer for the skin than bathing - a long hot bath is never friendly to the skin.

II. Topical Steroids

The principles for effective use of topical steroids for atopic eczema in the elderly are essentially the same as for younger patients: the correct strength needs to be used, for long enough. For acute eczema this can take several days to achieve, with increased use of emollient. For chronic eczema several weeks are required, with optimal use of emollient and habit reversal.

Worry over causing undesirable side-effects can lead to using a topical steroid that is too weak, leading to a failure to achieve desired therapeutic effect. Similar concern explains why topical steroids are not used for long enough. Stopping too soon, when healing looks complete, can result in early acute relapse: it is necessary to continue the treatment a while longer to ensure best results - a week more for chronic eczema, a few days more for acute eczema.

In old age the skin responds more slowly to the steroid. Chronic atopic eczema requires topical steroid treatment for one or two weeks longer than is required in younger adults - always combined with optimal use of emollient, and habit reversal. Acute atopic eczema in old age requires topical steroid treatment for two or three days longer, combined with increased use of emollient: then habit reversal is not required.

III. Habit Reversal

Assessment by use of a hand tally counter over one week establishes the frequency of scratching and rubbing, and its habitual nature. It is very unusual then for anyone with chronic atopic eczema to attribute all their scratching to itch. Habit reversal instruction focusses on what needs to be done, rather than what must be avoided - success in habit reversal is associated with positive advice. The specific instruction for when there is an impulse to scratch or rub - itch or otherwise - is to replace scratching and rubbing with light fist clenching for thirty seconds. Then if the skin is itching, the area that itches is lightly pinched, or pressed with a finger nail, until the itch goes - it always does (Figure 2).

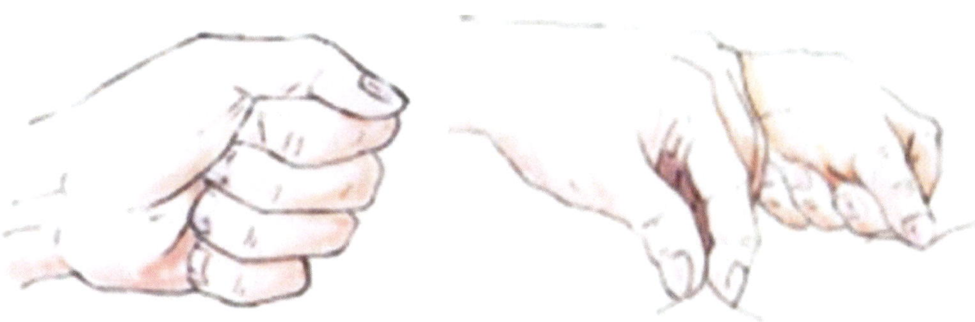

Figure 2. Fists, followed by pinch or pressure.

Otherwise an inventory of safe behaviours - doing things quickly, keeping the hands occupied - is assembled for particular situations when habitual scratching is predicted. As habit reversal succeeds and healing occurs the new behaviour becomes easier to achieve and habitual scratching ceases.

For the elderly involving others in habit reversal can be very important. This applies at all ages, but with the elderly it can be crucial if the habit reversal procedure is otherwise difficult to explain, or to remember. As with the very young (Bridgett, C 2014) in such circumstances those caring for the patient replace the hand tally counter, and habit reversal is enabled by observation and planned positive interventions using distraction and diversion. Even in the presence of cognitive impairment success with appropriate behavioural interventions is very feasible (Douglas, S et al. 2004) but greater time may be required.

Three Additional Dimensions

Attitudes of the Elderly

When introducing The Combined Approach to an elderly patient with atopic dermatitis it is particularly important to take account of attitude - the mindset that influences behaviour. It has been demonstrated that age stereotypes may influence recovery from disability (Levy, RL et al., 2012). Clinical experience suggests that spending time explaining the rationale of the treatment programme is particularly important for the elderly. A review with the patient of possible improvements in quality of life with effective treatment can also help instil the necessary motivation to follow the treatment programme.

Attitudes to the Elderly

A positive approach is infectious and an essential part of enabling successful behavioural change, especially in the elderly. Atopy, or the risk of getting eczema, is unavoidable, not the eczema itself. There is no need to encourage anyone, even when they are old, to "Live With Eczema".

Stress

Stress and eczema have a reciprocal relationship at all ages. In old age the experience of chronic eczema is stressful, while old age brings with it an increasing frequency of stressful experiences that can exacerbate the skin condition. The habitual scratching associated with chronic eczema is often not so much a manifestation of the eczema itself but a reaction to stressful circumstantial factors. Part of The Combined Approach should be to assess the part played by stress, and to introduce simple stress reduction strategies. The successful implementation of the treatment programme will be stress relieving in itself.

BOX 3. Key Points about Atopic Dermatitis in the elderly

- It can be a cause of significant adverse quality of life effects
- Recurrent acute eczema is often seen on a background of lichenification
- The Combined Approach is an effective treatment programme
- Topical treatment needs to be continued for longer
- Habit reversal for habitual scratching and rubbing may require the involvement of others

Conclusion

There is evidence of increasing chronic atopic dermatitis in the elderly. There is no need for this syndrome to go untreated: it responds very well indeed to The Combined Approach, a simple behavioural treatment programme that combines optimised topical treatment with a simple easy-to-use behaviour modification technique, *habit reversal.*

References

Bridgett, C *Habit reversal therapy: a behavioural approach to atopic eczema and other skin conditions in Practical Psychodermatology* Eds Bewley,A et al., Chichester,UK Wiley & Sons Ltd, 2014, Chapter 8, 66-71.

Bridgett, C Norén, P Staughton, R *Atopic Skin Disease: A Manual for Practitioners*. Bristol, PA: Wrightson Biomedical Publishing, Ltd, 1996.

Douglas, Simon, Ian James, and Clive Ballard. Non-pharmacological interventions in dementia. *Advances in Psychiatric Treatment* 10.3 (2004): 171-177.

Falk, Mari Helen Sandström, and Jan Faergemann. Atopic dermatitis in adults: Does it disappear with age?. *Acta dermato-venereologica* 86.2 (2006).

Farage, MA Miiler, KW Maibach, HI (Eds) *Textbook of Aging Skin Berlin*, Springer. 2010.

Levy BR, Slade MD, Murphy TE, Gill TM. Association Between Positive Age Stereotypes and Recovery From Disability in Older Persons. *JAMA*. 2012; 308(19):1972-1973. doi:10.1001/jama.2012.14541.

Norén P Habit reversal: a turning point in the treatment of atopic dermatitis 1995. *Clin. Exper. Derm*. 20 (1) 2-5.

Tanei, R Atopic Dermatitis in the Elderly 2009. *Inflamm Allergy Drug Targets Dec*; 8(5): 398-404.

www.atopicskindisease.com

In: Geriatric Psychodermatology
Editors: Mohammad Jafferany and Katlein França
ISBN: 978-1-63463-853-1

Chapter 11

Rosacea and Rhinophyma

Shailee Patel, BS and Jonette Keri*, M.D., Ph.D.

Introduction

Rosacea is a common and chronic inflammatory disease that primarily affects the centrofacial skin but can also include the forehead, nose, and chin. [1] It has been most frequently reported in patients of Celtic origin with fair skin, but can occur in men and women of all skin types and ethnicities. [2] Rosacea is not considered a part of normal aging but it is a chronic condition that steadily worsens with time. [3] Rosacea is diagnosed clinically and can present with various magnitudes and manifestations among different patients. [4-6] The current hypothesis is that during adulthood some individuals develop rosacea -prone skin, which is characterized by altered immune detection and reaction to a variety of triggers compared to facial skin of normal individuals. [6-9] These triggers, many of which are considered the most commonly implicated causes, stimulate cutaneous and neurosensory receptors, inciting an array of dysregulated neurovascular, angiogenic, and inflammatory responses. [7-13] This supports the theory that rosacea is an inflammatory disorder with numerous factors capable of stimulating potential pathways; leading to a flare of rosacea. [6, 8, 9, 12, 13]

The several factors that lead to a trigger of the innate immune system may explain the different findings in rosacea etiopathogenesis, which ultimately lead to heterogeneous clinical features including diffuse central facial erythema with or without inflammatory lesions among patients with rosacea. [6, 10, 14, 15] Part of the innate immunity response includes the release of cathelicidins antimicrobial peptides, which alter local inflammatory response, promote vascular permeability, and increase leukocyte chemotaxis. The only cathelicidin found in humans, LL-37, is expressed in the epithelial cells of the skin, the gastrointestinal and respiratory tract and in neutrophils, monocytes and natural killer cells. [2] Rosacea patients experience cathelicidin dysfunction by expressing 10 times increased levels in facial skin compared to normal facial skin. This coincides with increased levels of stratum corneum

* Corresponding author: Jonette Keri. Email: jkeri@med.miami.edu.

tryptic enzyme, kallikrein 5, the activator of cathelicidin, which is expressed only in the upper layers of epidermis in normal skin and throughout the whole epidermis in rosacea. [7, 8, 14, 16] Thus, proinflammatory cathelicidin LL-37 may play a key role in perpetuating the acute inflammation, angiogenic alterations, and vascular proliferation in the pathogenesis of this disease. [7, 16]

Although the cause of rosacea has yet to be elucidated, the potential pathophysiological mechanisms have been postulated and can be grouped into the following categories: vasculature hyperreactivity, matrix degeneration, pilosebaceous unit abnormalities, microbial organisms (proliferation of Demodex mites, Helicobacter pylori infection), and environmental exposure. [2, 6-8, 13, 14, 16, 17] Due to the paucity of basic science research of rosacea, the significance of each role of aforementioned causes is still an area of investigation.

2. Prevalence in Geriatric Population

Rosacea is a common dermatological disease of the elderly and most often affects patients with fair skin that have ancestry from North West Europe. [18] While Caucasians of Celtic origin appears to be most susceptible to this disorder, the condition has also been diagnosed in Asians and African Americans. [2] Many of the prevalence studies cannot be directly compared because of confounding variables in the study methodology and populations. Thus, the published prevalence statistics in Europe and the United States range from 1% to more than 20% adults affected. [17]

Similarly, the gender ratio has been variably documented with equal or female predominance. [19-23] A cross sectional study of a Greek outpatient clinic stratified the analysis by gender and age in which they found gender differences between the course and type of clinical patterns. In women, incidence of rosacea went up after age of 35 and the prevalence remained constant until peaking in the 61-65 age groups. In men, the incidence of rosacea increased after age of 50 and peaked in prevalence with the 76-80 year age group. [22]

Prevalence by subtype has been difficult to evaluate as studies have used a variety of definitions and in some cases even grouped subtypes together. In general population studies, subtype 1, erythematotelangiectatic rosacea, was four-fold more prevalent than subtype 2, papulopustular rosacea. [20-22] Subtype 3, phymatous rosacea, was rare but is predominantly seen in males. [21, 22, 24] And data on subtype 4, ocular rosacea, is questionable because the lack of definitive diagnostic criteria which leads to high false positive reporting ranging from 6% to 58%. [25] A more comprehensive body of epidemiological data that includes a broader variety of countries beyond Northern Europe and the United States, general population based demographics, and rosacea subtypes are necessary to better understand the patients affected by this disease process. [26]

3. Classification

In 2002, the National Rosacea Society Expert Committee (NRSEC) established a classification and staging system to help clinicians classify rosacea. [5] The diagnosis requires the presence of one or more of the following primary features localized to the convexities of the face: transient erythema, nontransient erythema, telangiectasia, papules and pustules. [5] There are four subtypes (erythematotelangiectatic, papulopustular, phymatous, and ocular) and one variant (granulomatous) of rosacea and based on the patterns of primary and secondary physical findings the patient may have more than one subtype. [5] Secondary findings may occur along with primary feature and independently in some cases, include burning or stinging, plaques, dry appearance, edema, peripheral locations, phymatous changes and ocular manifestations. [5] When the NRSEC developed these newer guidelines did not have enough scientific data to suggest one subtype progresses to another as previously proposed by the older classification system. The NRSEC stated that evolution from "one subtype to another may or may not occur" and as pathogenesis is elucidated the future definitions will be based on the cause rather than the morphology. [5]

Subtype 1: Erythematotelangiectatic Rosacea (ETR)

ETR is characterized by flushing and persistent central facial erythema. Telangiectases are associated but not essential for the diagnosis.

Subtype 2: Papulopustular Rosacea (PPR)

PPR is characterized by persistent central facial erythema with transient papule and/or pustules in a central facial distribution. Burning and stinging may also be reported.

Subtype 3: Phymatous Rosacea

Phymatous rosacea involves thickened skin with irregular surface nodularities and localized enlargement. Phymatous rosacea most commonly appears as rhinophyma but can occur on the chin, forehead, cheeks, and ears. Patulous, expressive follicles and telengiectases may be present in the phymatous region.

Subtype 4: Ocular Rosacea

Ocular rosacea is diagnosed based on 1 or more of the following: watery or blood shot appearance, foreign body sensation, burning or stinging, dryness, itching, light sensitivity, blurring of vision, conjuctival and marginal telangiectasia, lid or periocular erythema, blepharitis, conjunctivitis, chalazion, hordeolum, and corneal complications including corneal infiltrates ulcers and keratitis.

Variant: Granulomatous Rosacea

Granulomatous rosacea is characterized by discrete, firm, indurated, brownish-red papules or nodules.

4. Quality of Life and Psychosocial Impact

Clinicians are aware that a significant amount of dermatologic patients have psychosocial issues associated with their chief complaint; however both physicians and relatives tend to underestimate the effects of rosacea on the patients' quality of life (QoL). [27] Bar and Kuypers were the first to describe the patient with chronic blushing as timid, socially inhibited, and having diminished self-worth. Facial flushing due to central and autonomic response to social anxiety generates its own embarrassment and anxiety. This debilitating cycle causes the patient to avoid social situations that seem aggravating leading to poor social and sometimes poor family relationships. [28] These patients become withdrawn due to the chronicity of their disease and often have social phobia. [29] Facial involvement of not only flushing but also erythema, papules, pustules and telangiectasia provoke feelings of shame, guilt, and social stigmatization. The stress from stigmatization is due to the common misconception that rosacea is caused by excessive alcohol consumption. This fallacy is demonstrated in the cruel misnomer of "alcohol nose" for rhinophyma. [30]

As witnessed in other dermatological disorders, patients suffer from mental stress and decreased emotional well-being if visible areas are involved. [31,32] Therefore, rosacea patients may perceive a negative influence on their mental health resulting in psychological comorbidities including social anxiety disorder, depression, and body dysmorphic disorder. [33] Social anxiety stems from a considerable and persistent fear of social or performance situations in which humiliation may occur, and exposure to these settings consistently trigger an immediate reaction that can manifest as a panic attack. The patient senses their fear is excessive but is unable to control the symptoms, which include restlessness, dizziness, agitation, inability to relax, palpitations, shortness of breath, or sweating. Consequently, social or performance situations are avoided, producing a marked interference in a person's daily routine. [34] A depressive state may develop if the patient has longstanding history of rosacea features. Symptoms could include low energy or fatigue, poor appetite or overeating, poor concentration, insomnia, low interest, and feeling of hopelessness. This state becomes part of their new daily baseline and so it is often overlooked unless directly asked by the physician. [34] Body dysmorphic disorder, involves preoccupation with a "defect" in one's appearance no matter how small, is the most challenging psychological problem a patient with rosacea may develop. In terms of rosacea a few papules or telangiectasia may cause immense distress and hours may be spent fixating on their "defect" to the point that it dominates their lives. Significant impairment in functioning occurs as the self-consciousness about their "defect" leads to social avoidance and the frequent requests for reassurance leads to only momentary, if any, relief. [34]

The recurrent nature and the facial disfigurement of rosacea cause negative psychosocial functioning. [35] A Polish study assessing the psychosocial impact found that rosacea patients subjectively feel they receive poor social support, have difficulty in functioning in everyday life, have higher levels of anxiety and depression, and overall are less satisfied with their lives. [35] Using the Short Form 36 Health Survey, a Polish study evaluating the QoL in 40 rosacea patients compared to 40 healthy cohorts found the rosacea sufferers had reduced QoL in general health, emotional sphere, physical functioning, mental health, bodily pain, and vitality. [36] Studies have illustrated the marked psychosocial impact of rosacea, however very few have described the burden of disease among the specific subtypes of rosacea. [37] The RosaQol, a validated rosacea-tailored QoL instrument, was administered to 135 rosacea patients from the Emory Dermatology clinic in order to verify the symptomatic, emotional, and functional QoL impact among the ETR, PPR, and phymatous subtypes. The phymatous subtype had the worst symptomatic and emotional QoL in comparison to both ETR and PPR. There was no significant difference in symptomatic, emotional, and functional QoL impact between ETR and PPR. This supports the previous studies that have found the substantial QoL burden of rosacea to be analogous to that of leg ulcers, vitiligo, and occupational contact dermatitis. [38]

The effect of treating symptoms of rosacea on QoL was assessed by a Turkish study of 308 patients referred to a hospital dermatology clinic for treatment of rosacea. [39] Using the Dermatological Life Quality Index (DLQI), a validated instrument that investigates the impact of dermatological conditions on QoL in terms of symptoms, daily activities, leisure time, work, school, personal relations hip s, and response to treatment, health-related QoL was measure. [39] They found the negative effects of rosacea decreased after successful treatment of symptoms. [39] In summary, physicians treating rosacea patients should consider monitoring QoL parameters to include the patient's perspective in the treatment plan. And physicians managing patients with low QoL or those with worse general health perception should consider cooperating with a psychologist, recommending psychological co-treatment, and/or support groups to help improve overall outcome and patient satisfaction. [36, 40]

5. Medical Treatments

When considering a treatment option, patient's rosacea subtype, therapy effectiveness, and low risk profile should be taken into account. The four subtypes have different levels of response to therapy. ETR is the most resistant and responds poorly to topical and oral medications, while PPR is most responsive. [41, 42]

Avoid Triggers

It is important to identify factors that trigger signs and symptoms in rosacea patients. Patients have their unique triggers and these may change over time. They can include hot or cold temperatures, wind, hot drinks, alcohol, spicy food, exercise, emotions, topical products, and medications. It is also imperative to avoid sun exposure. Using sunscreen prepared with protective ingredients like silicone help to minimize erythema and stinging. Cosmetics can help conceal flushing, redness, and visible blood vessels but also can be the source of irritation and flare ups. When choosing skin -care and makeup products it is helpful to avoid ingredients like alcohol, fragrance, menthol, and exfoliating agents. Test a new product on a patch of skin in less noticeable area such as the neck to determine if the product is safe and tolerable. In addition, patients should be encouraged to apply a protective emollient to protect the face daily. [42]

Topical Therapies

Topical medications are the mainstay of treatment for many patients with rosacea. The three that are approved by Food and Drug Administration (FDA) for rosacea are metronidazole, sodium sulfacetamide with sulfur, and azelaic acid. There are other topical agents such as retinoids, clindamycin and calcineurin inhibitors that are used off label for rosacea. [41, 42]

Topical metronidazole is thought to act by inhibiting generation of reactive oxygen species as well as exhibiting other anti-inflammatory actions. [2] It comes in gel or ointment form with concentrations between 0.75% (twice daily application) and 1% (once daily application). It has shown to be effective in PPR by reducing the inflammatory lesions of papules and pustules and in some cases erythema. [43] It has been found to help reduce relapses after cessation of systemic treatment. [44] Side effects include dryness, burning and itching. [45]

Sodium sulfacetamide 10% with sulfur 5% was originally used for acne and seborrheic dermatitis. The combination of the antibacterial sulfacetamide with the antifungal and antibacterial sulfur provides improvement of PPR with a favorable safety profile. [2] Its use as lotion, cream, gel, and cleanser is more widespread since formulating the fragrance free version by successfully concealing the unpleasant odor of the sulfur component.

Azelaic acid is a dicarboxylic acid with anti-inflammatory, antimicrobial, and anti-keratinizing effects. [46] The mechanism of action is reported to inhibit generation of reactive oxygen species, inhibit serine protease activity of KLK5, and reduce activity of the cathelicidin pathway by decreasing gene expression of TLR2, KLK5, CAMP. [47] The approved form is available as a 15% gel (twice daily) formulation and is an effective therapy for PPR. It helps reduce papules, pustules, and erythema and does so without promoting bacterial resistance. Side effects include moderate facial burning, stinging, and pruritus which patients report to be tolerable. [48]

Topical clindamycin 1% and benzoyl peroxide 5% is an established acne medication that can also be used in rosacea. Clindamycin is a semisynthetic antibiotic and combined with benzoyl peroxide can reduce inflammatory lesions and erythema. [49]

Topical retinoids, including tretinoin, retinaldehyde, and adaplene, similar to oral retinoids appear to be useful in severe and recalcitrant rosacea. [50] Topical retinoids are not approved for treating rosacea due to limited evidence supporting their use. The main drawbacks are their irritant potential and their ability to aggregate angiogenesis, which can increase telangiectasia. [41, 42]

Topical calcineurin inhibitors include tacrolimus and pimecrolimus, which have been investigated for their anti-inflammatory effects by inhibiting T-cell activation and cytokine release. Studies have shown them to be effective in cases of steroid induced rosacea. [42, 51] Further studies are needed to provide support of their effectiveness in other types of rosacea.

Permethrin 5% cream is an antiparasitic and is considered for treatment of rosacea because it may target Demodex mites. [52] A few case studies have shown the utility of the topical form of a selective $\alpha 1$ agonist oxymetazoline that act as a potent vasoconstrictor that decreased erythema, and symptoms of stinging and burning. [53]

Systemic Therapies

Oral antibiotics have been used off label to treat rosacea for many years. In 2006, the FDA approved the only oral agent for rosacea, a modified-release anti-inflammatory dose of doxycycline 40mg daily capsule. [4] Doxycycline is a member of the Tetracycline family which is commonly used as oral treatment for rosacea and also includes non-FDA approved tetracycline and minocycline. [54] They are used especially for the PPR type as their clinical effectiveness is based more on their ability to reduce inflammatory response than on bacteriostatic effects. [55] Tetracyclines downregulate production of proinflammatory cytokines TNF -alpha and IL-1, inhibit reactive oxygen species, neutrophile chemotaxis, angiogenesis, and the matrix metalloproteinasesthat leads to a decrease in KLK5 activity and in turn LL-37. [45, 55, 56] Side effects of the tetracycline group include increased photosensitivity, changes in blood count, and discoloration of skin and nails. Tetracycline is an effective option; however the absorption may be reduced when taken with food. [54]

Macrolides antibiotics are effective for PPR and include first-generation erythromycin, second-generation clarithromycin and azithromycin. However their gastrointestinal side effects often limit their use for special cases of pregnancy, lactation, intolerance, allergy, and resistance to tetracyclines. Azithromycin, a second-generation macrolide, is thought to act as an antioxidant and has fewer gastrointestinal side effects making it a good choice for rosacea patients. [57]

Metronidazole as an oral agent is limited because of its need for alcohol avoidance, higher cost of new agents, and potential side effects of neuropathy and seizures. [55]

Isotretinoin is an option for severe and recalcitrant rosacea. It is one of the few medications that can treat more than one subtype. It can be used for ETR, PPR, rhinophyma and granulomatous rosacea. [41, 45, 55] It can help improve papule, pustules, and reduces facial cutaneous blood flow. Isotretinoin is contraindicated in women of childbearing potential due to its teratogenic effects and many patients have issues with compliance because it often causes dryness of lip and nose. [2, 58]

Other agents studied to improve flushing include nadolol, naloxone, ondansetron, propanalol, clonidine, and aspirin however there is a lack of clinical trial evidence for these potential treatments. [2]

Laser and Light Therapies

Topical and systemic therapies can improve the inflammatory component of rosacea but have little effect on the redness. [18] Lasers (e.g., pulsed dye laser) and intense pulsed light sources are effective treatment options for improving flushing, telangiectasia, and erythema. [42, 54] They remodel dystrophic dermal connective tissue, destruct excessive cutaneous vasculature associated with rosacea, and strengthen the epidermal barrier. Symptoms of burning and stinging are also alleviated by reducing cytokines and mediators such as substance P. [59] Numerous sessions are necessary to achieve satisfactory results and follow up sessions may be required later as the underlying disease process is still exists. Thus, lasers and intense pulsed light therapy have been crucial tools especially for managing ETR not amenable to other treatment options.

Treatment of Rhinophyma

Early phases of rhinophyma may respond to antibiotics or oral isotretinoin however later stages must be treated with surgical methods. The goal is to remove the hypertrophied glands and normalize the nasal contour. This can be accomplished using either complete excision or incomplete excision followed with reepithelialization from the remaining glandular tissue. [41] Incomplete excision includes dermabrasion, laser ablation, electrosurgery, cryosurgery, ultrasonic surgery, or carbon dioxide laser vaporization. [41, 54, 60-62]

Treatment of Ocular Rosacea

Treatment options for ocular rosacea have varied widely and patients are recommended to consult an ophthalmologist. Artificial tears can help manage dry eyes. [41] Topical metronidazole, fucidic acid, and corticosteroids combined with antibiotics are applied to the lid margins for treatment of mild ocular rosacea. [18] For more severe cases of blepharitis with erythema, adding systemic antibiotics like doxycycline may be helpful. [41]

Important Factors for Treating the Elderly

Management should be tailored to severity, subtype, comorbidities, and patient preferences. Geriatric patients are more likely to have multiple medical issues leading to risk of complication from polypharmacy. It is important to keep the medication regimen as simple as possible and to communicate with all other health care providers which medications are being prescribed. It is important to also share with other health care providers if the patient is undergoing laser or light therapy in order to avoid drugs that could cause photosensitivity. [63] These principles will ensure the patient centered care and minimize preventable adverse reactions to treatment.

6. Psychological Treatments

Psychological interventions can help improve the distress associated with dermatological symptoms. [30] Psychocutaneous diseases can present as primary psychiatric diseases such delusions of parasitosis or as secondary psychiatric disorders such as anxiety and depression that are exacerbated by the appearance of skin disease as psoriasis, alopecia areata, and rosacea. [64] About 30% of dermatology patients have psychiatric comorbidities. [65] A large survey from 1995 to 2002 among rosacea patients from data collected in the US calculated an odd ratio for depressive disorders was 4.81. [66] Understanding the clinical implications of comorbidity of skin disorders and psychiatric disease is on the forefront of the field of dermatology. The brain and skin share a common ectodermal origin and remain connected by a neuro-immuno-cutaneous-endocrine network throughout life. [67] Thus, using pharmacological and nonpharmacological psychotherapy to treat the complex somatopsychosocial issues may improve the skin condition and overall health.

Based on the current understanding, psychotherapy should be provided to patients with rosacea that have developed depression, social anxiety, or body dysmorphic disorder. [68] Stress and other emotional factors can flare papular inflammation and facial flushing in rosacea. [29] It is important to determine how much of the stress is from the skin condition and how much is from external events. Nonpharmacological interventions, such as hypnosis or relaxation training, help reduce stress which can in turn lead to enhanced efficacy of standard dermatological treatments and in some cases reduction in drug dosage treatment duration. [69] Hypnosis has been studied as complementary therapy for treating rosacea. The hypnotic trance can help in reducing the stinging and burning sensations while concurrently inducing favorable alterations in heart rate, muscle tension, and other physiologic changes. [70] Relaxation training involves different techniques that help with the main goal of minimizing sympathetic reactivity and enhancing parasympathetic function. Included in this group is breathing techniques or meditation techniques that can help the patient feel of sense of control and help with global stress reduction. [30]

For patients with anxiety that do not have time to learn relaxation exercises and stress management, the use of anxiolytic medication may be of benefit. [29] Dermatologists can use two types of anti-anxiety medications: agents from the benzodiazepine family (alazopram, lorazepam, and diazepam) and an azapirone (buspirone). Benzodiazepines have risk of addiction, have sedative effects, and if suddenly discontinued the patient can have recurrence of symptoms. Thus, it's important to restrict its use to 2 to 3 weeks, slowly increase does until therapeutic benefit is achieved, and taper when discontinuing. Alazopram may be the preferable option of the benzodiazepine family because the half-life is short and predictable. If the patient requires long term anxiolytic therapy, buspirone, a serotonin agonist, is a good choice as it is not addictive or sedating. Its disadvantage is that is has delayed onset of action of about 2 weeks and it is not useful for an "as needed" basis. [64]

If the patient is suffering from depression, there are many antidepressants to choose from if the patient is willing to be treated. Selective serotonin reuptake inhibitors (SSRIs) (citalopram, escitalopram, fluoxetine, fluvoxamine, paroxetine, sertraline, and venlafaxine), tricyclic antidepressants (amitriptyline, clomipramine, doxepin, imipramine, nortriptyline, protryptyline, and trimipramine), and less commonly norepinephrine and dopamine reuptake inhibitor (bupropion) can be used for treating depression. SSRIs are better tolerated compared to tricyclic antidepressants. Side effects of SSRIs include GI disturbances, sexual dysfunction, insomnia, and sedation most of which resolve after a few weeks. SSRIs should be started at a low dose and increased also there is a delayed onset of about 3 to 6 weeks. Tricyclic antidepressants have side effects such as dry mouth, urinary retention, blurry vision, constipation, and orthostatic hypotension. Similar to SSRIs the dose should be started low and increased slowly over a few weeks. [64]

Body dysmorphic disorder is considered a delusional disorder and patients should be managed the same way to treat a patient with delusions of parasitosis. Antipsychotic options include the typical or dopamine receptor antagonist (haloperidol and pimozide) and atypical or serotonine-dopamine antagonist (risperidone, olanzapine, and ziprasidone). The atypical antipsychotic medications are preferred as there are less extrapyramidal side effects like stiffness and restlessness. Having good communication and having the patient trust the physician is important in these cases as medication compliance can be challenging with patients suffering from body dysmorphic disorder. [29, 64]

The clinician must consider the physical and mental distress of a patient dealing with the recurrent and chronic nature of rosacea. Thus, managing rosacea dermatologically and psychologically will improve outcomes and patient satisfaction. When dealing with an older patient population it is important to keep in mind the age -related cognitive impairment s, subtle mental changes, and functional disabilities that may affect the psychodermatologic therapy such as compliance. [71] In addition, psychiatric therapies such as antidepressants may be less effective in cognitively impaired geriatric patients. [72] So it is imperative to provide special attention to the geriatric patients with rosacea associated with psychiatric disorders to ensure they receive appropriate care for both their primary skin condition and their secondary psychological disorder.

Conclusion

Rosacea is a complex inflammatory facial skin disorder that affects the elderly population. Recent research has provided some insight into the mechanisms of pathogenesis; however there are still many large gaps in the understanding of the disease. Avoiding triggers, sun protection, emollients, topical and systemic therapies help manage many of the symptoms. Relaxation techniques and psychotherapeutic medications can alleviate some of the mental distress caused by rosacea. Treatment should be carefully tailored based on severity and type of the disease as well as accounting for the patients' comorbidities. It is likely as we learn more about the pathophysiology of rosacea, newer developments in therapy and management will also emerge.

References

[1] Del Rosso JQ, Thiboutot D, Gallo R, Webster G, Tanghetti E, Eichenfield L, et al. Consensus recommendations from the American Acne & Rosacea Society on the management of rosacea, part 1: a status report on the disease state, general measures, and adjunctive skin care. *Cutis*. 2013;92(5):234-40.

[2] Elewski BE, Draelos Z, Dreno B, Jansen T, Layton A, Picardo M. Rosacea - global diversity and optimized outcome: proposed international consensus from the Rosacea International Expert Group. *Journal of the European Academy of Dermatology and Venereology: JEADV*. 2011;25(2):188-200.

[3] Papadakis MA, Lawrence M. Tierney, and Stephen J. McPhee. Current medical diagnosis & treatment. New York, NY: Lanfe Medical Books / *McGraw-Hill;* 2000.

[4] Del Rosso JQ, Baldwin H, Webster G, American A, Rosacea S. American Acne & Rosacea Society rosacea medical management guidelines. *Journal of Drugs in Dermatology:* JDD. 2008;7(6):531-3.

[5] Wilkin J, Dahl M, Detmar M, Drake L, Feinstein A, Odom R, et al. Standard classification of rosacea: Report of the National Rosacea Society Expert Committee on the Classification and Staging of Rosacea. *Journal of the American Academy of Dermatology.* 2002;46(4):584-7.

[6] Crawford GH, Pelle MT, James WD. Rosacea: I. Etiology, pathogenesis, and subtype classification. *Journal of the American Academy of Dermatology.* 2004;51(3):327-41; quiz 42-4.

[7] Yamasaki K, Di Nardo A, Bardan A, Murakami M, Ohtake T, Coda A, et al. Increased serine protease activity and cathelicidin promotes skin inflammation in rosacea. *Nature medicine.* 2007;13(8):975-80.

[8] Yamasaki K, Gallo RL. The molecular pathology of rosacea. *Journal of Dermatological Science.* 2009;55(2):77-81.

[9] Fleischer AB, Jr. Inflammation in rosacea and acne: Implications for patient care. *Journal of Drugs in Dermatology:* JDD. 2011;10(6):614-20.

[10] Steinhoff M, Buddenkotte J, Aubert J, Sulk M, Novak P, Schwab VD, et al. Clinical, cellular, and molecular aspects in the pathophysiology of rosacea. *The Journal of Investigative Dermatology Symposium proceedings*/the Society for Investigative Dermatology, Inc [and] European Society for Dermatological Research. 2011;15(1): 2-11.

[11] Del Rosso JQ, Gallo RL, Kircik L, Thiboutot D, Baldwin HE, Cohen D. Why is rosacea considered to be an inflammatory disorder? The primary role, clinical relevance, and therapeutic correlations of abnormal innate immune response in rosacea-prone skin. *Journal of Drugs in Dermatology*: JDD. 2012;11(6):694-700.

[12] Bevins CL, Liu FT. Rosacea: skin innate immunity gone awry? *Nature Medicine.* 2007;13(8):904-6.

[13] Del Rosso JQ. Advances in understanding and managing rosacea: part 2: the central role, evaluation, and medical management of diffuse and persistent facial erythema of rosacea. *The Journal of Clinical and Aesthetic Dermatology.* 2012;5(3):26-36.

[14] Del Rosso JQ, Gallo RL, Tanghetti E, Webster G, Thiboutot D. An evaluation of potential correlations between pathophysiologic mechanisms, clinical manifestations, and management of rosacea. *Cutis. 2013*;91(3 Suppl):1-8.

[15] Del Rosso JQ. Advances in understanding and managing rosacea: part 1: connecting the dots between pathophysiological mechanisms and common clinical features of rosacea with emphasis on vascular changes and facial erythema. *The Journal of Clinical and Aesthetic Dermatology.* 2012;5(3):16-25.

[16] Schauber J, Gallo RL. Antimicrobial peptides and the skin immune defense system. *The Journal of Allergy and Clinical Immunology.* 2009;124(3 Suppl 2):R13-8.

[17] Buechner SA. Rosacea: an update. *Dermatology.* 2005;210(2):100-8.

[18] Powell FC. Clinical practice. Rosacea. *The New England Journal of Medicine.* 2005;352(8):793-803.

[19] Augustin M, Herberger K, Hintzen S, Heigel H, Franzke N, Schafer I. Prevalence of skin lesions and need for treatment in a cohort of 90 880 workers. *The British Journal of Dermatology.* 2011;165(4):865-73.

[20] Berg M, Liden S. An epidemiological study of rosacea. *Acta Dermato-venereologica.* 1989;69(5):419-23.

[21] Abram K, Silm H, Oona M. Prevalence of rosacea in an Estonian working population using a standard classification. *Acta Dermato-venereologica.* 2010;90(3):269-73.

[22] Kyriakis KP, Palamaras I, Terzoudi S, Emmanuelides S, Michailides C, Pagana G. Epidemiologic aspects of rosacea. *Journal of the American Academy of Dermatology.* 2005;53(5):918-9.

[23] Spoendlin J, Voegel JJ, Jick SS, Meier CR. A study on the epidemiology of rosacea in the U.K. *The British Journal of Dermatology.* 2012;167(3):598-605.

[24] Lazaridou E, Fotiadou C, Ziakas NG, Giannopoulou C, Apalla Z, Ioannides D. Clinical and laboratory study of ocular rosacea in northern Greece. *Journal of the European Academy of Dermatology and Venereology: JEADV.* 2011;25(12):1428-31.

[25] Michel JL, Cabibel F. [Frequency, severity and treatment of ocular rosacea during cutaneous rosacea]. *Annales de dermatologie et de venereologie.* 2003;130(1 Pt 1):20-4.

[26] Tan J, Berg M. Rosacea: current state of epidemiology. *Journal of the American Academy of Dermatology.* 2013;69(6 Suppl 1):S27-35.

[27] Beikert FC, Langenbruch AK, Radtke MA, Augustin M. Willingness to pay and quality of life in patients with rosacea. *Journal of the European Academy of Dermatology and Venereology: JEADV.* 2013;27(6):734-8.

[28] Bar LH, Kuypers BR. Behaviour therapy in dermatological practice. *The British Journal of Dermatology.* 1973;88(6):591-8.

[29] Garnis-Jones S. Psychological aspects of rosacea. *Journal of Cutaneous Medicine and Surgery.* 1998;2 Suppl 4:S4-16-9.

[30] Fried RG. Nonpharmacologic treatments in psychodermatology. *Dermatologic Clinics.* 2002;20(1):177-85.

[31] Shuster S, Fisher GH, Harris E, Binnell D. The effect of skin disease on self image [proceedings]. *The British Journal of Dermatology.* 1978;99(Suppl 16):18-9.

[32] Roosta N, Black DS, Peng D, Riley LW. Skin disease and stigma in emerging adulthood: impact on healthy development. *Journal of Cutaneous Medicine and Surgery.* 2010;14(6):285-90.

[33] Obermeyer M. Psychocutaneous medicine. *Springfield, IL:* CC Thomas; 1995.

[34] Lundberg L, Johannesson M, Silverdahl M, Hermansson C, Lindberg M. Quality of life, health -state utilities and willingness to pay in patients with psoriasis and atopic eczema. *The British Journal of Dermatology.* 1999;141(6):1067-75.

[35] Chodkiewicz J, Salamon M, Miniszewska J, Wozniacka A. [Psychosocial impact of rosacea]. *Przeglad lekarski.* 2007;64(12):997-1001.

[36] Salamon M, Chodkiewicz J, Sysa-Jedrzejowska A, Wozniacka A. [Quality of life in patients with rosacea]. *Przeglad lekarski.* 2008;65(9):385-9.

[37] Kini SP, Nicholson K, DeLong LK, Dannemann T, Estaris J, Foster J, et al. A pilot study in discrepancies in quality of life among three cutaneous types of rosacea. *Journal of the American Academy of Dermatology.* 2010;62(6):1069-71.

[38] Lewis V, Finlay AY. 10 years experience of the Dermatology Life Quality Index (DLQI). *The journal of investigative dermatology Symposium proceedings / the Society for Investigative Dermatology,* Inc [and] European Society for Dermatological Research. 2004;9(2):169-80.

[39] Aksoy B, Altaykan-Hapa A, Egemen D, Karagoz F, Atakan N. The impact of rosacea on quality of life: effects of demographic and clinical characteristics and various treatment modalities. *The British Journal of Dermatology. 2010*;163(4):719-25.

[40] Bohm D, Schwanitz P, Stock Gissendanner S, Schmid-Ott G, Schulz W. Symptom severity and psychological sequelae in rosacea: Results of a survey. *Psychology, Health & Medicine*. 2013.
[41] Gupta AK, Chaudhry MM. Rosacea and its management: an overview. Journal of the European Academy of Dermatology and Venereology: *JEADV*. 2005;19(3):273-85.
[42] Pelle MT, Crawford GH, James WD. Rosacea: II. Therapy. *Journal of the American Academy of Dermatology*. 2004;51(4):499-512; quiz 3-4.
[43] McClellan KJ, Noble S. Topical metronidazole. A review of its use in rosacea. *American Journal of Clinical Dermatology. 2000*;1(3):191-9.
[44] Dahl MV, Katz HI, Krueger GG, Millikan LE, Odom RB, Parker F, et al. Topical metronidazole maintains remissions of rosacea. *Archives of Dermatology*. 1998;134(6):679-83.
[45] Korting HC, Schollmann C. Current topical and systemic approaches to treatment of rosacea. *Journal of the European Academy of Dermatology and Venereology: JEADV*. 2009;23(8):876-82.
[46] Del Rosso JQ, Baum EW, Draelos ZD, Elewski BE, Fleischer AB, Jr., Kakita LS, et al. Azelaic acid gel 15%: clinical versatility in the treatment of rosacea. *Cutis*. 2006;78(5 Suppl):6-19.
[47] Del Rosso JQ. Update on rosacea pathogenesis and correlation with medical therapeutic agents. *Cutis*. 2006;78(2):97-100.
[48] Thiboutot D, Thieroff-Ekerdt R, Graupe K. Efficacy and safety of azelaic acid (15%) gel as a new treatment for papulopustular rosacea: results from two vehicle-controlled, randomized phase III studies. *Journal of the American Academy of Dermatology*. 2003;48(6):836-45.
[49] Breneman D, Savin R, VandePol C, Vamvakias G, Levy S, Leyden J. Double-blind, randomized, vehicle-controlled clinical trial of once-daily benzoyl peroxide /clindamycin topical gel in the treatment of patients with moderate to severe rosacea. *International Journal of Dermatology*. 2004;43(5):381-7.
[50] Ertl GA, Levine N, Kligman AM. A comparison of the efficacy of topical tretinoin and low-dose oral isotretinoin in rosacea. *Archives of Dermatology*. 1994;130(3):319-24.
[51] Lee DH, Li K, Suh DH. Pimecrolimus 1% cream for the treatment of steroid-induced rosacea: an 8-week split-face clinical trial. *The British Journal of Dermatology*. 2008;158(5):1069-76.
[52] Gooderham M. Rosacea and its topical management. *Skin Therapy Letter*. 2009;14(2):1-3.
[53] Shanler SD, Ondo AL. Successful treatment of the erythema and flushing of rosacea using a topically applied selective alpha1-adrenergic receptor agonist, oxymetazoline. *Archives of Dermatology*. 2007;143(11):1369-71.
[54] Wollina U. Rosacea and rhinophyma in the elderly. *Clinics in Dermatology*. 2011;29(1):61-8.
[55] Baldwin HE. Systemic therapy for rosacea. *Skin therapy letter*. 2007;12(2):1-5, 9.
[56] Kanada KN, Nakatsuji T, Gallo RL. Doxycycline indirectly inhibits proteolytic activation of tryptic kallikrein-related peptidases and activation of cathelicidin. *The Journal of Investigative Dermatology*. 2012;132(5):1435-42.

[57] Bakar O, Demircay Z, Yuksel M, Haklar G, Sanisoglu Y. The effect of azithromycin on reactive oxygen species in rosacea. *Clinical and Experimental Dermatology.* 2007;32(2):197-200.

[58] Park H, Del Rosso JQ. Use of oral isotretinoin in the management of rosacea. *The Journal of Clinical and Aesthetic Dermatology.* 2011;4(9):54-61.

[59] Lonne-Rahm S, Nordlind K, Edstrom DW, Ros AM, Berg M. Laser treatment of rosacea: a pathoetiological study. *Archives of Dermatology.* 2004;140(11):1345-9.

[60] Rordam OM, Guldbakke K. Rhinophyma: big problem, simple solution. *Acta Dermato-venereologica.* 2011;91(2):188-9.

[61] Aferzon M, Millman B. Excision of rhinophyma with high-frequency electrosurgery. Dermatologic surgery: official publication for American Society for Dermatologic Surgery [et al]. 2002;28(8):735-8.

[62] Lim SW, Lim SW, Bekhor P. Rhinophyma: Carbon dioxide laser with computerized scanner is still an outstanding treatment. *The Australasian Journal of Dermatology.* 2009;50(4):289-93.

[63] Fuller D, Martin S. Rosacea. *Journal of Midwifery & Women's Health.* 2012;57(4):403-9.

[64] Shenefelt PD. Psychological interventions in the management of common skin conditions. *Psychology Research and Behavior Management.* 2010;3:51-63.

[65] Gupta MA, Gupta AK, Ellis CN, Koblenzer CS. Psychiatric evaluation of the dermatology patient. *Dermatologic Clinics.* 2005;23(4):591-9.

[66] Gupta MA, Gupta AK, Chen SJ, Johnson AM. Comorbidity of rosacea and depression: an analysis of the National Ambulatory Medical Care Survey and National Hospital Ambulatory Care Survey--Outpatient Department data collected by the U.S. National Center for Health Statistics from 1995 to 2002. *The British Journal of Dermatology.* 2005;153(6):1176-81.

[67] Brazzini B, Ghersetich I, Hercogova J, Lotti T. The neuro-immuno-cutaneous-endocrine network: relationship between mind and skin. *Dermatologic Therapy.* 2003;16(2):123-31.

[68] Harth W. Clinical management in psychodermatology Berlin; Heidelberg *Springe;* 2009.

[69] Koo JY, Do JH, Lee CS. Psychodermatology. *Journal of the American Academy of Dermatology.* 2000;43(5 Pt 1):848-53.

[70] Shenefelt PD. Hypnosis in dermatology. *Archives of Dermatology.* 2000;136(3):393-9.

[71] Wilkins VM, Kiosses D, Ravdin LD. Late-life depression with comorbid cognitive impairment and disability: nonpharmacological interventions. *Clinical Interventions in Aging.* 2010;5:323-31.

[72] Rajji TK, Mulsant BH, Lotrich FE, Lokker C, Reynolds CF, 3rd. Use of antidepressants in late-life depression. *Drugs & Aging.* 2008;25(10):841-53.

In: Geriatric Psychodermatology
Editors: Mohammad Jafferany and Katlein França

ISBN: 978-1-63463-853-1

Chapter 12

Hyperhidrosis

Tulsie Patel, BS, Shailee Patel, BS and Katlein França*, M.D., MSc

Introduction

Hyperhidrosis is a condition characterized by excessive sweating. [1] It is characterized by the fact that it leads to sweating beyond what is necessary for thermoregulation, the normal function of this process. [2] It is an autonomic disorder that is known most often for its associated psychological, physical, social, and emotional challenges. [1] Hyperhidrosis is regulated by acetylcholine. [3] It occurs in areas where there are a large number of eccrine (sweat) glands. Common areas include the axillae, palms, and soles. [1] Apocrine glands may also be involved, especially in cases of axillary hyperhidrosis in younger patients. [3] It is believed that nearly 3% of the population of the United States is dealing with this life-altering condition. [3]

The true pathophysiology of this condition is not certain. [2] Patients have a normal amount of eccrine glands; however, they produce excess sebum. [2] Histology of the eccrine glands and the sympathetic chain has been shown to be normal in these patients. [3] It has been found that activation of these glands may stem from emotional and environmental stimuli including exercise, alcohol, and anxiety. [2] There are various presentations of this disorder. [2] The most commonly affected area is the axillae. [2] In descending order of prevalence, the palms, soles, scalp, and groin are then affected. [2]

There are a variety of classifications of this disease. [1] Primary hyperhidrosis is focal condition that tends to present symmetrically. [2] It most often begins in childhood. [1] It has been shown to have a genetic component. [1] For example, autosomal dominant inheritance is displayed in some cases as a familial variant has been shown. [1] The abnormality is present on chromosome 14q. [1] Secondary hyperhidrosis is due to another underlying condition such as infection, drugs /toxins, and endocrine and neurological illnesses. [1, 2] It tends to be more

* Corresponding author: Katlein França. Email: k.franca@med.miami.edu

generalized, occurs at night, and is often associated with systemic symptoms. [2] This type is commonly found among geriatric patients. Compensatory hyperhidrosis, on the other hand, is excessive sweating in a new and unrelated location after treatment to the site of the focal, primary hyperhidrosis. [1]

Table 1. Classification of Hyperhidrosis [1-6]

Type of Hyperhidrosis	Etiology	Distribution	Location	Characteristics
Primary hyperhidrosis	Idiopathic	More commonly focal	Most commonly axillae, palms, soles, craniofacial region, inguinal area	Bilateral and symmetric, does not occur at night, onset at a young age, depreciation of daily activities, family history
Secondary hyperhidrosis	Drugs/toxins, systemic dysfunctions (neurological, endocrine, cardiovascular, respiratory), infection, neoplasm, hereditary conditions	More commonly generalized	Dependent on the etiology	Occurs at night
Compensatory hyperhidrosis	Develops as a result of treatment for hyperhidrosis elsewhere	Related to the level of the sympathectomy	Most commonly lower back, buttocks, groin, and thighs	Reactive mechanism, commonly results after sympathetic denervation, severity dependent on location of procedure (usually around T2-4)

Hyperhidrosis is a condition that affects patients throughout their lives. [7] In the United States, the disease tends to affect men and women equally. [7] However, the group that is most often recorded is that of Caucasian females. [2] Based on a survey, this condition has been found to affect children under the age of 12 the least. [7] The disease most often begins around 25 years old and affects patients between 25 and 64 years old the most. [7] The mean age of affected patients tends to be around 40 years old. [7] The specific presentations of the condition tend to vary by demographics as well. [7] Men tend to be more affected by axillary hyperhidrosis. [7] Women are more likely to seek medical attention. [7] In patients older than the onset of puberty, the elderly (65+) tend to experience axillary hyperhidrosis the least. [7] Older patients, such as those over the age of 35, have also been found to experience greater rates of compensatory hyperhidrosis as a result of other comorbidities. [6] Other studies have found that it tends to be much less common in the elderly, thus illustrating a spontaneous regression with age. [2]

Secondary hyperhidrosis is the most common type to affect the geriatric population. Although sweating typically decreases with age, secondary hyperhidrosis can occur due to hypertension, diabetes, and Parkinson's disease, which are ailments that often occur with increased age. [6] Other sources of hyperhidrosis in elderly patients include endocrine causes such as postmenopausal hyperhidrosis and hyperthyroidism. [8] Malignancies that may affect geriatric patients such as myeloproliferative syndromes and Hodgkin's disease are also associated with generalized hyperhidrosis. [9] Antidepressants, such as fluoxetine, venlafaxine, and doxepin, have also been implicated as a cause of hyperhidrosis. [10] It is crucial to keep these possible causes of secondary hyperhidrosis in mind when approaching an elderly patient with hyperhidrosis.

Hyperhidrosis is a very complex disorder. [2] It affects various aspects of a patient's life. [2] It has been stated that compared to other skin conditions, such as psoriasis, hyperhidrosis has a much greater impact on one's quality of life. [11] Thus, subjective and personal opinions of this disorder and its impact on one's life often lead to complications in its true understanding, diagnosis, and treatment. [2] These complications also lead to it being a highly underreported condition. [2] For example, patients suffering from this condition often wait years before reporting their symptoms to a physician. [2] It has been found that the condition often occurs around the onset of puberty at the age of 14, but that medical attention is not sought for another 15 years, on average. [2] The embarrassment that many patients feel leads to its heightened underreporting. [2] It has been found that only about 38% of patients with symptoms actually sought medical treatment for their hyperhidrosis. [2]

Diagnosis

A variety of factors are included in the proper diagnosis of this condition. [1] The diagnosis of primary hyperhidrosis is very specific. [1] A patient must experience excessive sweating of an unknown etiology for at least six months. [1] The patient must also experience two of the following symptoms: bilateral and symmetric pattern of symptoms that occurs at least once a week, symptoms that start before the age of 25, cessation of sweating with sleep and at night, a positive family history, and a depreciation of daily activities. [1]

Quality of Life

Patients suffering from hyperhidrosis, no matter the location, often face psychological and social challenges with dealing with their condition. [12, 13] Many patients complain of the debilitating effects this condition has on their ability to deal with social situations and career goals. [14] Hyperhidrosis, in conjunction with social/emotional challenges, lead to an overall decrease in the quality of life of these patients. [15]

Improvement of quality of life in these patients is most often linked to treatment of their hyperhidrosis. [13] Regardless of the area involved in their condition, patients have indicated an improvement in their quality of life after treatment. [11, 13] This was recently indicated in studies following patient's perspective of their quality of life both before and after treatment with botulinum toxin. [11, 13] Patients indicated a marked increase in their quality of life after treatment. [11, 13] This was further elucidated on a study that characterized a patient's perspective of his/her quality of life before and after treatment of palmar hyperhidrosis using thorascopic sympathetctomy. [16] This study found an irrefutable difference and improvement of social functioning in postoperative patients. [16] It is thought that this stems from a decrease in the psychological stress of the patient after successful treatment of their hyperhidrosis. [16]

The presence of complications, such as anxiety, are commonly found and reported in hyperhidrosis patients, but they are not necessarily causative of the condition. [17] No correlation has been found between the presence and severity of these features and the outcomes of treatments and chances for recurrence in hyperhidrosis patients. [17] Further, hyperhidrosis continues to be characterized as a physiological disorder and not a psychological one. [14] For example, the disorder has been found in the neonatal period, indicating that it is more than just a responsive, emotional disorder. [14]

However, even though psychiatric and psychological disorders may not be catalysts for this condition, they are important markers of a patient's overall wellbeing. [12] Treatment of these conditions, and not just the hyperhidrosis, could undoubtedly help the exacerbation of hyperhidrosis that may occur if a patient is faced with psychological stress ors or trauma such as social and intimate circumstances that draw attention to the symptoms of the disease. [12, 18] Patients whose symptoms stem from a social anxiety may require anti-depressants and psychiatric care. [14]

Diazepam has been used to help hyperhidrosis patients whose symptoms stem from social, anxiety -producing events. [14] Of note, there is some data that has found age -related increase in sensitivity to diazepam. This is related to the increased volume of distribution which could lead to a higher plasma concentration of the same dose in older adults compared to younger patients. Diazepam can impair memory, and psychomotor performance causing sedation in geriatric patients hence the dosing should be started as low as possible and increased as needed and tolerated. [19]

Medical Treatments

Numerous medical therapies are available for the treatment of hyperhidrosis. [18] These include topical antiperspirants, tap-water iontophoresis, botulinum toxin injections, oral medications, surgical technique s, sympathectomy and laser. [18] Although there are a variety of modalities to choose from, one draw-back remains that many of these treatments require constant follow-up and treatment, such as iontophoresis. [20]

Topical treatments are commonly as initial treatment of axillary, palmar, and plantar hyperhidrosis. [3, 14] The most common treatment for axillary hyperhidrosis is aluminum chloride. [14] These treatments work by inhibiting the secretory ducts of the eccrine glands in the area treated. [3] Most patients are able to use over-the-counter products but more severe cases require the use of aluminum chloride hexahydrate dissolved in anhydrous ethyl alcohol. [14] The product is to be applied to dry skin and is most efficient when used at night. [14] Palmar and plantar cases are also initially treated topically using prescription strength antiperspirant. [14] Treatment is usually ongoing and may be reduced, but still continued, once symptoms have decreased. [3] The most common side effect is irritation to the skin in the area treated. [3] Toxicity from these products is rare but should be considered in elderly patients with accompanying renal failure. [3] Studies are still being done to prove the true effectiveness and wide application of other topical treatments such as anticholinergic agents and local anesthetic s. [3]

Oral treatments are also often used. [3] To counteract the effects of the muscarinic receptorsin sweat glands, anticholinergic drugs have been used to treat idiopathic hyperhidrosis. [3] However, the use of these is limited by the fact that they are associated with numerous side effects, systemically. [3] Beta-blockers, such as propranolol, have also been used as an anxiolytic agent in the hopes of decreasing symptoms associated with hyperhidrosis. [3] Beta-blockers are often the first-line treatment for craniofacial hyperhidrosis. [3]

New studies have shown the efficacy of psychotherapy. [21] One study shows how biofeedback can be used to reduce sweating. [21] These examples focus on the development of behavioral skills that allow the patient to control their level of anxiety and emotion in the hopes of controlling their hyperhidrosis. [21] However, these treatments stem from the idea that these emotional stimuli are somewhat causative of the condition. [21] Although patients experienced an improvement of their symptoms in the clinical setting, most were not able to recreate that effect on their own. [21] Patients who were most successful were those who suffered from focal hyperhidrosis. [21, 22]

Another viable treatment option is iontophoresis. [14] It is often the preferred second-line treatment option for palmar and plantar hyperhidrosis. [3] This method involves the application of an ionized substance to the patient's skin through a direct current. [14] Most patients undergo tap-water iontophoresis but more severe cases may require an anticholinergic supplement. [14] It is most effective in the treatment of palmar and plantar hyperhidrosis cases. [14] It has also been found to be associated with associated resolution of plantar hyperhidrosis after iontophoretic treatment to just the palms. [3] Some patients may suffer from side effects such as pain and redness. [23] Another complication is the time required for proper treatment using this method. [23] However, unlike other treatments such as sympathectomy, iontophoresis is not associated with the development of compensatory hyperhidrosis. [3] Iontophoresis treatment is not currently applied to axillary hyperhidrosis cases as it leads to numerous side effects including irritation. [14] Numerous contraindications are present for iontophoresis including pregnancy, glaucoma, and cardiovascular conditions. [3]

A therapy that has been shown to be effective is the use of botulinum toxin for the treatment of hyperhidrosis. [14] Botulinum toxin works by blocking the release of acetylcholine, and thus blocks the activity of the eccrine glands. [3] It is accompanied by few side effects and is therefore a commonly used treatment option, today. [14] Botulinum toxin A is most often used for the treatment of hyperhidrosis. [3] Botulinum B is reserved for patients who are resistant to type A and often involves more side effects. [3] Botulinum toxin is applied as an injection. [14] However, the use of injections is often considered painful and must therefore be associated with pain -control remedies. [24] Some patients apply ice for skin cooling prior to the injection. [24] New studies, however, have found efficacy in using a lidocaine-diluted botulinum toxin A solution. [24] This method is preferred as it is much less painful than the previously accepted saline-diluted method, especially for the treatment of axillary hyperhidrosis. [24] Botulinum toxin is most often applied in the treatment of craniofacial hyperhidrosis. [14] This technique varies from that used for the treatment of other facial conditions such as wrinkles. [14] Here, the technique is more uniform and superficial. [14] Injections tend to be placed just a couple centimeters apart and the effects of toxin radiate out to a distance of 1 centimeter. [3] It has also been found to be extremely useful in the treatment of axillary hyperhidrosis as it targets eccrine gland secretions at various levels physiologically. [14] It is often the next treatment option for patients suffering from axillary hyperhidrosis who have not found results through topical remedies. [3] Further, the results of this procedure can last up to six months, for normal doses. [14] It has also been shown to be effective in the treatment of palmar and plantar hyperhidrosis. [14] However, these cases require higher doses, can be associated with muscle weakness, and require sufficient anesthesia before application. [14] The pay-off, however, remains that the efficacy of the treatment could last up to a year. [14]

Surgical ablation is also an option for some hyperhidrosis patients. [14] This technique is used to treat axillary hyperhidrosis. [14] It is a very viable treatment and can be adjusted based on the severity of the condition. [14] Some of the surgical modalities include simple excision, arthroscopic shaving, and subcutaneous liposuction. [14]

Sympathectomy is another treatment option that offers incredible success ratesin the treatment of palmar and craniofacial hyperhidrosis. [14] Sympathectomy involves the removal of specific sympathetic ganglia. [23] Different techniques that can be used include cauterization and clipping. [3] Though the treatment is aimed at palmar hyperhidrosis, it has been reported that plantar hyperhidrosis may also be relieved. [23] Though the cause for this is unknown, it is hypothesized that it may stem from the decrease in emotional stress that previously triggered some of the patient's hyperhidrosis symptoms. [23] In recent years, bilateral endoscopic thoracic sympathectomy has grown increasingly popular. [3] The quick results of this procedure have helped spread its application. [3] It is often used to treat axillary and palmar hyperhidrosis. [3] Although treatment is very effective, it is also associated with various side effects including compensatory hyperhidrosis, infection, and recurrence. [14] New techniques have been adopted, however, the rates of compensatory hyperhidrosis remain high. [14] Bilateral lumbar sympathectomy is also an effective treatment and may be used as second-line treatment for craniofacial hyperhidrosis and as treatment for plantar hyperhidrosis. [3]

It is important to evaluate the risk to benefit ratio when recommending a procedure. This is especially crucial when assessing elective surgeries that may be recommended to an elderly patient as they have limited physiologic reserve and may have difficulties in the perioperative setting. Advanced age increases the risk of post-surgical complications but this is more related to comorbidities and not age alone. Thus, procedures should only be recommended to fit candidates to try to minimize risks and ultimately improve outcome. [25]

Special Cases

Numerous factors come into play when considering hyperhidrosis. [8] One special case that has been greatly studied involves the presence of secondary hyperhidrosis in elderly patients. [8] For example, postmenopausal hyperhidrosis, a form of secondary hyperhidrosis, is generalized and excessive sweating that affects many elderly women. [8] Although the true physiological mechanism behind this presentation is unknown, it relates to the patient's passage through menopause. [8] Various treatments have been used to help counter the excessive night sweats and decreased quality of life associated with this condition. [8] Hormone-replacement therapy and other medications such as anticholinergics, selective serotonin reuptake inhibitor s, and gabapentin have been used. [8] Alternative methods such as herbal remedies and acupuncture have also been used to treat these patients. [8] Patients who find the use of hormonal therapies successful indicate that the instigating problem may be the change in estrogen levels in the patient. [8] However, most patients are cautious about using hormonal therapies due to its many possible side effects. [8] A commonly used anticholinergic is oxybutynin. [8] This drug is preferred because it does not cross the blood - brain barrier and therefore leads to decreased chances of side effects. [8] Oxybutynin has been found to be successful in the treatment of postmenopausal hyperhidrosis in many cases. [8]

Conclusion

Hyperhidrosis is a complex condition that stems from a malfunction of the sympathetic nervous system. It is a very serious condition and it affects millions of Americans. Although this condition of excessive sweating stems from a physiological basis, it often goes hand-in-hand with psychological features that may exacerbate the condition. Due to the varying nature of this disorder, numerous treatment options are available. New treatments continue to come about in the hopes of helping solve the many facets of this life-altering disease.

References

[1] Lakraj AA, Moghimi N, Jabbari B. Hyperhidrosis: anatomy, pathophysiology and treatment with emphasis on the role of botulinum toxins. *Toxins.* 2013 Apr;5(4):821-40.

[2] Benson RA, Palin R, Holt PJ, Loftus IM. Diagnosis and management of hyperhidrosis. *BMJ.* 2013;347:f6800.

[3] Callejas MA, Grimalt R, Cladellas E. [Hyperhydrosis update]. *Actas Dermo-sifiliograficas.* 2010 Mar;101(2):110-8.

[4] Walling HW. Clinical differentiation of primary from secondary hyperhidrosis. *Journal of the American Academy of Dermatology.* 2011 Apr;64(4):690-5.

[5] Hoorens I, Ongenae K. Primary focal hyperhidrosis: current treatment options and a step-by-step approach. *Journal of the European Academy of Dermatology and Venereology: JEADV.* 2012 Jan;26(1):1-8.

[6] Miller DL, Bryant AS, Force SD, Miller JI, Jr. Effect of sympathectomy level on the incidence of compensatory hyperhidrosis after sympathectomy for palmar hyperhidrosis. *The Journal of Thoracic and Cardiovascular Surgery.* 2009 Sep;138(3):581-5.

[7] Strutton DR, Kowalski JW, Glaser DA, Stang PE. US prevalence of hyperhidrosis and impact on individuals with axillary hyperhidrosis: results from a national survey. *Journal of the American Academy of Dermatology.* 2004 Aug;51(2):241-8.

[8] Kim WO, Kil HK, Yoon KB, Yoo JH. Treatment of generalized hyperhidrosis with oxybutynin in post-menopausal patients. *Acta Dermato-venereologica.* 2010 May;90(3):291-3.

[9] Haider A, Solish N. Focal hyperhidrosis: diagnosis and management. CMAJ: Canadian Medical Association journal = journal de l'Association medicale canadienne. 2005 Jan 4;172(1):69-75.

[10] Boni R. Generalized hyperhidrosis and its systemic treatment. *Current Problems in Dermatology*. 2002;30:44-7.

[11] Weber A, Heger S, Sinkgraven R, Heckmann M, Elsner P, Rzany B. Psychosocial aspects of patients with focal hyperhidrosis. Marked reduction of social phobia, anxiety and depression and increased quality of life after treatment with botulinum toxin A. *The British Journal of Dermatology*. 2005 Feb;152(2):342-5.

[12] Ak M, Dincer D, Haciomeroglu B, Akarsu S, Cinar A, Lapsekili N. Temperament and character properties of primary focal hyperhidrosis patients. *Health and Quality of Life Outcomes*. 2013;11:5.

[13] Campanati A, Penna L, Guzzo T, Menotta L, Silvestri B, Lagalla G, et al. Quality-of-life assessment in patients with hyperhidrosis before and after treatment with botulinum toxin: results of an open-label study. *Clinical Therapeutics*. 2003 Jan;25(1):298-308.

[14] Stolman LP. Hyperhidrosis: medical and surgical treatment. *Eplasty*. 2008;8:e22.

[15] Ramos R, Moya J, Turon V, Perez J, Villalonga R, Morera R, et al. [Primary hyperhidrosis and anxiety: a prospective preoperative survey of 158 patients]. *Archivos de Bronconeumologia*. 2005 Feb;41(2):88-92.

[16] Kumagai K, Kawase H, Kawanishi M. Health-related quality of life after thoracoscopic sympathectomy for palmar hyperhidrosis. *The Annals of Thoracic Surgery*. 2005 Aug;80(2):461-6.

[17] Ruchinskas RA, Narayan RK, Meagher RJ, Furukawa S. The relationship of psychopathology and hyperhidrosis. *The British Journal of Dermatology*. 2002 Oct;147(4):733-5.

[18] Schneier FR, Heimberg RG, Liebowitz MR, Blanco C, Gorenstein LA. Social anxiety and functional impairment in patients seeking surgical evaluation for hyperhidrosis. *Comprehensive Psychiatry*. 2012 Nov;53(8):1181-6.

[19] Pomara N, Stanley B, Block R, Berchou RC, Stanley M, Greenblatt DJ, et al. Increased sensitivity of the elderly to the central depressant effects of diazepam. *The Journal of Clinical Psychiatry*. 1985 May;46(5):185-7.

[20] Taylor CJ, He R, Bartlett PF. The role of the N-methyl-D-aspartate receptor in the proliferation of adult hippocampal neural stem and precursor cells. *Science China Life Sciences*. 2014 Apr;57(4):403-11.

[21] Connolly M, de Berker D. Management of primary hyperhidrosis: a summary of the different treatment modalities. *American Journal of Clinical Dermatology*. 2003;4(10):681-97.

[22] Duller P, Gentry WD. Use of biofeedback in treating chronic hyperhidrosis: a preliminary report. *The British Journal of Dermatology*. 1980 Aug;103(2):143-6.

[23] Schlereth T, Dieterich M, Birklein F. Hyperhidrosis--causes and treatment of enhanced sweating. *Deutsches Arzteblatt International*. 2009 Jan;106(3):32-7.

[24] Gulec AT. Dilution of botulinum toxin A in lidocaine vs. in normal saline for the treatment of primary axillary hyperhidrosis: a double-blind, randomized, comparative preliminary study. *Journal of the European Academy of Dermatology and Venereology: JEADV*. 2012 Mar;26(3):314-8.

[25] Stefan M, Iglesia Lino L, Fernandez G. Medical consultation and best practices for preoperative evaluation of elderly patients. *Hospital Practice*. 2011 Feb;39(1):41-51.

In: Geriatric Psychodermatology
Editors: Mohammad Jafferany and Katlein França

ISBN: 978-1-63463-853-1

Chapter 13

Seborrheic Dermatitis in Geriatric Psychodermatology

Shailee Patel, BS, Tulsie Patel, BS and Katlein França, M.D., MSc*

Introduction

Seborrheic dermatitis (SD) is a chronic, inflammatory, superficial skin disease that often presents with greasy scaling, erythema, and pruritus [1]. This disorder involves the head and trunk in regions of the body with high density of sebaceous glands such as the scalp, eyebrows, nasolabial folds, over the ears, presternal and intrascapular areas, axillae, intergluteal region, and pubic region [1, 2]. The lesions are characterized as macules or thin plaques with a yellow, pink or erythematous hue, with dry, flakey white or oily, yellow scales [3]. The amount, density, and diffuseness of flaking and erythema can vary from patient to patient [4]. This condition has bimodal incidence peaks, the first in the initial 3 months of life and the second around 30-60 years of age [5]. SD as with other common geriatric diseases, although it rarely causes serious complications, can produce chronic distress in the geriatric population [6]. Although it is a relapsing disease, it tends to manifest during the winter and early spring and remits in the summer months [5]. The worldwide prevalence of SD ranges between 3 to 5% [1]. Despite its prevalence, the pathogenesis remains controversial.

The precise pathophysiology of SD is yet to be determined however the disorder is associated with the affected individuals' genetic, hormonal, and immunological profile along with presence of lipophilic *Malassezia* yeasts on their skin [7]. Yeast from the genus *Malassezia* are known to be present on all human skin but in terms SD affected skin it is thought to be an abnormal reaction to the presence of the yeast and not necessarily related to the its quantity [8-10]. Research shows that patients with the disorder have higher *Malassezia* counts compared to healthy controls but there is some disagreement upon this finding [7]. The

*Corresponding author: Katlein França. Email: k.franca@med.miami.edu

exact role of the yeast has yet to be elucidated; however the fact that there is response to antifungal therapy and the *Malassezia* counts decrease as the condition improves suggests the involvement in disease progression [11, 12].

Others have proposed that sebum in the skin is metabolized by the *Malassezia* yeasts into free fatty acids and possibly activating the alternative complement pathway leading to an inflammatory response [1, 13]. This response manifests as scaling, erythema, and inflammation. Thus, it's not the amount of *Malassezia* present but rather the amount of lipids on the surface of the skin and an abnormal host immune response to the presence of the *Malassezia* [14]. Some researchers believe the increased incidence of SD in immunocompromised patients, provides evidence the dysregulated immune response is key component in etiology [4]. While others argue that a study of biopsies from patients with SD showed an increased number of natural killer cell s, CD16 cells, complement activation which may reveal a response from irritation rather than immune deficiency [15].

The basis for suggesting the immune system is important for the pathogenesis of SD stems from the significantly higher SD prevalence (34-83%) in patients with HIV /AIDS compared to the general population (3%) [16, 17]. Other immunosuppressed groups in which SD is more common includes patients with hepatitis C, chronic alcoholic pancreatitis, and various malignancies [18-20]. SD occurs more often in patients with neurological, mood, and genetic disorders, including Parkinson's disease, tardive dyskinesia, epilepsy, traumatic spinal cord injury, cerebrovascular accidents, depression, Down syndrome, and Hailey-Hailey disease [21-26]. The association in the aforementioned groups is unclear and may have to do with altered hygiene habits [27].

There is also a possible hormonal link because SD is more prevalent in males than females in all age groups. This may be explained by the effect of androgens on the pilosebaceous unit [3, 7]. Patients with Parkinson's disease also have a higher incidence of SD due to elevated circulating α-melanocyte stimulating hormone, which may alter sebum levels [28]. Patients with Parkinson's treated with L-dopa restore the ability to make MSH-inhibiting factor which in turn reduces sebum secretion and the patients experience an improvement of SD [29, 30]. Many medications have been implicated in inducing or worsening SD (see table 1) [1]. Increased stress or fatigue can exacerbate SD [31].

Prevalence

SD affects 3-5% of the general population while dandruff, a mild variant of this disorder, has a prevalence of 15 to 20% [1, 13]. SD occurs in all ethnicities and has a predilection for men [3]. Having a bimodal distribution, SD tends to occur during the first in the initial 3 months of life and around 30-60 years of age [5]. SD has a prevalence of about 31% in the elderly but tends to appear less severe in this group [1, 32].

The estimates of greater prevalence of SD in elderly people than in the general population led a group from Italy to hypothesize if factors involved in senescence have some influence on the progression of the disease. They evaluated the association between SD and gender, coexisting non-cutaneous conditions, degree of loss of self-sufficiency in activities of daily living (ADL index) for 186 patients over the age of 65. The ADL index includes tasks of hygiene, dressing and undressing, mobility, ability to go to the toilet, bowel and bladder continence, and food intake.

Table 1. Medications that can induce or worsen Seborrheic Dermatitis

Aurothioglucose
Buspirone
Chlorpromazine
Cimetidine
Ethionamide
Gold
Griseofulvin
Haloperidol
Hydrochloride
Interferon alpha
Lithium
Methoxsalen
Methyldopa
Phenothiazine
Psoralen
Stanozolol
Thiothixene
Trioxsalen

They detected 43 cases of SD or 23.1% of their study population had SD. They found age and ADL<5 (subject with two or more dependencies) had increased predictive ability in association with SD (odds ratio [OR] of 1.14 (95% confidence interval [95% CI]: 1.04 – 1.25; p<0.001 and OR of 30.15 (95% CI: 5.83 – 155.95; p<0.0001 respectively) [33]. This coincides with previously published data that SD is common among nursing home residents [1]. They did not find a statistically significant predictive ability for (male) gender or coexisting non-cutaneous conditions [33]. These findings suggest that the elderly population may be more susceptible to developing SD as they age and lose functionality and thus caretakers should be vigilant to watch for symptoms to help manage this special at risk population.

Quality of Life and Psychosocial Impact

It is thought that about one-third of dermatological conditions are associated with emotional factors [34]. Many skin disorders, including SD, may begin or flare with psychological stress [7]. The course of SD often fluctuates from periods of remission to exacerbation, despite therapeutic management [35]. Flare-ups frequently occur during times of emotional stress, depression, and fatigue [36]. While the condition is non-threatening, it can lead to severe esthetic decline generating emotional and social distress for the affected individual. Regardless of the prevalence of SD, only a small number of studies have partially explored its effect on patients' quality of life (QoL) [35, 37-39].

One of the first studies assessing QoL in patients with SD included surveys to measure predisposition for psychiatric symptoms and dermatology life quality index (DLQI) in 30 patients from an outpatient clinic in Turkey [37]. When compared to 30 healthy age - and sex -matched volunteers, the study found an increased predisposition to depression in SD patients. This supports Maietta et al. results of a high prevalence of SD in patients with mood depression [24]. The study also showed a statistically significant decrease of DLQI in the SD group. This likely stems from the social stigma and rejection due to the excessive itching of the scalp and the scales seen in the collarette area that the patient experiences [37]. Though this was a small study, it introduced the association of reduced QoL in SD patients and the link with depression [37]. A study done by Misery et al. from Paris specifically looked at the triggering event, location of disease, and prognosis found that from their 82 SD patients stress was the main triggering factor. They found that depression was more common among patients affected on the face, which was the second (33%) after scalp (82%) for location of disease involvement. And cases with SD preceded by stress correlated with poor prognosis. This was the first study to illustrate the connection between stressful life events with outbreaks of SD [38].

A larger study including 2,159 patients with SD performed in Spain by Peyri et al. evaluated intensity of symptoms and impact on QoL using the Skindex-29 questionnaire. Their patient population had more cases with the facial involvement (88%) followed by scalp (70%). Stress/depression /fatigue (76%) and seasonal variation (44%) were the most common triggers for episodes. Differences in severity of symptoms were appreciated in the patients aged over 60 years compared to the overall group with an average age of 44 years.

The patients aged over 60 years reported more severe erythema, infiltration, and pruritus with less severe oily skin compared to the overall group. Interestingly, despite describing more severe symptoms overall in patients over 60 years, they reported less negative impact on QoL compared to their younger counterparts ($p<.05$).

However, when taking all patients into account those with severe symptoms had a significantly greater negative impact on QoL ($p<.0001$). Women were also found to experience greater effect of impairment of QoL [35]. Utilizing the Skindex-29, Patients with SD are less emotionally affected (20.5 score on Skindex-29) than patients with acne (39.2) and psoriasis (38.9) [35, 40]. In terms of functioning and symptoms, patients with SD (14.9 and 30.1) were similar to patients with acne (14.9 and 29.5) but less impacted than patients with psoriasis (22.8 and 42.1). Thus, SD does affect QoL but only modestly with a score of 20.5 on a scale of 0 to 100 (with 100 being the maximum impact on QoL) [35].

Similar trends were observed in a study performed in Poland on 2,075 patients with SD that analyzed modulation of QoL due to SD using DLQI and socioeconomic factors that could affect the patients' QoL. The older participants were significantly less impacted in QoL compared with the younger participants as with the Peyri et al. study [35, 39]. Overall they found that younger, female, and patients with higher education had the most negative impact on QoL. Younger patients with higher education may be more socially active and have more opportunities to have their skin observed by others and feel more embarrassed [39]. While the finding about older patients being less affected may be due to better acceptance of their disease process by this group compared to their younger counterparts [35]. This study was the first to consider the socioeconomic factors that may play into QoL.

Based on the few aforementioned studies SD does have some negative effect on QoL but this has been found to be even less when assessing the geriatric population. Nevertheless, just because SD does not severely debilitate geriatric patients does not mean the psychosocial impact can be overlooked. Stress has been shown to worsen flaking and pruritus of SD [41].

To our knowledge there is no data for psychotherapeutic management of SD. There is only a vague suggestion of stress management potentially through self-hypnosis in SD patients [42]. Medical hypnotherapy guides the patient into a trance state of focused awareness, selective wakefulness, and heightened suggestibility for a certain goal such as relaxation, habit modification or pruritus reduction. Hypnosis has helped improve or clear atopic dermatitis, hyperhidrosis, lichen planus, psoriasis, rosacea, and trichotillomania [43, 44]. Thus, as the field of psychodermatology expands more studies may include methods to help improve outcomes and overall QoL in patients with SD.

Medical Treatments

The goals of therapy in SD are to improve lesions, decrease symptoms (pruritus, flaking, erythema), and prevent relapses or outbreaks. Counseling patients about the persistent, recurring, and chronic nature of the inflammatory skin disease is important to help with compliance and long term management [45]. Lifelong therapy may be necessary in some cases to maintain disease suppression. Based on the current knowledge of the etiology of SD the objectives of treatment include monitoring the inflammation and proliferation of the *Malassezia* yeasts. There are many fast acting and effective treatments including antifungals and anti-inflammatory agents [4].

Topical Therapy

Topical therapies are the mainstay of the skin disorder as they are well tolerated and patients usually have good response.

Antifungal Medications

Antifungals are a first line option with their ability to inhibit growth of *Malassezia* yeasts that are implicated in the pathogenesis of SD. Azole class of antimycotic agents are lanosterol 14 α-demethylase inhibitors, which are very effective at inhibiting *Malassezia* yeasts growth. Of the azoles, ketoconazole is used first line as its variety of vehicles (cream, foam, gel, and shampoo) has proved better results, it is well tolerated, and has mild anti-inflammatory effects [46-48]. Ketoconazole shampoo 2% can be very effective if used twice weekly for treatment of scalp SD or once weekly for maintenance [48].

The cream formulation of ketoconazole 2% improves lesions of facial and body SD when used twice daily as effectively as hydrocortisone 1% cream.

Bifonazole 1% cream is a good option for treating scalp and facial lesions of SD and has a convenient once daily application [49]. An ointment of bifonazole in combination with 40% urea has been found to help with SD of the scalp and face [50]. Miconazole is alternative azole that can be used alone or in combination with hydrocortisone [51]. Ciclopirox olamine, a broad-spectrum antifungal agent, has anti-inflammatory properties and its 1.5% shampoo was shown to be as effective as 2% ketoconazole shampoo in scalp SD [52, 53]. Ciclopirox 1% cream reduces symptoms of facial SD when used twice daily [54].

Corticosteroids

In severe SD cases, low to moderate potency topical corticosteroids help with quick improvement in symptoms and visible signs. They should be used judiciously with avoidance of prolonged use as their side effects include atrophy, hypertrichosis, and telangiectasias [55]. Topical corticosteroids can be used as monotherapy or in combination with antifungal medications. Antifungal treatments are still first line for SD due to studies that have shown better reduction of symptoms and number of *Malassezia* yeasts with ketoconazole 2% foaming gel compared to betamethasone diproprionate 0.05% lotion [56]. Thus, topical corticosteroids are ideally utilized in short-term setting to relieve pruritus, erythema, and desquamation [3].

Calcineurin Inhibitors

Topical calcineurin inhibitors include pimecrolimus 1% cream, tacrolimus 0.03% and 0.1% ointment. They decrease cutaneous inflammation by inhibiting T-lymphocyte associated cytokine production [11]. Both types exert anti-inflammatory effects on SD that are greater than or equal to low potency topical corticosteroids. Other benefits include a prolonged remission time and avoidance of side effects caused by corticosteroids [57]. Pimecrolimus 1% cream was effective and well tolerated in trials for facial SD [58]. In two randomized clinical trials, pimecrolimus 1% demonstrated equal effectiveness as topical corticosteroids (hydrocortisone acetate 1% cream or betamethasone 17-valerate 0.1% cream) [59, 60]. Although similar efficacy was observed in comparison to ketoconazole 2% cream, more side effects were reported with pimecrolimus 1% cream [57].

Metronidazole

Topical metronidazole is a well-known treatment for rosacea, however its utility for SD is equivocal. Only a few trials have been performed and the findings are contradictory.

In two trials, metronidazole 0.75% gel showed better efficacy than placebo and equal to ketoconazole 2% cream [61, 62]. In contrast, two studies found it not to be better than placebo [63, 64].

Lithium Salts

Topical lithium succinate and lithium gluconate are effective at treating SD likely due to their anti-inflammatory effects. Lithium succinate 8% ointment has been shown to be more effective than placebo and has demonstrated positive results in HIV patients with facial SD [65, 66]. Similarly, lithium gluconate 8% ointment proved to be more effective than placebo in a randomized clinical trial [67]. Furthermore, another study found it to be more effective than ketoconazole 2% emulsion [68].

Zinc Pyrithione

Many over the counter anti-dandruff shampoos contain zinc pyrithione (1% or 2%) as an active ingredient as it has both antifungal and antimicrobial effects [69]. Zinc pyrithione 1% shampoo has shown to be less effective than ketoconazole 2% shampoo in a few trials. However, it may be effective to clear the appearance of the disease when used alone or in combination with ketoconazole [70].

Selenium Sulfide

Selenium sulfate shampoo comes in either 1% or 2.5%. A randomized double blind trial compared selenium sulfate 2.5%, ketoconazole 2%, and placebo in moderate to severe dandruff. The selenium sulfate 2.5%, and ketoconazole 2% were more effective than placebo but the ketoconazole was better tolerated [71].

Tar/Tea Tree

Tea tree oil, extracted from *Melaleuca alternifolia* leaves, based soaps and shampoo are effective treatments for SD due to their antifungal abilities [72].

Coal Tar

Coal tar shampoos are thought to work in SD because of its anti-proliferative, anti-inflammatory, antifungal actions, and inhibition of sebum secretion [73]. In a randomized double blind study 4% coal tar shampoo was found to significantly reduce SD compared to placebo and substantially more when it was combined with ciclopirox [74].

Systemic Medications

Orally administered treatment is mainly used for SD cases that are extensive, severe or refractory to topical medication. The oral antifungal drugs used are ketoconazole, itraconazole, and terbinafine. Most of the studies are performed on a small number of patients and at times the data is unclear. In a randomized placebo controlled study, ketoconazole 200mg daily for four weeks showed significant improvement [75]. In a noncomparative study, itraconazole given at an initial dose of 200mg daily for 1 week followed by a single dose of 200mg every two weeks help improve symptoms in patients with moderate to severe SD [76]. In a randomized placebo controlled study oral terbinafine of 250mg for six weeks was more effective than placebo in all areas except the face [77]. Monitoring liver function is necessary during long-term usage of oral antifungals.

Phototherapy

Patients report improvement of symptoms during the summer months. The direct inhibition of *Malassezia* yeasts culture from skin has been shown by experimentation with UVA and UVB light [78].

UVB

Using phototherapy is an option for severe recalcitrant SD. A study followed 18 patients treated with narrow-band UVB three times per week until clearance or 2 months of therapy. All the patients responded well to the therapy with the median number of treatment sessions was 23 and the median cumulative UVB dose was 9.8J/cm2. Some of the drawbacks to this form of treatment are frequent visits to the phototherapy unit, rapid relapse after 2-6 weeks post treatment, and risk associated with exceeded maximum lifetime cumulative dose [79].

Psoralen Plus Ultraviolet A (PUVA)

Five patients with HIV were administered systemic PUVA over two-4-week periods, 2 months apart. The total irradiation ranged from 30 to 262 J/cm2. The patients cleared all their skin lesions, including therapy -resistant psoriasis vulgaris, seborrheic dermatitis, folliculitis, and chronic urticaria, cleared during the first weeks of PUVA [80].

In addition to the psychotherapy and medical treatment, physicians must also consider the sociophysiologic characteristics when managing SD in the elderly population [6]. Geriatric patients frequently experience dementia, memory loss, impaired vision, decreased hearing and limited mobility [81]. And they may lack caregivers, appropriate nutrition, or the physical ability to comply with a therapy regimen. Thus, physicians should ensure that compliance with therapy is realistic and they are carefully monitoring possible dangerous medication interactions due to polypharmacy [81, 82].

Conclusion

SD is a common chronic relapsing inflammatory skin disorder that affects the geriatric population [1, 6]. The exact pathogenesis has yet to be elucidated but involves presence of *Malassezia* yeasts on the skin of susceptible patients that undergo an abnormal reaction leading to greasy scaling, erythema, and pruritus of regions involved [53]. There are many medical treatment options, mostly topical therapies that are generally well tolerated and help resolve SD lesions.

Having effective topical treatment alleviates some of the dangers associated with systemic polypharmacy in the vulnerable elderly population [81, 82]. Ideally, a patient will be controlled with long-term maintenance to avoid recurrence however the patient should be educated that relapse are possible regardless of therapy. Understanding that stress or fatigue may worsen symptoms may help patients seek out stress management techniques to avoid the triggers [41-44].

References

[1] Schwartz, R. A., Janusz, C. A., Janniger, C. K. Seborrheic dermatitis: an overview. *American Family Physician*. 2006 Jul. 1;74(1):125-30.

[2] Stefanaki, I., Katsambas, A. Therapeutic update on seborrheic dermatitis. *Skin Therapy Letter*. 2010 May;15(5):1-4.

[3] Sampaio, A. L., Mameri, A. C., Vargas, T. J., Ramos-e-Silva, M., Nunes, A. P., Carneiro, S. C. Seborrheic dermatitis. *Anais Brasileiros de Dermatologia*. 2011 Nov.-Dec.;86(6):1061-71; quiz 72-4.

[4] Elewski, B. E. Safe and effective treatment of seborrheic dermatitis. *Cutis*. 2009 Jun.; 83(6):333-8.

[5] Gupta, A. K., Madzia, S. E., Batra, R. Etiology and management of Seborrheic dermatitis. *Dermatology*. 2004;208(2):89-93.

[6] Farage, M. A., Miller, K. W., Berardesca, E., Maibach, H. I. Clinical implications of aging skin: cutaneous disorders in the elderly. *American Journal of Clinical Dermatology*. 2009;10(2):73-86.

[7] Gupta, A. K., Bluhm, R. Seborrheic dermatitis. *Journal of the European Academy of Dermatology and Venereology: JEADV*. 2004 Jan.;18(1):13-26; quiz 19-20.

[8] Faergemann, J., Fredriksson, T. Tinea versicolor with regard to seborrheic dermatitis. An epidemiological investigation. *Archives of dermatology*. 1979 Aug.;115(8):966-8.

[9] McGinley, K. J., Leyden, J. J., Marples, R. R., Kligman, A. M. Quantitative microbiology of the scalp in non-dandruff, dandruff, and seborrheic dermatitis. *The Journal of Investigative Dermatology*. 1975 Jun.;64(6):401-5.

[10] Faergemann, J. Tinea versicolor and Pityrosporum orbiculare: mycological investigations, experimental infections and epidemiological surveys. *Acta Dermato-venereologica Supplementum*. 1979 (86):1-23.

[11] Cook, B. A., Warshaw, E. M. Role of topical calcineurin inhibitors in the treatment of seborrheic dermatitis: a review of pathophysiology, safety, and efficacy. *American Journal of Clinical Dermatology*. 2009;10(2):103-18.

[12] Bergbrant, I. M. Seborrhoeic dermatitis and Pityrosporum yeasts. *Current Topics in Medical Mycology*. 1995;6:95-112.

[13] Naldi, L., Rebora, A. Clinical practice. Seborrheic dermatitis. *The New England Journal of Medicine*. 2009 Jan. 22;360(4):387-96.

[14] Terui, T., Kudo, K., Tagami, H. [Cutaneous immune and inflammatory reactions to Malassezia furfur]. *Nihon Ishinkin Gakkai zasshi = Japanese journal of medical mycology.* 1999;40(2):63-7.

[15] Bikowski, J. Facial seborrheic dermatitis: a report on current status and therapeutic horizons. *Journal of Drugs in Dermatology: JDD*. 2009 Feb.;8(2):125-33.

[16] Marino, C. T., McDonald, E., Romano, J. F. Seborrheic dermatitis in acquired immunodeficiency syndrome. *Cutis*. 1991 Sep.;48(3):217-8.

[17] Mathes, B. M., Douglass, M. C. Seborrheic dermatitis in patients with acquired immunodeficiency syndrome. *Journal of the American Academy of Dermatology*. 1985 Dec.;13(6):947-51.

[18] Barba, A., Piubello, W., Vantini, I., Caliari, S., Cocchetto, R., Vallaperta, P., et al. Skin lesions in chronic alcoholic pancreatitis. *Dermatologica*. 1982 May;164(5):322-6.

[19] Cribier, B., Samain, F., Vetter, D., Heid, E., Grosshans, E. Systematic cutaneous examination in hepatitis C virus infected patients. *Acta Dermato-venereologica*. 1998 Sep.;78(5):355-7.

[20] Clift, D. C., Dodd, H. J., Kirby, J. D., Midgley, G., Noble, W. C. Seborrheic dermatitis and malignancy. An investigation of the skin flora. *Acta Dermato-venereologica*. 1988; 68(1):48-52.

[21] Binder, R. L., Jonelis, F. J. Seborrheic dermatitis in neuroleptic-induced parkinsonism. *Archives of Dermatology*. 1983 Jun.;119(6):473-5.

[22] Sandyk, R. Seborrhea and persistent tardive dyskinesia. *The International Journal of Neuroscience*. 1990 Feb.;50(3-4):223-6.

[23] Rubin-Asher, D., Zeilig, G., Klieger, M., Adunsky, A., Weingarden, H. Dermatological findings following acute traumatic spinal cord injury. *Spinal cord*. 2005 Mar.;43 (3): 175-8.

[24] Maietta, G., Fornaro, P., Rongioletti, F., Rebora, A. Patients with mood depression have a high prevalence of seborrhoeic dermatitis. *Acta Dermato-venereologica*. 1990;70(5): 432-4.

[25] Ercis, M., Balci, S., Atakan, N. Dermatological manifestations of 71 Down syndrome children admitted to a clinical genetics unit. *Clinical genetics*. 1996 Nov.;50(5):317-20.

[26] Marren, P., Burge, S. Seborrhoeic dermatitis of the scalp--a manifestation of Hailey-Hailey disease in a predisposed individual? *The British Journal of Dermatology*. 1992 Mar.;126(3):294-6.

[27] Bukvic Mokos, Z., Kralj, M., Basta-Juzbasic, A., Lakos Jukic, I. Seborrheic dermatitis: an update. *Acta Dermatovenerologica Croatica: ADC*. 2012;20(2):98-104.

[28] Shuster, S., Thody, A. J., Goolamali, S. K., Burton, J. L., Plummer, N., Bates, D. Melanocyte-stimulating hormone and parkinsonism. *Lancet*. 1973 Mar. 3;1(7801): 463-4.

[29] Burton, J. L., Shuster, S. Effect of L-dopa on seborrhoea of parkinsonism. *Lancet*. 1970 Jul. 4;2(7662):19-20.

[30] Potter, J., Wyburn-Mason, R. Effect of L-dopa on seborrhoea of parkinsonism. *Lancet*. 1970 Sep. 26;2(7674):660.

[31] Carter, D. M., Balin, A. K. Dermatological aspects of aging. *The Medical Clinics of North America*. 1983 Mar.;67(2):531-43.

[32] Fitzpatrick, J. E. Common inflammatory skin diseases of the elderly. *Geriatrics*. 1989 Jul.;44(7):40-6.

[33] Mastrolonardo, M., Diaferio, A., Vendemiale, G., Lopalco, P. Seborrhoeic dermatitis in the elderly: inferences on the possible role of disability and loss of self-sufficiency. *Acta Dermato-venereologica*. 2004;84(4):285-7.

[34] Gupta, M. A., Voorhees, J. J. Psychosomatic dermatology. Is it relevant? *Archives of Dermatology*. 1990 Jan.;126(1):90-3.

[35] Peyri, J., Lleonart, M., Grupo espanol del Estudio S. [Clinical and therapeutic profile and quality of life of patients with seborrheic dermatitis]. *Actas dermo-sifiliograficas*. 2007 Sep.;98(7):476-82.

[36] Picardi, A., Abeni, D. Stressful life events and skin diseases: disentangling evidence from myth. *Psychotherapy and Psychosomatics*. 2001 May-Jun.;70(3):118-36.

[37] Oztas, P., Calikoglu, E., Cetin, I. Psychiatric tests in seborrhoeic dermatitis. *Acta Dermato-venereologica*. 2005;85(1):68-9.

[38] Misery, L., Touboul, S., Vincot, C., Dutray, S., Rolland-Jacob, G., Consoli, S. G., et al. [Stress and seborrheic dermatitis]. *Annales de Dermatologie et de Venereologie*. 2007 Nov.;134(11):833-7.

[39] Szepietowski, J. C., Reich, A., Wesolowska-Szepietowska, E., Baran, E., National Quality of Life in Dermatology G. Quality of life in patients suffering from seborrheic dermatitis: influence of age, gender and education level. *Mycoses*. 2009 Jul.;52(4):357-63.

[40] Lasek, R. J., Chren, M. M. Acne vulgaris and the quality of life of adult dermatology patients. *Archives of Dermatology*. 1998 Apr.;134(4):454-8.

[41] Arck, P., Paus, R. From the brain -skin connection: the neuroendocrine-immune misalliance of stress and itch. *Neuroimmunomodulation*. 2006;13(5-6):347-56.

[42] MJ, S. *Hypnosis in Skin and Allergic Diseases*. Springfield, IL: Thomas Publisher; 1960.

[43] Shenefelt, P. D. Psychological interventions in the management of common skin conditions. *Psychology Research and Behavior Management*. 2010;3:51-63.

[44] Shenefelt, P. D. Hypnosis in dermatology. *Archives of Dermatology*. 2000 Mar.;136(3): 393-9.

[45] Bhatia, N. Treating seborrheic dermatitis: review of mechanisms and therapeutic options. *Journal of Drugs in Dermatology: JDD*. 2013 Jul. 1;12(7):796-8.

[46] Elewski, B., Ling, M. R., Phillips, T. J. Efficacy and safety of a new once-daily topical ketoconazole 2% gel in the treatment of seborrheic dermatitis: a phase III trial. *Journal of Drugs in Dermatology: JDD*. 2006 Jul.-Aug.;5(7):646-50.

[47] Elewski, B. E., Abramovits, W., Kempers, S., Schlessinger, J., Rosen, T., Gupta, A. K., et al. A novel foam formulation of ketoconazole 2% for the treatment of seborrheic dermatitis on multiple body regions. *Journal of Drugs in Dermatology: JDD*. 2007 Oct.; 6(10):1001-8.

[48] Peter, R. U., Richarz-Barthauer, U. Successful treatment and prophylaxis of scalp seborrhoeic dermatitis and dandruff with 2% ketoconazole shampoo: results of a multicentre, double-blind, placebo -controlled trial. *The British Journal of Dermatology*. 1995 Mar.;132(3):441-5.

[49] Segal, R., David, M., Ingber, A., Lurie, R., Sandbank, M. Treatment with bifonazole shampoo for seborrhea and seborrheic dermatitis: a randomized, double-blind study. *Acta Dermato-venereologica*. 1992 Nov.;72(6):454-5.

[50] Shemer, A., Nathansohn, N., Kaplan, B., Weiss, G., Newman, N., Trau, H. Treatment of scalp seborrheic dermatitis and psoriasis with an ointment of 40% urea and 1% bifonazole. *International Journal of Dermatology*. 2000 Jul.;39(7):532-4.

[51] Faergemann, J. Seborrhoeic dermatitis and Pityrosporum orbiculare: treatment of seborrhoeic dermatitis of the scalp with miconazole-hydrocortisone (Daktacort), miconazole and hydrocortisone. *The British Journal of Dermatology*. 1986 Jun.;114(6): 695-700.

[52] Ratnavel, R. C., Squire, R. A., Boorman, G. C. Clinical efficacies of shampoos containing ciclopirox olamine (1.5%) and ketoconazole (2.0%) in the treatment of seborrhoeic dermatitis. *The Journal of dermatological treatment*. 2007;18(2):88-96.

[53] Gupta, A. K., Bluhm, R. Ciclopirox (Loprox) gel for superficial fungal infection s. *Skin Therapy Letter*. 2004 Aug.-Sep.;9(7):4-5, 9.

[54] Dupuy, P., Maurette, C., Amoric, J. C., Chosidow, O., Study Investigator G. Randomized, placebo -controlled, double-blind study on clinical efficacy of ciclopiroxolamine 1% cream in facial seborrhoeic dermatitis. *The British Journal of Dermatology*. 2001 May;144(5):1033-7.

[55] Del Rosso, J. Q. Adult seborrheic dermatitis: a status report on practical topical management. *The Journal of Clinical and Aesthetic Dermatology*. 2011 May;4(5):32-8.

[56] Ortonne, J. P., Lacour, J. P., Vitetta, A., Le Fichoux, Y. Comparative study of ketoconazole 2% foaming gel and betamethasone dipropionate 0.05% lotion in the treatment of seborrhoeic dermatitis in adults. *Dermatology*. 1992;184(4):275-80.

[57] Shin, H., Kwon, O. S., Won, C. H., Kim, B. J., Lee, Y. W., Choe, Y. B., et al. Clinical efficacies of topical agents for the treatment of seborrheic dermatitis of the scalp: a comparative study. *The Journal of Dermatology*. 2009 Mar.;36(3):131-7.

[58] Rigopoulos, D., Ioannides, D., Kalogeromitros, D., Gregoriou, S., Katsambas, A. Pimecrolimus cream 1% vs. betamethasone 17-valerate 0.1% cream in the treatment of seborrhoeic dermatitis. A randomized open-label clinical trial. *The British Journal of Dermatology*. 2004 Nov.;151(5):1071-5.

[59] Firooz, A., Solhpour, A., Gorouhi, F., Daneshpazhooh, M., Balighi, K., Farsinejad, K., et al. Pimecrolimus cream, 1%, vs hydrocortisone acetate cream, 1%, in the treatment of facial seborrheic dermatitis: a randomized, investigator-blind, clinical trial. *Archives of Dermatology*. 2006 Aug.;142(8):1066-7.

[60] Koc, E., Arca, E., Kose, O., Akar, A. An open, randomized, prospective, comparative study of topical pimecrolimus 1% cream and topical ketoconazole 2% cream in the treatment of seborrheic dermatitis. *The Journal of Dermatological Treatment*. 2009;20 (1):4-9.

[61] Parsad, D., Pandhi, R., Negi, K. S., Kumar, B. Topical metronidazole in seborrheic dermatitis --a double-blind study. *Dermatology*. 2001;202(1):35-7.

[62] Seckin, D., Gurbuz, O., Akin, O. Metronidazole 0.75% gel vs. ketoconazole 2% cream in the treatment of facial seborrheic dermatitis: a randomized, double-blind study. *Journal of the European Academy of Dermatology and Venereology: JEADV*. 2007 Mar.;21(3):345-50.

[63] Koca, R., Altinyazar, H. C., Esturk, E. Is topical metronidazole effective in seborrheic dermatitis? A double-blind study. *International Journal of Dermatology*. 2003 Aug.;42 (8):632-5.

[64] Ozcan, H., Seyhan, M., Yologlu, S. Is metronidazole 0.75% gel effective in the treatment of seborrhoeic dermatitis? A double-blind, placebo controlled study. *European Journal of Dermatology: EJD*. 2007 Jul.-Aug.;17(4):313-6.

[65] Dreno, B., Moyse, D. Lithium gluconate in the treatment of seborrhoeic dermatitis: a multicenter, randomised, double-blind study versus placebo. *European Journal of Dermatology: EJD*. 2002 Nov.-Dec.;12(6):549-52.

[66] Langtry, J. A., Rowland Payne, C. M., Staughton, R. C., Stewart, J. C., Horrobin, D. F. Topical lithium succinate ointment (Efalith) in the treatment of AIDS -related seborrhoeic dermatitis. *Clinical and Experimental Dermatology*. 1997 Sep.;22(5):216-9.

[67] Warshaw, E. M., Wohlhuter, R. J., Liu, A., Zeller, S. A., Wenner, R. A., Bowers, S., et al. Results of a randomized, double-blind, vehicle-controlled efficacy trial of pimecrolimus cream 1% for the treatment of moderate to severe facial seborrheic dermatitis. *Journal of the American Academy of Dermatology*. 2007 Aug.;57(2):257-64.

[68] Dreno, B., Chosidow, O., Revuz, J., Moyse, D., Study Investigator G. Lithium gluconate 8% vs ketoconazole 2% in the treatment of seborrhoeic dermatitis: a multicentre, randomized study. *The British Journal of Dermatology*. 2003 Jun.;148(6): 1230-6.

[69] Opdyke, D. L., Burnett, C. M., Brauer, E. W. Anti-seborrhoeic qualities of zinc pyrithione in a cream vehicle. II. Safety evaluation. *Food and Cosmetics Toxicology*. 1967 Aug.;5(3):321-6.

[70] Pierard-Franchimont, C., Goffin, V., Decroix, J., Pierard, G. E. A multicenter randomized trial of ketoconazole 2% and zinc pyrithione 1% shampoos in severe dandruff and seborrheic dermatitis. *Skin Pharmacology and Applied Skin Physiology*. 2002 Nov.-Dec.;15(6):434-41.

[71] Danby, F. W., Maddin, W. S., Margesson, L. J., Rosenthal, D. A randomized, double-blind, placebo -controlled trial of ketoconazole 2% shampoo versus selenium sulfide 2.5% shampoo in the treatment of moderate to severe dandruff. *Journal of the American Academy of Dermatology*. 1993 Dec.;29(6):1008-12.

[72] Satchell, A. C., Saurajen, A., Bell, C., Barnetson, R. S. Treatment of dandruff with 5% tea tree oil shampoo. *Journal of the American Academy of Dermatology*. 2002 Dec.;47 (6):852-5.

[73] Paghdal, K. V., Schwartz, R. A. Topical tar: back to the future. *Journal of the American Academy of Dermatology*. 2009 Aug.;61(2):294-302.

[74] Davies, D. B. B. G., Shuttleworth, D. Comparative efficacy of shampoos containing coal tar (4.0% w/w; TarmedTM), coal tar (4.0% w/w) plus ciclopirox olamine (1.0% w/w; TarmedTM AF) and ketoconazole (2.0% w/w; Nizoral®) for the treatment of dandruff /seborrhoeic dermatitis. *J. Dermatol. Treat*. 1999;10:177–83.

[75] Ford, G. P., Farr, P. M., Ive, F. A., Shuster, S. The response of seborrhoeic dermatitis to ketoconazole. *The British Journal of Dermatology*. 1984 Nov.;111(5):603-7.

[76] Shemer, A., Kaplan, B., Nathansohn, N., Grunwald, M. H., Amichai, B., Trau, H. Treatment of moderate to severe facial seborrheic dermatitis with itraconazole: an open non-comparative study. *The Israel Medical Association Journal: IMAJ*. 2008 Jun.;10 (6):417-8.

[77] Vena, G. A., Micali, G., Santoianni, P., Cassano, N., Peruzzi, E. Oral terbinafine in the treatment of multi-site seborrhoic dermatitis: a multicenter, double-blind placebo -

controlled study. *International Journal of Immunopathology and Pharmacology*. 2005 Oct.-Dec.;18(4):745-53.

[78] Wikler, J. R., Janssen, N., Bruynzeel, D. P., Nieboer, C. The effect of UV -light on pityrosporum yeasts: ultrastructural changes and inhibition of growth. *Acta Dermato-Venereologica*. 1990;70(1):69-71.

[79] Pirkhammer, D., Seeber, A., Honigsmann, H., Tanew, A. Narrow-band ultraviolet B (ATL-01) phototherapy is an effective and safe treatment option for patients with severe seborrhoeic dermatitis. *The British Journal of Dermatology*. 2000 Nov.;143(5): 964-8.

[80] Ranki, A., Puska, P., Mattinen, S., Lagerstedt, A., Krohn, K. Effect of PUVA on immunologic and virologic findings in HIV -infected patients. *Journal of the American Academy of Dermatology*. 1991 Mar.;24(3):404-10.

[81] Bleiker, T. O., Graham-Brown, R. A. Diagnosing skin disease in the elderly. *The Practitioner*. 2000 Nov.;244(1616):974-81.

[82] Smoker, A. Skin care in old age. *Nursing standard*. 1999 Aug. 18-24;13(48):47-53.

In: Geriatric Psychodermatology
Editors: Mohammad Jafferany and Katlein França
ISBN: 978-1-63463-853-1

Chapter 14

Urticaria and Elderly

Ilknur Altunay, M.D.* and Sibel Mercan, M.D.

Introduction

Definition

Urticaria is a vascular reaction to various stimuli and covers a heterogenous group of diseases with many subtypes. It is characterized by the wheals, white or red transient edematous papules and plaques. A typical lesion is called wheal or hive with edematous, pale central area and erythematous surrounding area. If the edema in the superficial dermis in urticarial lesions, involves the deep dermis or is subcutaneous, then the term 'angioedema ' is used. Based on the duration, it is considered to occur as two types: acute (AU) and chronic urticaria (CU). This differentiation is only about its duration not about the severity of urticaria. Acute urticaria is defined as the presence of wheals and/or angioedema < 6 weeks. When daily or recurrent lesions last > 6 weeks, it is referred to as CU.

Epidemiology

Urticaria is a worldwide disease and may present at any age. In fact, ratios change with respect to age range, sampling methods and urticaria subtypes. Acute urticaria is one of the most common skin disorders; 15-25% of individuals have at least one episode of acute urticaria in their lifetime [1, 2]. Lifetime prevalance of chronic urticaria is estimated at 1-4% with a predominance of middle age female [3, 4]. Some epidemiological studies report a prevalance rate of 0.5-1[3, 4]. There are some survey studies including both acute and chronic urticaria patients. A nationwide survey study conducted for dermatologic disorders in Japan indicated that among 67448 patients, urticaria/angioedema was one of the most common four

* Corresponding author: Ilknur Altunay. Email: ialtunay@gmail.com

diseases [5]. In Cairo, urticaria was at a rate of 7.4% among 7528 dermatology patients, which was considered among the most common diagnoses [6].

Despite all these community based data, there are scarce and unreliable epidemiological studies for urticaria in elderly people A more spesific study carried out in 5961 elderly patients who were admitted to a dermatology outpatient clinic in Turkey, showed that urticaria was diagnosed at 449 patients (7.5%) and it was considered among top four dermatologic diseases [7]. Another study consisting of 874 geriatric patients reported a urticaria prevalance rate of 2.4% [8]. A recent epidemiological survey indicates that prevalance rates of chronic urticaria in elderly are actually similar to those of adult population; however, female predominance, which is characteristic of adult patients, is not present in elderly patients [4]. Apparently, most of studies state that urticaria is one of uncommon hospital referral problems in elderly [9-11]. Although elderly people have somewhat decreased histamin induced skin reactivity and the lower occurrence of auto-reactivity associated with immunosenescence, the increase of systemic diseases, use of multiple medications and some psychosocial factors due to aging can cause to occur the occurrence of urticarial reactions [4,12-15].

Etiological Factors

Numerous etiological factors exist in urticaria and/or angioedema. They are responsible for both AU and CU.

Drugs: Penicillin and related antibiotics, aspirin and sulfonamids are the most frequent offenders. NSAID's (including aspirin and salicylate containing drugs) and ACE inhibitors that are mostly prescribed for geriatric population are blamed for angioedema without wheals and exacerbations of chronic urticaria [16]. Also, drugs such as morphine, curare, quinine, codein, dextran, etc. cause mast cells to liberate histamin non immunologically, and thus lead to acute urticaria attacks [17].

Foods: Fish, sellfish, eggs, chocolate, strawberries, cheese, yeast, tomato, soya, peanut are the most blamed foods in particularly acute urticaria while they are infrequent reasons in chronic urticaria. Food-related etiology is actually rare in older people when compared to young people [18-20].

Infections, infestations: Localized infections of the sinuses, gallbladder, bladder, prostate and kidney, and systemic viral infectionssuch as hepatitis B and C and uncommonly parasitic infectionscan cause urticaria [17].

Inhalants: Pollens, grass, house dust mites, animal dander, aerosols, and molds can cause urticaria.

Systemic /metabolic diseases /neoplasms: Increased thyroid autoantibodies can be found in patients with CU, even if there is no evidence of thyroid malfunction. Patients with collagen vascular disease, particularly in systemic lupus erythematosus and Sjogren syndrome occasionally present with urticarial attacks. Urticarial reactions can be seen in acute rheumatic fever or acute rheumatoid arthritis.

Carcinomas, Hodgkin lymphoma and chronic lymphocytic leukemia can be considered in this context.

Psychological Factors and Psychiatric Associations about Etiology

The idea that there is an intimate relationship between body and mind has been around since antiquity. The recognition of the psychogenic aspects of asthma has been attributed to Hippocrates, who supposedly warned that asthmatic patients must guard against anger. Regarding urticaria,a pure psychological origin previously was almost unquestionable. Today, new knowledge from a variety of disciplines affirms the existence of a complex, fascinating, and intricately entangled mind–body factors and there is growing evidence that psychological factors play a role in the etiology of particularly chronic urticaria [21-23]. Nevertheless, some debate and controversy are still ongoing, because there are a few studies fulfilling reliable methodologic standards to assess the link between stress and urticaria [24-26]. Also, a lack of formal studies comparing drug and 'mind- body' treatment outcomes will continue to impact negatively the adoption of 'mind- body' approaches in CU [27].

Data regarding the fact that stressful life events may contribute to the onset or exacerbation of CU, are gradually continuing to cumulate. Some recent controlled studies have reported stressful life events that within six months/1 year preceding the onset or flare up of urticaria attack, may be the major triggering factors. In literature, stressful life events have been described as death or illness of a close person, financial loss or problems, physical or emotional injuries, traumas or sexual problems, etc. [28-35]. Kimyai-Asadi and Usman noticed some isolated cases of urticaria occurring after earthquakes and dental procedures [36]. Rees reported that stressful life events were associated with onset of symptoms in 51% of 100 patients with CU/angioedema as compared to 8% of surgical control patients[29]. In a study, 90% of patients with CU had a history of stressful life experiences before disease onset and suffered from depression and anxiety [30]. A survey of 43 patients of CU found that increased mental tension and fatique may be precipitating factors in 77% of the cohort [37]. Engin et al. proposed that anxiety and depressive symptoms secondary to stressful life events may precipitate emergence of urticarial symptoms in susceptible subjects and also the severity of urticaria is not indicative for higher scores of depression and anxiety [34].

Table 1. Etiological Classification of Psychogenic Urticaria
(*Adapted from Iamandescu ref. 41*)

Psychogenic Urticaria
1 - *Apparently exclusive psychological factors (rare cases, without other proven etiology)*
2 - *Constantly psychologically triggered urticaria associated with other etiology*
Cholinergic urticaria
Adreneregic urticaria
Psychological itching
3- *Optionally psychologically triggered urticaria*
Spontaneous acute urticaria
Spontaneous chronic urticaria
Dermographic urticaria
Cold contact urticaria

Some clinical subtypes of urticaria such as symptomatic dermographism, cholinergic and adrenergic urticaria have been reported to be associated with preceding emotional distress [33, 38]. Czubalski and Rudzki postulated that frustrating situations are associated with 80% of dermographism and 75% of adrenergic urticaria cases [39]. On the other hand, Weller et al., found that anxiety and depression appear less frequently in patients with auto-reactive CU which is a distinct urticaria group [40].

Iamandescu and Florea have suggested a classification of urticaria and/or angioedema with psychogenic etiology [41]. (Table 1).

According to this classification, pure psychogenic etiology /pure psychogenic urticaria is very rare. As diagnostic investigation expands, other causal factors will also be revealed. The certainty of the psychological etiology may be reasonable to approve in the event of awareness of the patient himself that urticarial attacks are repeatedly associated with psychogenic stress. In these cases, prolonged psychic stress, although shares the responsibility with other etiological factors, has a constant and regular effect on attacks. Additionally, chronic emotional stress may occasionally be a triggering factor for attacks in CU wherein different etiologic factors may also play a role. It should be kept in mind that psychogenic label should be considered in the case of the predominance or presence of the psychic factors within multi-factorial etiology [41].

Considering other psychiatric factors that contribute to CU etiology, discussion has rather intensified on obsessive compulsive disorder, personality traits, somatization disordersand post traumatic stress disorder as well as triggering stressful events associated with depression and anxiety symptoms in this context [30, 42-51].

In some studies, obsessive-compulsive disorder, alexythymic trait, neuroticism and introversion have been highlighted [42, 45, 47-51]. Patients with dilemma without solutions, competitive individuals, patients having resentment, hostility or insecure attachment scale have been reported to be prone to develop urticaria [43]. Insecure attachment style was emphasized to potentiate the occurrence of anxiety in CU [48]. In a study, passive aggressive trait was found significantly higher in women [42]. It has also been suggested that post-traumatic stress disorder resulting from traumatic memories or emotions is possibly manifested via CU and favorable improvement of CU may not take place without treatment of post- traumatic stress disorder [49, 50]. Meanwhile, it should be kept in mind that depression can affect clinical picture reducing the threshold for itching [52].

Despite all these evidence, the issue of whether the underlying depression /anxiety or the personality trait increases stress perception is still controversial. Similarly, the matter of whether psychiatric conditions predispose an individual to develop CU or co-exist with CU, has not yet been concluded.

When geriatric period is focused on, one can see that this age group has particular problems and stressors. Lots of stress including illnesses, loss of physical and mental abilities, economic downturn s, multiple or expensive medical treatments, changes of life style etc. can lead to depression in seniors. Several population studies across the world have examined its prevalence, with results ranging from 1 to 20%, however, methodological differences may account for this variability [53]. Suicide rates are the highest in old age in almost every country in the world. The failure to deal with social stress ors may play an important role in suicidal behavior, and suicide attempters report difficulties in resolving social problems. It is conceivable that a misperception of others' emotions can undermine social problem solving, leading to feelings of hopelessness in the face of losses, conflict, and dependence on caregivers [54, 55]. Deficits in emotion recognition may lead to low levels of social connectedness and belonging, to known risk factors for suicide attempt and death by suicide in late life [56]. It appears that geriatric population has adequate stressors to trigger urticaria.

Case Samples and Psychoanalytic Explanations

In some patients, causes of the onset or exacarbation of urticaria could be disclosed by only psychoanalytically oriented interviews. Sometimes, chronic urticaria might even be healed simply by solving social stress or. Here are some examples from our cases and literature:

Patient A, 66 years old male had the story of urticaria several years ago. There was no reason to describe his attacks and he was resistant to all medications. Dermatologists could not find the solution and at the end, his family physician recommended him to divorce. He had a very problematic marriage which made his life a torture. He was aware of his wife's unfair behaviors but was actually blamed as 'paranoid person' by his wife. When he was trying to control his feelings, he was having urticaria attacks. After divorce, his urticaria symptoms had subsided.

When he applied for psychiatric help, he had similar problems with his girlfriend. He was stuck in the relationship and was blamed for being paranoid. Even though there were clues about other men in his girlfriend's life, he could not solve this problem or leave the relationship. He ended his marriage with the help of this girlfriend; Once, at one of psychotherapy sessions, he had nasal bleeding when he was talking his guilt about divorce and the new relationship. He had high blood pressure during these times. He had stroke after talking about his grandfather's unfair relationship, which was his secret for years. He heard fights of his grandparents and his grandmother's cries for years. He knew why she was crying, but preferred not to tell anyone. He felt responsible about keeping his grandfather's secret. On one hand, he was feeling guilty about that and on the other hand, he was repeating the similar behavior with his new girlfriend. His grandmother passed away during his therapy. He dreamt about his grandmother crying. The following day, he had stroke and doctors again couldn't find the underlying reason At the end of all physical examination, his physician said that he might have atrial fibrillation during the sleep. His atrial fibrillation might be reaction to his conflictual feelings.

Patient B, 65 year-old female patient had first urticaria attack 14 years ago. She has been married for 29 years and has two sons *of* 22 and 27 years old. Her marriage was problematic and had unresolved conflictswith her husband and his parents since the first years of the marriage. Her husband *was* alcoholic and she has been subjected to physical violence. The first urticaria attack has emerged during an argument between her husband and her son. During psychoanalytic session, she disclosed that she was disgusted with him and could not tolerate him any more. Whenever she felt her husband's intimacy or an argument occured between him and her sons, she has an urticarial attack. She implied that she was very angry with him and had a problem in anger management. However, she could not leave him. She also constantly emphasized her fondness for her sons.

The patient had depressive periods with sleeping problems, crying seizures and social isolation in the past. Her psychiatric examination and test revealed the presence of depression, anxiety and hyperthimic temperament. Kinesthetic responses in Rorscharch test included agressive impulses. In addition, need for the other and imaginations referring to symbotic relationships were remarkable.

Here is another example from Taylor's paper [57]. He summarized the story about the Greek philosopher, writer Kazanstakis.

Kazantzakis left his house and went to Vienna. He met with Frieda and he wanted to spend the night with her. She invited him not that evening but the following day. When he went back to his hotel his face was swollen. He postponed this meeting with Frieda and he sent a telegram to her. He repeated sending it everyday. He couldn't be relieved from his illness for several weeks. He consulted his illness to Stekel. Stekel made the diagnosis of ascetics' disease, a rare disorder but one recorded in the legends of the saints. In this condition, the man's soul or psyche believes that sleeping with a woman is a mortal sin. For that reason, the soul refuses to permit his body to commit this sin. Stekel did not offer to analyze Kazantzakis; instead, he told him that he would be cured as soon as he departed from Vienna and left Frieda behind him. He refused to do so at first. But after several weeks, he couldn't find any other solution to his illness and so he left the city. By the time he went to the railway station, his swelling had subsided [57]. Taylor pointed out another story in the autobiography of Kazantzakis, which was about his guilty feelings towards his religion teacher He hated his teacher and wanted to send him away. He wrote a personal note and said that the teacher's mother was sick and he could go back hometown as soon as possible. The teacher left for several days. When the teacher returned he was depressed and unrecognizable. "His face was bloated and disfigured by an eczema which reached to his throat and armpits. He scratched himself continually, turned fiery red, and was unable to speak ..." [58]. For three months the teacher remained bedridden. Kazantzakis repressed his own shame and guilt over this incident for many years. Kazantzakis describes his illness in his adulthood as eczema but there is no itching or scratching as seen in allergic reaction s. According to his description, his illness might be angioedema.

When we look at these patient stories, it might seem that symptom formation is not symbolization of unconscious conflicts. Fonagy and his colleagues [59] have clarified the function of mentalization as a psychic container for bodily experience. Without it, the physiological correlates of unmetabolized affect, such as stress, arousal, fear, and anger, must be managed by the body alone and may reflect themselves in illness or in physical acting out. Mr. A and Kazantzakis might be complaining about unmetabolized feelings and symptom formation at the end. It is highly possible they have attachment problems with their mothers in their early childhood. There is no information about the mother of Kazantzakis but some clues about Mr. A's mother. She was distant and highly fragile and it was a puzzle for Mr. A to understand her feelings. Everything might hurt her and she might stop talking to even 3 years old grandchild for a simple reason. We can think about French psychosomaticians explaining psychosomatic illness with Freud's economic principles of energy for the functioning of the mind. Before the development of the mind structures, they describe libidinized maternal care taking environment that both supplies and protects the infant's reservoir of libidinal energy. This ideal libidinal ecology facilitates a turn from the milieu interne to the external environment. They suggested that the retention of libido, rather than being innate, presupposed that the individual had attained a level of organization leading to desomatization. In the absence of such organization, promoted by the libidinal energy stemming from the interaction with the caretaking environment, distress takes the form of action leading to exhaustion and apathy and/or somatization resulting in illness [60].

Contemporary psychoanalysts have much to say about the multi-faceted and very stressful psychosomatic disorders, especially about the dynamics of cognition, affect, attachment patterns, interpersonal relations hip, and psychophysiology that play such salient roles in the inception and maintenance of somatic disease like some skin diseases [57]. The interconnections between psychic and physiological functioning are highly complex, rarely if ever linear, and are shaped by multiple factors that they still do not fully understand. Psychodynamic formulation is not capable of understanding all these illnesses alone. But it might be helpful to understand medical intervention in unexplained syndromes and phenomena [61].

One of the most significant shapers of our articulated theories about psychosomatics, Alexander [62], made recommendations for the psychotherapy of patients with somatic disturbances, stating: "The knowledge of the central emotional conflict situations which are more or less specific in the different forms of the vegetative disturbances, makes it possible for the therapist to make faster progress in the treatment". Taylor reviewed theoretical reasons for conceptualizing somatization and conversion as distinctly different processes that require very different modes of psychotherapy [57]. In patients with somatization symptoms, emotions are not well represented symbolically and there is a lack of underlying fantasy activity. In these patients, the symptoms begin in the body and follow somatic laws. Somatization symptoms involve lower order physiological perturbations, a passive phenomenon, namely, a failure to symbolize states of emotional and instinctual arousal, which therefore escape psychic elaboration and affect the soma directly. If conflict is present in somatization, it evokes chronic states of emotional arousal rather than being expressed symbolically in the body [63].

According to Koblenzer (a dermatologist and psychoanalyst), it seems that any specific unconcious conflict is expressed in the somatic symptom of urticaria, but rather idiosynchratic unconcious motivating factors will choose this expression when genetic and environmental factors are appropriate [64]. As Wittkower and Russell refer to repressed aggressiveness somatized to the skin, Panconesi and Hautmann highlight symbolic characteristics of urticarial lesions /symptoms [65, 66]. Itching, burning or irritation of abruptly arising lesions correspond to emotional responses on the anger spectrum which consist of anger, rage, irritation, frustration and resentment.

Mr. A's psychoanalytic work has claimed to uncover about his unconscious conflicts, which are expressed by his information—his self-hatred, his identification with his unfaithful grandfather, his guilt and belief in deserved punishment etc. It was clear that his physical illnesses including urticaria are strongly related to his psychiatric situation. After working through all these traumatic life events, his symptom formation ceased and he could stay in a stable, self affirming relationship.

Mrs A's psychoanalytic work demonstrated conflicted emotions of anger and dependency on her husband and extreme fondnessof her sons. Every argument between them triggered her inner conflicts and thus urticarial attacks.

Pathogenesis

A typical hive or wheal results from localized edema following vasodilatation and increased capillary permeability with diffusion of proteins and fluids into the dermis. Degranulation of cutaneous mast cells and increased release of histamin are of major importance in pathogenetic march. Also other substances as well as histamin are released and lead to capillary permeability and vasodilatation to increase. These substances are prostoglandins (D_2), leukotriens (C_4, D_4 E_4) bradykinin and various other kinins, cytokins (tumour necrosis factor α (TNF α), interleukins (IL-3, IL-4,IL-6, IL-8,IL-10,IL-13), granulocyte-macrophage colony-stimulating factor. A variety of immunological, non-immunological, physical and chemical stimuli trigger mast cells to release all these substances into the surrounding tissue and circulation. Vascular permeability in the skin is yielded by the interaction of both H1 and H2 receptors [67-73].

Type I (classical immediate or anaphylactic hypersensitivity) reactions are probably responsible for mostly acute urticaria. Circulating antigens including food, food additives, infectious agents, drugs bind receptor-bound specific IgE and lead to degranulation of mast cells to liberate histamine. Reaction takes 15-30 minutes from the time of exposure to antigen, albeit a delayed onset [10-12 hours) is sometimes possible.

Type III hypersensivity (immun-complex mediated hipersensivity) reactions involve compleman-mediated or immun-complex mediated urticaria. They occur with deposition of insoluble immun complexes in vessel wall. IgG or IgM composes with culprit antigen and C3a-C5a as potent histamin releasers occur. CU in many patients may be an immune mediated inflammatory disease. Urticaria in serum sickness, systemic lupus erythematosus, urticarial vasculitis can occur via this mechanism.

Nonimmunologic reactions (pseudoallergic reactions) are caused by some pharmacologic agents such as acetylcholine, opiates, polymyxine B, some neuropeptides [e.g.Substance P, Vasoactive intestinal peptide (VIP] aspirin/NSAI, radiocontrast agents and some foods like strawberry shellfish, chocolate, etc. They bind spesific receptors, independent of the FcεRI [68].

Although these mechanisms are suggested for both AU and CU and mast cells play a role in CU, exact pathogenesis of CU is still unclear [71]. Some physicians share the idea of its being a chronic inflammatory disease rather than an allergic disease [72].Thus, it remains a major problem regarding etio-pathogenesis, investigation and therapy. In fact CU can be considered as two subgrups: truly idiopathic and turning to autoimmune from idiopathic. The latter may be also called auto-reactive CU and recognized by a positive autolog intradermal test. This test is expression of auto-antibodies directed against the high-affinity receptor for IgE (anti-FcεRI) of mast cells or IgE (anti-IgE) is accounted for this phenomenon [73, 74]. The former group is a diagnosis by exclusion.

Physical urticarias are a distinct and heterogenous subgroup of chronic urticarias and they should be examined separately. They comprise up to 25% of CU and occur more frequently in young adults than the elderly. A specific physical stimulus induces a reproducible wheal. In physical urticarias, increased mast cell numbers are not evident and also their activation mode is poorly understood. Nevertheless, in some dermographism, cold urticaria and solar urticaria patients, a IgE–like factor has been identified. It has been hypothesized that this factor may prompt a neo-antigen that can leads to production of IgE. Thus activation of mast cells and then mediator release would occur on rechallenge. Increased SP and VIP have been elicited from particularly dermographic and cold urticarial lesions [74-76].

Psychopathogenesis

The new multidisciplinary field of psychoneuro-immunology deals with the role of endocrine, nervous, and immune systemsin psychogenic stress and events. The body's response to stress is mediated by hypothalamus, pituitary, cerebral cortex, and the limbic system, in addition to the adrenal gland, as proposed by Selye [77]. Recent studies suggest that urticaria, particularly stress induced CU, may arise from these interactions between the brain, nervous and immune systems and skin wherein hypothalamic-pituitary-adrenocortical axis, the symphathetic and adrenomedullary system and local cutaneous nerve fibres may play a role [28, 41, 46, 66]. Researchers could not find any provoking antigen in some chronic recalcitrant cases. An emotional allergy may perhaps be assumed in these patients [66]

Although conclusive data are nonexistent, several independent lines of evidence postulate a significant role of mast cells regarding psychoneuro-immunological mechanisms. Mast cells are potent inducers of tissue inflammation and their activation is the key process in urticaria. Depression and anxiety may lead to mast cell degranulation via psychoneuro-immunological pathways and various chemical mediators cause urticarial lesions [41, 78-80]. In addition, pruritus severity of urticaria increases with increasing severity of depressive symptoms [52). Investigations on these chemicals in urticaria, appear to be more informative in the future.

Anatomically, mast cells are closely related to peripheric sensory nervous system within various tissues. There are some reports that indicate an intense bidirectional communication between mast cells and sensory nerves in the skin. Mast cells are often co-localized with substans P (SP) and calcitonin gene related peptid (CGRP) expressing nerve fibres. SP among neurotransmitters is one of the most important mediators that play a role in neurogenic and non-neurogenic inflammation [81-83].Neurogenic inflammation is an inflammatory response that occurs with electrical, chemical, heat and mechanical stimulation of somatic nerves including unmyelinated C fibres leading to vasodilatation of arterioles (flares) and the extravasation of plasma from postcapillary venules (wheals). Both SP and its binding location, neurokinin 1 receptor are found in the brain areas where response and processing to physiological and psychological stress are developed. Mast cells are potently activated by sensory nerve products such as SP and endothelin 1. Thus, degranulation of mast cells and liberation of vasoactive peptides including histamin as well as other mediators such as IL-4, IL-5, IFN -γ and TNF α are resulted in neurogenic inflammation [84]. Conversely, aforementioned products activate sensory nerves and raise inflammation.

Animal models have shown that acute psychological stress results in cutaneous mast cell activation and evokes the expression of corticotropin releasing factor (CRF) receptors. Human in vitro studies also reveal that basophils in CU patients have heightened responses to CRF and adrenocorticotropic hormone. Also serum cortisol levels are higher in CU patients [85, 86].

One possible mediator in the relationship between stress and urticaria is dehydroepiandrosteronesulfate (DHEAS) which plays an important role in modulating the vulnerability of the organism to negative effects of stress (87]. Some patients with CU have been shown to have lower serum levels of DHEAS during the active form of the disease [88]. Low DHEAS levels were associated with greater psychological distress and higher anxiety and depression levels [89].

Among physical urticarias, cholinergic and adrenergic urticarias have a particular relevance to emotional stress. Nonetheless, literature is yet inadequate. Brief emotions provoked symptoms in three quarters of patients in a study [39]. Iamendescou and Florea hypothesized that anxiety or psychogenic stress may lead to the release of acetylcholine [41]. In fact, how the release of acetylcholine from the nerve endings causes to mast cell activation is still unknown [90]. A significant proportion of patients with adrenergic urticaria reported in literature were noted to have a history of psychiatric diagnosis or stress/anxiety during their attack. In the case of stress, locus coeruleus liberates norepinephrine through neuronal projections into the limbic system that triggers symphathetic activation and catecholamine release into the bloodstream [38]. Several studies noted that chronic stress causes norepinephrine mediated β_1 adrenergic receptor activation eventuated with excessive emotional and symphathetic response to learned stressors.

Clinical Presentations and Symptoms

Lesions develop rapidly, frequently in minutes. They usually last for 4-6 hours up to 48 hours and then clear leaving clinically normal skin. Eruption is often generalized and rarely localized with erythematous macules, papules and/or plaques from numerous to simply a few in number. Their size can vary from a few milimeters to more than 30 cm. Central clearing within plaques goes with annular patterns, Polycyclic patterns may occur when papules and plaques are confluent. Intense edema may lead to bullae or purpura. Itching, stinging and sometimes pricking sensations are associated symptoms. Itching associated with urticaria is usually most severe as the hives develop and in the evenings due to predominant role of parasymphaetic nervous system. Lesions are not scratched, thus excoriations are unusual [67, 90, 91].

Angioedema is slightly different than urticaria. It occurs alone or is associated with the wheals in the 40-50% of urticaria patients, involving the eyelids, lips, mouth and occasionally respiratory and gastrointestinal tractswith symptoms such as hoarseness or sore throat, asthma, abdominal pain, etc. Its resolution may last up to 72 hours. Anaphylaxis and hypotension may also be seen in severe reactions. Symptoms of urticarial lesions are milder in angioedema because fewer sensory nerve endings exist in the deep dermis in comparison to the superficial dermis [67, 90, 91].

In a study where the clinical features of urticaria in elderly and adult patients are compared, more severe pruritus, fewer wheals and lower incidence of angioedema are noted in the elderly. Some factors such as low humidity, immunosenesence characterized by decreased histamin reactivity and mast cell number or aged mast cells might account for these different clinical presentation s. In addition concomitant physical urticarias are proposed to be at lower incidence [4].

Clinical Subtypes of Urticaria

The latest GA^{2}LEN/EAACI/WAO/EDF guideline offers a classification system based on clinical symptoms, duration and frequency [92]. Hence, the term "chronic urticaria " is reserved for spontaneous appearance of wheals *(chronic spontaneous urticaria)*, but it does not mean that subtypes of physical urticaria (wheals can be elicited by only physical stimulus) are not chronic. This classification facilitates diagnosis and therapy of this heterogeneous disease. (Table 2)

Some conditions formerly classified as urticaria are no longer considered to be subtypes of urticaria according to this guideline. These include urticaria pigmentosa (cutaneous mastocytosis), urticarial vasculitis, familial cold urticaria, and non-histaminergic angioedema (hereditary or acquired angioedema).

Table 2. Urticaria Classification / Subtypes *(adapted from ref. 92)*

Type	Subtype
Spontaneous Urticaria	Acute spontaneous urticaria
	Chronic spontaneous urticaria
Physical Urticaria	Cold contact urticaria
	Delayed pressure urticaria
	Heat contact urticaria
	Solar urticaria
	Dermographic urticaria
	Vibratory urticaria
Other types of urticaria	Aquagenic urticaria
	Contact urticaria
	Cholinergic urticaria
	Exercise-induced anaphylaxia /urticaria

Psychiatric Symptoms

An important dimension of psychiatric morbidities related to CU is the impairment of health related quality of life and secondary emotional disturbances. Herein, one should discuss chronicity and unclear pathogenesis of the disease, ambiguity of potential triggers as well as difficulties in treatment. All these factors impact emotional status of individual with CU negatively and may accompany dermatologic clinic symptoms.

CU often lasts for many years and only 35-55% of patients improve with spontaneous remission within five years [71]. Thus, it can reduce health related quality of life (HRQOL) of patients by impairing physical and emotional functioning. Recently, CU-specific quality of life questionnaries have been developed in several countries, because determination of simply urticaria activity scores and/or rating of pruritus do not seem to be adequate. These questionnaries provide a better assessment facility in effectiveness of treatments [45, 93-97].

Generally speaking, patients with CU experience difficulties with terms of work, home, social and sex life, supporting the family, hobbies and holidays. Energy loss, sleep disturbance and emotional upset occur as significant negative effects impairing daily life [95-98]. Itching creates discomfort by disturbing sleep cycle and predisposing to other complaints to appear. Insomnia from constant pruritus, fatique due to antihistamines and lack of sleep quality, recurrent pain syndromes (tension headachesand fibromyalgia -like pain) cause mood disorderssuch as depression, anxiety and irritability to develop. Both occurrence and recurrence of physical symptoms (e.g., itching, burning) may cause increased emotional tension resulting in distress and anxiety. The occurrence of lesions on visible body parts can lead to disturbed body image. However, this factor may not affect geriatric patients as much as their young counterparts.

Regarding physical urticarias, patients with delayed pressure urticaria have the greatest disabilities in work, leisure and sports. Cholinergic urticaria impairs mostly leisure, sporting and sexual activities [94]. With regard to factors related to QoL, some demographic variables including age, sex and income levels as well as disease duration, concurrent angioedema were found not to affect the severity of QoL impairment, while the presence of psychiatric co-morbidities has significant impact on it [35, 45, 95]. CU patients often suffer depression, anxiety and somatoform disorders [45]. Zachariae et al. state that it is not the disease itself, but its impact on daily activities and social relations hips, which are associated with, increased psychiatric co-morbidity [99]. Uguz et al., demonstrated a considerable effect of Axis I and Axis II disorders on QoL [100].

In fact, psychiatric symptoms can appear both before and after the onset of urticaria symptoms. According to Iamandescu and Florea, psychiatric symptoms preceding urticaria are an expression of affective-behavioral structure of the patient, whereas those that subsequently occur, particularly depression and anxiety, rather refer to an expression of psychiatric syndrome co-existing with urticaria or induced by urticaria [41].

Discussing the emotional impact of CU increases a patient's satisfaction with treatment and trust in their physician [101]. Treatment should be planned comprehensively in these patients.

Diagnosis

A detailed history is crucial for determination of potential triggers as causative factors. Hence, etiological factors should be attentively inquired and necessary laboratory tests should be performed. In the case of the predominance or presence of any psychic factor accompying other trigger factors, whether primary or secondary, psychological investigations may be needed for required therapuetic interventions. Information of the onset, duration and course of the disease is also helpful regarding this issue.

The location, numbers and morphological characteristics of lesions are usually not helpful in differentiating urticarias, but cholinergic, adrenergic urticarias and dermographism, which are frequently associated with psychological factors, have diagnostic clues in dermatological examinations [17, 68, 73, 75].

Treatment

Principally, elimination of specific triggers that may be displayed by the history and/or laboratory investigations should be aimed as the first step. If any trigger including emotional stress can be identified, there are many ways to exclude culprit agent. Drugs can be discontinued or changed. Foods, although rare in geriatrics, can be removed from the diet. Bacterial, fungal, parasitic or viral infection s, if present, should be treated. Therapies for auto-immune syndromes and malignancies should be organized. However, multifactorial and heterogeneous nature of disease makes each patient peculiar. Conventional drug therapies for urticaria associated with psychiatric co-morbidity may not work, or stress management in a patient having stress induced urticarial attacks may not provide benefit because of the presence of other factors. Even when all possible triggers are eliminated, secondary psychiatric associations due to impaired quality of life may continue to affect the patient negatively. Thus, treatment modalities/outcomes change from case to case.

Conventional therapy of CU is made by first and second-generation H_1 receptor antagonists [102]. Occasionally, combination of H1 and H2 receptor blockers, leukotriene antagonists such as montelukast or zileuton may be considered. Actually, the most recent treatment guidelines all state that CU should be treated with non-sedating second generation antihistaminics that appear to be relatively safe for elderly patients. Recalcitrant cases are subject to another therapy options such as potent antiinflammatory and immunosuppressive agents (e.g., cyclosporine, omalizumab, rituximab [103-105].When CU is associated with any stress or psychiatric co-morbidity, especially H_1 receptor antagonists such as hydroxysizine with significant sedative and anticholinergic effects may be of interest to contribute to the treatment of CU [102, 103]. Nevertheless, antimuscarinic and anticholinergic side effects of first generation antihistaminics may be observed with caution in geriatric patients [104, 106, 107].

Antidepressant medication appears to be effective for the treatment of chronic idiopathic urticaria in controlled studies Tricyclic antidepressants, selective serotonin reuptake inhibitors, serotonin noradrenalin reuptake inhibitors might be preferred to treat their anxiety or depression. Tricyclic antidepressants are well-known for antipruritic and antihistaminic effects [105]. Doksepin and amytriptilin particularly have antagonistic effects on H_1, H_2, muscarinic, α_1 and α_2 receptors. However, side effects of these medications, similar to other H1 receptor blocker antihistaminics, that arise from anti-muscarinic, antihistaminic and anti-adrenergic activities limit their use in older urticaria patients. Geriatric patients may need lower dosing or slower titration [105, 107, 108].

Selective serotonin reuptake inhibitors (SSRI), (eg, fluoxetine) probably should be first-line agents nowadays. SSRIs selectively inhibit presynaptic serotonin reuptake with minimal or no effect in the reuptake of norepinephrine or dopamine. The adverse effect profile of SSRIs is less prominent, improved compliance is promoted and they are preferred more. Cardiac arrhythmia risk is lower than tricyclic antidepressants. Arrhythmia risk is especially pertinent in overdose. Half dose is usually preferred for older population [108].

Recently mirtazapin, as a noradrenergic and specific serotonergic antidepressant (NaSSA), is recommended in selected cases of severe urticaria It is the only tetracyclic antidepressant that has been approved by the Food and Drug Administration to treat depression. Mirtazapine is also effective in the treatment of severe chronic urticaria patients

[109-111]. It demonstrates a significant effect on H1 receptor and has antipruritic activity. Also, safety profile of mirtazapine is better than tricyclic antidepressants. Nevertheless, prospective, controlled and large patient series are needed to prove its efficiency.

In literature reviews of CU, stress reduction is sometimes recommended, but biological aspects of disease are always prioritized. As a matter of fact, the link between psychological factors and urticaria is simply neglected in some reports. [27].On the other hand, some authors strongly suggest a complementary treatment because of the high frequency of psychological symptoms. [112].

Although systematic and comperative studies of stress reducing therapies for urticaria do not exist, some individual reports can encourage dermatologists to consider such therapies that consist of psychotherapies, hypnosis, cognitive- behavorial techniques and biofeedback. Herein, cumulative clinical experience predominates comperative studies. Biofeedback of muscle tension by EMG can be used to increase the teaching of relaxation. Exacerbation of urticaria due to psychosomatic triggering was emoliorated in a female patient using cognitive-behavorial therapy with specific talk and relaxation techniques [113]. Out of 15 patients with CU, 6 patients were cleared in within 14 months by hypnosis with relaxation therapy [114]. Eye movement desensitizaton and reprocessing techniques appear to be useful in urticaria associated with post-traumatic stress [115].

All these therapies can be considered complementary to other urticaria medications or as an alternative therapy for selected cases of CU.

Conclusion

An issue to be addressed is that physicians should not approach a geriatric patient with CU ignoring possible hidden psychiatric problems or remains unfocused on their emotional well- being. Evaluating a patient's emotional status and helping her/him to manage the impact of CU on her/him daily life, enhances a patient's satisfaction of treatment and trust in the physician.

References

[1] Zuberbier, T; Balke, M; Worm, M; Edenharter, G; Maurer, M. Epidemiology of urticaria: a representative cross-sectional population survey. *Clin Exp Dermatol*, 2010 35, 869-873.

[2] Ballmer-Weber, BK; Kündig, TM. Urticaria - the most frequent dermatological disease. *Ther Umsch,* 2010 67, 167-173.

[3] Weller, K; Altrichter, S; Ardelean, E; Krause, K; Magerl, M; Metz, M; Siebenhaar, F; Maurer, M. Chronic urticaria. Prevalence, course, prognostic factors and impact. *Hautarzt,* 2010 61, 750-757.

[4] Magen, E; Mishal, J; Schlesinger, M. Clinical and laboratory features of chronic idiopathic urticaria in the elderly. *Int J Dermatol,* 2013 52, 1387-1391.

[5] Furue, M; Yamazaki, S; Jimbow, K; Tsuchida, T; Amagai, M; Tanaka, T; Matsunaga, K; Muto, M; Morita, E; Akiyama, M; Soma, Y; Terui, T; Manabe, M. Prevalence of

dermatological disorders in Japan: a nationwide, cross-sectional, seasonal, multicenter, hospital-based study. *J Dermatol*, 2011 38, 353-363.

[6] El-Khateeb, EA; Imam, AA; Sallam, MA. Pattern of skin diseases in Cairo, Egypt. *Int J Dermatol*, 2011- 50, 844-853.

[7] Bilgili SG, Karadag AS, Ozkol HU, Calka O, Akdeniz N. The prevalence of skin diseases among the geriatric patients in eastern *Turkey.J Pak Med Assoc,* 2012-62, 535-539.

[8] SacarT, Sacar H. Prevalence of dermatoses in the geriatric population in Izmir region. *Turk Geriatri Dergisi,* 2011-,14, 231-237.

[9] Yap KB,Siew MG, Goh CL. Pattern of skin diseases in the elderly seen at the National Skin Centre (Singopore 1990). *Singapore Med J* 1994- 35,147-150.

[10] Yalçın B, Tamer E, Toy GG, Oztaş P,Hayran M, Allı N. The prevalence of skin diseases in the elderly: analysis of 4099 geriatric patients. *Int J Dermatol* 2006- 45: 672-676.

[11] Rubegni P, Poggiali S, Nami N, Rubengi M, Fimiani M. Skin diseases in geriatric patients: our experience from a public skin outpatient clinic in Siena *G Ital Dermatol Venereol,* 2012- 147, 631-636.

[12] Ramos-Romey C, López-Malpica F, Nazario S, Jiménez-Válezques IZ. Urticaria in the elderly. *Bol Asoc Med P* R 2008,100,32-35.

[13] Song WJ, Lee SM, Kim MH, Kim SH, Kim KW, Cho SH, Min KU, Chang YS. Histamine and allergen skin reactivity in the elderly population: results from the Korean Longitudinal Study on Health and Aging. *Ann Allergy Asthma Immuno,l* 2011-107:347-352.

[14] Skassa-Brociek W, Manderscheid JC, Michel FB, Bousquet J.Skin test reactivity to histamine from infancy to old age. *J Allergy Clin Immunol* 1987-80:711-716.

[15] Roupe G. Skin of the aging human being. *Lakartidningen* 2001-98:1091-1095.

[16] Aftin, LB. Nonhistaminergic idiopathic angioedema may be a presentation of mast cell activation syndrome. *J Investig Allergol Clin Immunol.*2013-23(3), 212.

[17] Odom, RB; James, WD; Berger, TG. *Andrew's Diseases of The Skin.* 9th.Edition. Philadelphia: W.B Saunders Company; 2000.

[18] Sicherer SH, Sampson HA. Food allergy: epidemiology, pathogenesis,diagnosis and therapy. *J Allergy Clin Immunol* 2014-133(2):291-307.

[19] Zuberbier T, Edenharter G,Worm M, Ehlers I,Reimann S, Hantke T, Roehr CC, Bergmann KE, Niggemann B. Prevalance of adverse reactions to food in Germany - a population study. *Allergy* 2004-59: 338-345.

[20] Ventura,MT; Napolitano, S;Buguicchio, C;Cecere, R;Arsieni,A. An approach to urticaria in elderly patients. *Immunopharmacol Immunotoxicol.* 2012,34(3),530-533.

[21] Sloate P., Kohutis E. *Prologue.* Psychoanal Inq, 2010- 30:377-379.

[22] Pasaoglu G, Bavbek S, Tugcu H, Abadoglu O, Mısırlıgil Z. Psychological status of patients with chronic urticaria. *J Dermatol* 2006-33: 765-771.

[23] Sberber J, Shaw J, Bruce S. Psychological components and the role of adjunctive interventions of chronic idiopathic urticaria. *Psychoter Psychosom* 1989;52:135-141.

[24] Consoli SG. Psychological factors in urticaria. *Ann Dermatol Venereol* 2003- 130 Spec No 1:1: 73-77.

[25] Picardi, A., Abeni, D., Melchi, C., Puddu, P., Pasquini, P. Psychiatric morbidity in dermatologic outpatients:an issue to be recognized. *Br J Dermatol* 2000 -143:983-991.

[26] Buffet, M. Management of psychologic factors in chronic urticaria. When and how? *Ann Dermatol Venereol* 2003- 130 Spec No 1:1: 145-159.

[27] Broom, B.C. A reappraisal of the role of 'mindbody' factors in chronic urticaria. *Postgrad Med J* 201086, 365-370.

[28] Malhotra, SK; Mehta, V. Role of stressful life events in induction or exacerbation of psoriasis and chronic urticaria. *Indian J Dermatol Venereol Leprol*, 2008 74, 594-599.

[29] Rees, L. An etiological study of chronic urticaria and angioneurotic oedema. *J Psychosom Res*,1957 3,172-189.

[30] Fava, GA; Perini, GI; Santonastaso, P; Fornaso, C. Life events and psychological distress in dermatologic disorders: Psoriasis,chronic urticaria and fungal infection s. *Br J Med Psy chol*,1980 53,277-282.

[31] Wallengren, J; Isaksson, A. Urticarial dermographism: clinical features and response to psychosocial stress. *Acta Derm Venereol*, 2007, 87, 493-498.

[32] Sukan, M; Maner, F. Stressful life events in vitiligo and chronic urticaria. *Klinik Psikiyatri Dergisi*, 2006 9, 17-26.

[33] -. Badoux, A;Levy, D. Psychological symptoms in asthma and chronic urticaria. *Ann Allergy,* 1994, 72 (3), 229-234

[34] Engin, B., Uguz, F., Yilmaz, E., Ozdemir, M., Mevlitoglu, I. The levels of depression, anxiety and quality of life in patients with chronic idiopathic urticaria. *J Eur Acad Dermatol Venereol*. 200822(1),36-40.

[35] Chung,MC; Simons, C, Gilliam,J; Kaminski,ER. Stress, psychiatric co-morbidity and coping in patients with chronic idiopathic urticaria. *Psychol Health.* 2010 25(4),477-490.

[36] Kimyai-Asadi, A;Usman, A. The role of psychological stress in skin disease. *J Cutan Med Surg* 2001 5,140-145.

[37] Michaelsson,G. Chronic urticaria. *Acta Derm Venereol*,1969 49, 404-416.

[38] Hogan, SR; Mandrell, J; Eilers, D. Adrenergic urticaria: review of the literature and proposed mechanism. *J Am Acad Dermatol,* 2014 70, 763-766.

[39] Czubalski, K; Rudzki, E. Neuropsychic factors in physical urticaria. *Dermatologica,* 1977 154, 1-4.

[40] Weller, K; Koti, I; Makris, M; Maurer, M. Anxiety and depression seem less common in patients with autoreactive chronic spontaneous urticaria. *Clin Exp Dermatol,* 2013 38, 870-873.

[41] Iamandescu, IB; Florea, D. Urticaria,angioedema and their psychogenic triggers -a clinical approach. In: Iamendescu IB, editor. *Psychoneuroallergology*. Bucuresti: Amaltea Medical Publishing House; 2007309-322.

[42] Topal, IO; Altunay, IK; Mercan, S. Personality disorders, anxiety and depression in patients with chronic urticaria. *Klinik Psikiyatri Dergisi,* 2004 7, 199-209.

[43] Champion,RH;Roberts, SOB; Carpenter, RG. Urticaria and angioedema: a review of 554 patients. *Br J Dermatol* 1969 81,558-597.

[44] Menninger, WC; Kemp, J. Psychogenic urticaria. *J Allergy*,1935 6,467-473.

[45] Staubach, P; Eckhardt-Henn, A; Dechene, M; Vonend, A; Metz, M; Magerl, M; Breuer, P,Maurer,M. Quality of life in patients with chronic urticaria is differentially impaired and determined by psychiatric comorbidity. *Br J Dermatol,* 2006 154, 294-298.

[46] Gupta, MA. Stress and urticaria. In: Granstein, RD; Luger, TA, editors. *Neuroimmunology of the Skin.* Berlin: Springer; 2009;209-217.

[47] Unal, S; Berksun, O; Kinikli, G; Kaya, E. Psychological symptoms in patients with chronic urticaria and allergic rhinitis. *Türk Psikiyatri Dergisi,*19912,289-293.
[48] Barbosa, F; Freitas, J; Barbosa, A. Alexithymia in chronic urticaria patients. *Psychol Health Med*, 2011 16, 215-224.
[49] Chung, MC; Symons, C; Gilliam, J; Kaminski, ER. The relationship between posttraumatic stress disorder, psychiatric comorbidity, and personality traits among patients with chronic idiopathic urticaria. *Compr Psychiatry*, 2010 51, 55-63.
[50] Gupta, MA, Gupta, AK. Chronic idiopathic urticaria and post-traumatic stress disorder (PTSD): an under-recognized comorbidity. *Clin Dermatol,* 2012, 30 (3),.351-354
[51] Lindemayer, H; Gathmann, P; Cermak T;Grunberger, J. Is chronic recurrent urticaria a psychosomatic disease? *Z Hautkr,*1981 56,28-40.
[52] Gupta, MA; Gupta, AK; Schork, NJ; Ellis, CN. Depression modulates pruritus perception: a study of pruritus in psoriasis, atopic dermatitis, and chronic idiopathic urticaria. *Psychosomatic Medicine*, 199456, 36-40.
[53] Barua, A; Kar, N. Screening for depression in elderly Indian population. *Indian J Psychiatry,* 2010 52, 150-3.
[54] Pollock, LR; Williams, JM. Problem solving and suicidal behavior. *Suicide Life Threat Behav,* 199828,375–387.
[55] Gibbs, LM; Dombrovski, AY; Morse, J; Siegle, GJ; Houck, PR; Szanto, K. When the solution is part of the problem: problem solving in elderly suicide attempters. *Int J Geriatr Psychiatry,* 2009- 24(12),1396–1404.
[56] Duberstein, PR; Conwell, Y; Conner, KR; Eberly, S; Evinger, J.S; Caine, E.D. Poor social integration and suicide: fact or artefact? A case-control study. *Psychol Med,* 2004- 34,1331–1337.
[57] Taylor, GJ. Somatization and conversion: Distinct or overlapping constructs? *J Amer Acad Psychoanal*, 2003- 31,487-508.
[58] Kazantzakis, N. *Report to Greco*. New York: Simon and Schuster,1965.
[59] Fonagy, P; Gergely, G; Jurist, E; Target, M. *Affect Regulation, Mentalization, and the Development of the Self.* New York: Other Press;2004.
[60] Oliner, MM. The minefield of emotions. *Psychoanal Inq,* 2010,30,405-415.
[61] Bergner, S. The Analytic Environment in Times of Bodily Dysfunction: The Effect of Psychoanalytic Psychosomatic Theories. *Psychoanal Psychol*, 200926,362-378.
[62] Alexander, F. *Psychosomatic Medicine: Its Principles and Applications*. New York: Norton,1950.
[63] Kirmayer, LJ; Santhanam, R. The anthropology of hysteria. In Halligan, PW; Bass, C; and Marshall, JC, editors. *Contemporary Approaches to Hysteria*. Oxford: Oxford University Press;2001; 251-270.
[64] Koblenzer, CS. *Psychocutaneous Disease*.Orlando: Grune &Stratton, Inc.;1987.
[65] Wittkower E, Russell B. Emotional factors in skin disease. New York: Paul B Hoeber; 1953.
[66] Panconesi, E; Hautmann, G. Psychophysiology of stress in dermatology. The psychobiological patern of psychosomatics. *Dermatol Clin*, 1996- 14,399-421.
[67] Sachdeva, S; Gupta, V; Amin, SS; Tahseen, M. Chronic urticaria. *Indian J Dermatol,* 2011-56(6), 622-628.
[68] Grattan, C. Urticarias: pathophysiology and management. *Clin Med.* 2012, 12(2),164-167.

[69] Charlesworth,N. Urticaria and angioedema. *Allergy Asthma Proc*. 2002- 23(5),341-345.
[70] Papadopoulos, J;Karpouzis, A;Tentes, J;Kouskoukis C. Assessment of interleukins IL-4, IL6, IL-8, IL10 in acute urticaria. *J Clin Med Res,* 2014-,6 (2),133-137.
[71] Ben-Shoshan, M; Blinderman, I; Raz, A. Psychosocial factors and chronic spontaneous urticaria: a systematic review. *Allergy*, 2013- 68, 131-141.
[72] Augey,F; Gunera-Saad, N;Bensaid,B; Nosbaum,A; Berard,F; Nicolas,JF. Chronic spontaneous urticaria is not an allergic disease. *Eur J Dermatol*, 2011, 21, 349-353.
[73] Wedi, B. Urticaria. *J Dtsch Dermatol Ges*, 2008- 6,306-317.
[74] Patil, S; Sharma, N; Godse, K. Autologous serum therapy in chronic urticaria. *Indian J Dermatol,* 2013 58, 225-226.
[75] Grattan, CEH & Black K. Urticaria and mastocytosis. In: Burns, T, Breatnach, S; Cox, N; Griffiths C.(Eds.), *Rook's Textbook of Dermatology.*Italy, Blackwell-Publishing, 2004.
[76] Abajian, M; Mlynek, A; Maurer, M. Physical urticaria. *Curr Allergy Asthma Rep,* 2014,- 12(4),281-287.
[77] Selye, H. The general adaptation syndrome and the diseases of adaptation. *J Clin Endocrinol*,1946, 6,117-230.
[78] Moore, RY; Bloom, FE. Central catecholamine neuron systems: anatomy and physiology of the norepinephrine and epinephrine systems. *Annu Rev Neurosci*, 1979-22,113-168.
[79] Zane, TL. Psychoneuroendocrinimmunodermatology.Pathophysiological mechanisms of stress in cutaneous disease. In: Koo, JYM; Lee, CS. (Eds.), *Psychocutaneous Medicine.* New-York: Marcel-Dekker Inc; 2003; 65-95.
[80] Grippo, aj, Scotti, MLA. Stress and neuroinflammation. In: Halaris,A; Leonard, BE. (Eds.), *Inflammation in Psychiatry*. Basel: Karger; 2013- 20-31.
[81] Siebenhaar, F; Magerl, M; Peters, EMJ; Hendrix, S; Metz, M; Maurer,M. Mast cell-driven skin inflammation is impaired in the absence of sensory nerves. *J Allergy Clin Immunol,* 2008- 121, 955-961.
[82] Arck, PC; Paus, R. From the brain -skin connection: the neuroendocrine-immune misalliance of stress and itch. *Neuroimmunomodulation,* 2006-, 13,347-356.
[83] Urpe, M; Buggiani, G; Lotti, T. Stress and psychoneuroimmunologic factors in dermatology. *Dermatol Clin*, 2005 23, 609-617.
[84] Arck, PC; Slominski A; Theoharides, TC; Peters EM; Paus,R. Neurommunology of stress:skin takes central stage. *J Invest Dermatol,* 2006-,126,1697-1704.
[85] Theoharides, TC; Donelan, JM; Papadopoulou, N; Cao, J; Kempura, D; Conti, P. Mast cells as targets of corticotropin -releasing factor and releated factors. *Trends Pharmacol,* 2004-, 25, 5668.
[86] Dyke, SM; Carey, BS; Kaminski, ER. Effect of stress on basophil function in chronic idiopathic urticaria *Clin Exp Allergy,* 2008-38.86-92.
[87] Morgan, CA; Sauthwick, S; Hazlett, G; Rasmusson, A; Hoyt, G; Zimolo, Z., Charney, D. Relationship with plasma dehydroepiandrosteronesulfate and cortisol levels, symptoms of dissociation, and objective performance in humans exposed to acute stress. *Arch Gen Psychiatry,* 2004- 61,819-825.
[88] Kasperska-Zajac, A.; Brzoza, Z; Rogala, B. Lower serum dehydroepiandros--terone sulfate concentration in chronic idiopathic urticaria: a secondary transient phenomenon? *Br J Dermatol*,2008, 159:743-744.

[89] Brzoza, Z; Kasperska-Zajac, A; Badura-Brzoza, K; Matysiakiewicz, J; Hese, RT; Rogala, B. Decline in dehydroepiandrosterone sulfate observed in chronic urticaria is associated with psychological distress. *Psychosom Med*, 2008-, 70(6):723-8.
[90] Grattan, CHH. Urticaria and angioedema. In: Bolognia, JL; Jorizzo, JL; Schaffer, JV. (Eds.), Dermatology, China: Elsevier; 2012; 291-306.
[91] Grabbe, J. Urticaria and angioedema. In: Burgdorf, WHC; Plewig, G; Wolf, HH; Lanthaler, M. (Eds.), *Braun-Falco's Dermatology.*Heidelberg: Springer;2009 359-376.
[92] Zuberbier, T. Classification of urticaria. *Indian J Dermatol*, 201358, 208-210.
[93] Ye, YM; Park, JW; Kim, SH; Choi, JH; Hur, GY; Lee, HY; Lee, EH; Park, HS. Clinical evaluation of the computarized chronic urticaria -spesific quality of life questionnaire in Korean patients with chronic urticaria. *Clin Exp Dermatol*, 2012 37, 722-728.
[94] Kocaturk, E; Weller, K; Martus, P; Aktas, S; Kavala, M; Sarıgul, Ş; Baiardini, I; Canonica, GW; Brzoza, Z; Kalogeromitros, D; Maurer, M. Turkish version of the chronic urticaria quality of life questionnaire: cultural adaptation, assessment of reliability and validity. *Acta Derm Venereol*, 2012 92, 419-425.
[95] Weldon, DR. Quality of life in patients with urticaria. *Allergy Asthma Proc*, 2006 27, 96-99.
[96] Baiardini, I; Pasquali, M; Braido, F; Fumagalli, F; Guerra, L, Campalati, E; Braga, M; Lombardi,C. A new tool to evaluate the impact of chronic urticaria on quality of life: chronic urticaria quality of life questionnary (CU-QoL). *Allergy*, 2005 60 (8),1073-1078.
[97] O'Donnell, BF; Lawlor, F; Simpson, J; Morgan, M; Greaves, MW. The impact of chronic urticaria on the quality of life. *Br J Dermatol,* 1997 136, 197-201.
[98] Yang, HY; Sun, CC; Wu, YC; Wang, JD. Stress, insomnia, and chronic idiopathic urticaria - a case control study. *J Formos Med Assoc,* 2005 104:254-63.
[99] Zachariae, R; Zachariae, C; Ibsen, HH; Mortensen, JT; Wulf, HC. Psychological comorbidity and quality of life in dermatology outpatients and hospitalized dermatology patients. *Acta Dermato Venereol*, 2004 84(3), 205-212.
[100] Uguz,F; Engin,B; Yılmaz, E. Quality of life in patients with chronic idiopathic urticaria: the impact of Axis I and Axis II psychiatric disorders. *Gen Hosp Psychiatry*, 2008 30(5),453-457.
[101] Maurer, M; Ortonne, JP; Zuberbier, T. Chronic urticaria:a patient survey on quality of life, treatment usage and doctor-patient relation. *Allergy* 2009 64, 581-588.
[102] Goetz DW; Jacobson,JM; Murname, JE; Reid,MJ;Repperger, DW; Goodyear, C. Prolongation of simple and choice reaction times in a double-blind comparison of twice-daily hydroxyzine versus terfenadine. *J Allergy Clin Immunol,* 1989 84:316-322.
[103] Kalogeromitros, D; Papageorgiou, C; Gregoriou, S; Chatziantonakis, N; Makris, M; Spanoudaki, N; Rabavilas, A; Rigopoulos, D; Theoharides, TC. Depressive symptoms in urticaria patients treated with first- or second-generation histamine 1 receptor antagonists. *J Clin Psychopharmacol*, 200727, 404-406.
[104] Kozel, MM; Sabroe, RA. Chronic urticaria: aetiology, management, current and future treatment options. *Drugs,* 2004 64 (22),2515-2536.
[105] Tennyson,H; Levine, L. Neurotropic and psychotropic drugs in dermatology. *Dermatol Clin*, 2001 19,179-197.
[106] Dreyfus, DH. Urticaria and angioedema: a rational approach to diagnosis and therapy. *Skin Therapy Lett*, 2013 18, 4-9.

[107] Endo, JO; Wong, JW; Norman, RA; Chang, AL. Geriatric dermatology: Part I. Geriatric pharmacology for the dermatologist. *J Am Acad Dermatol*, 201368, 521.e1-10.

[108] Wiese, B.S. Geriatric depression: The use of antidepressants in the elderly. *BC Medical Journal,* 2011 53, 341-347.

[109] Kulaç, Ş; Karaca, Ş; Özbulut, Ö; Çetişli, A. Oral mirtazapine in persistent chronic urticaria. *Turkderm,* 2008 42, 31-33.

[110] Bigatà, X; Sais, G; Soler, F. Severe chronic urticaria: response to mirtazapine. *J Am Acad Dermatol,* 2005 53, 916-917.

[111] Thormann, H; Bindslev-Jensen, C. Mirtazapine for chronic urticaria. *Acta Derm Venereol,* 2004 84, 482-483.

[112] Ozkan,M; Oflaz SB; Kocaman, N; Ozseker, F; Gelincik, A; Buyukozturk, S; Ozkan S. Psychiatric morbidity and quality of life in patients with chronic idiopathic urticaria. *Ann Allergy Asthma Immunol.* 200799, 29-33.

[113] Fried, RG. Nonpharmacological treatments in psychodermatology. *Dermatol Clinic* 2002 20, 177-185.

[114] Shertzer, CL; Lookingbill, DP.Effects of relaxation therapy and hipnotizability in chronic urticaria. *Arch Dermatol*1987 123, 913-916.

[115] Gupta,MA;Gupta,AK. Use of eye movement desentizisation and reprocessing (EMDR) in the treatment of dermatological disorders. *J Cutan Med Surg*2002 6 (5),415-421.

In: Geriatric Psychodermatology
Editors: Mohammad Jafferany and Katlein França

ISBN: 978-1-63463-853-1

Chapter 15

Psoriasis: Psychological Burden and Quality of Life Implications

Susana Coimbra, Ph.D., Alice Santos-Silva, Ph.D. and Américo Figueiredo, M.D., Ph.D.*

Introduction

Psoriasis is a chronic, recurrent, immune-mediated erythematosquamous dermatitis that affects approximately 2–3% of the Caucasian population. It can affect the skin, nails and the joints. Psoriasis vulgaris or chronic plaque psoriasis is the most common form of psoriasis presentation. It is characterized by papulosquamous plaques well-defined from surrounding normal skin. These plaques are red or salmon pink, covered by white or silvery scales, and the plaques may be thick, thin, large or small. Histologically, psoriasis vulgaris presents epidermal hyperplasia (acanthosis), dilated and prominent blood vessels in the dermis, and an inflammatory infiltrate of leukocytes, predominantly in the dermis [1]. It is, usually, symptomatic, with patients complaining of intense pruritus or burning; about 30% of the patients suffer from itch and pain, mostly due to the dryness and cracking of the psoriatic area [2]. The other forms of psoriasis include guttate, erythrodermic and pustular psoriasis. Psoriatic arthritis is a seronegative inflammatory arthritis that occurs in the presence of psoriasis vulgaris. About 10-30% of patients with psoriasis vulgaris develop psoriatic arthritis [3]. Psoriatic nail disease is most commonly found in patients with psoriatic arthritis. Fingernails are more commonly affected than toenails, and the clinical manifestations range from pitting, yellowish discoloration, and paronychia, to subungual hyperkeratosis, onycholysis, and severe onychodystrophy [4].

Patients with psoriasis require an individual management and long-term planning of therapeutic strategies. The main goal of psoriatic therapies is to try to control the disease and its clinical manifestations, contributing to improve the quality of life of the patient. A chronic,

* Corresponding author: Américo Figueiredo. Email: amcfigueiredo@ci.uc.pt

unpredictable course of the disease and the need of periodical alternation of drugs or classesof drugs, make difficult to treat psoriasis and to increase the quality of life of the patients.

Psoriasis has been associated with several comorbidities, such as hypertension, dyslipidemia, obesity, type 2 diabetes mellitus and cardiovascular diseases, as well as with a decreased quality of life and with depression. Indeed, in addition to the physical impact, psoriasis can have a profound impact on patients' psychosocial wellbeing. It is known to deeply affect the well-being of the patients and their emotional and social lives [5]. Psoriatic patients often manifest, not only a profound psychosocial disability, but also a significant impairment of quality of life (QOL) [6, 7]. Indeed, a major component of the assessment of psoriasis is the measurement of QOL, because improving patient's quality of life is the primary goal of psoriatic therapy.

Assessing Quality of Life and Psychological Burden

In clinical practice, broad global assessments of psoriasis activity and how it affects patient's quality of life are used to define the severity of patient's disease and to define the more appropriate treatment. In clinical trials, it is crucial to measure the efficacy of the treatment under study, by comparing the severity of disease before and after the treatment.

The severity of psoriasis can be defined by the percentage of body surface area involved. In mild cases, the lesions cover less than 10% of the body surface, in moderate cases 10-20% and in the severe cases the lesions affect more than 20% of skin surface [8].

There are several other approaches to measure the severity of psoriasis, which consider besides the affected skin surface, the degree of scaling and the type of infiltration. The Psoriasis Area and Severity Index (PASI) is the prototype for such measures, and is the most widely used tool to assess psoriasis severity in clinical trials and in clinical practice [9]. The PASI score ranges from 0 to 72. It combines the assessment of four body areas: head and neck, upper limbs, trunk and lower limbs. To assess affected body surface area, the proportion of skin affected in each area is given by a numerical score representing the proportion involved. Within each area the severity of the lesions is assessed by three signs, erythema, thickness/induration, and desquamation/scaling, using a five-point scale. Finally, the PASI score is calculated according to an appropriate formula. A PASI score below 10 defines psoriasis as mild, between 10 and 20 as moderate, and above 20 as severe [8].

Another traditional assessment tool to evaluate psoriasis severity is the Physician's Global Assessment (PGA), a simple instrument that provides a subjective global evaluation. There are several variants for PGA. Typically, the patient is asked to rate the disease, using a scale of seven categories, "clear", "almost clear", "mild", "mild to moderate", "moderate", "moderate to severe" and "severe". It is less objective than PASI, but the result is more easily understood by the patient [10].

The Lattice System Physician's Global Assessment (LS-PGA), formerly known as Lattice System Global Psoriasis Scale, applies a more objective approach to global assessment of disease severity than PGA, because it considers the body surface area involved and the morphological characteristics of the plaques (10). Total body surface area involved is estimated using a scale of seven categories (0, 1-3, 4-9, 10-20, 21-29, 30-50, ≥ 51%). Then, using a matrix system, the average of plaque characteristics (elevation, erythema and scaling) will be evaluated. The categories, on an eight-point scale, are: "clear", "almost clear", "mild", "mild to moderate", "moderate", "moderate to severe", "severe", and "very severe".

There are also other important psoriasis measurement tools, namely those that also measure the patient's perception of well-being. The National Psoriasis Foundation (NPF) developed the National Psoriasis Foundation Psoriasis Score, a responder index, that include six subdomains: induration at two target sites, current and baseline body surface area, physician global assessment, patient global assessment, and patient assessment of itch [11]. Recently, the Psoriasis Symptom Inventory (PSI) was developed as a patient-reported measure of psoriasis symptoms [12].

Most of these tools do not include a measure about the quality of life or considers the patient's perception of well-being; direct information about psychological and/or social disease consequences is not provided. The evaluation of psoriasis severity should consider the impact of the disease on physical discomfort, but also the impact in social life and self-perception. The improvement in patients' lives is the primary goal of therapy, therefore, a major component in the assessment of psoriasis should be the measurement of the quality of life. The term quality of life refers to a quantitative estimation of the global impact of a disease on physical, social, and psychological well-being of a patient. Indeed, the correlation between the QOL and the severity of the disease is not always strong. For instance, the visibility of psoriatic lesions or the impairment of daily activities may incapacitate a patient to work and reduce self-esteem; itch and pain may cause also severe impairment of QOL.

The estimation of quality of life is obtained through standardized questionnaires exploring the relevant dimensions of the patient's life that may be affected by the disease. Non-specific queries, such as the Medical Outcome Survey Short Form 36 (SF-36) and the Euro QOL, are used to assess patients' overall quality of life [13, 14].

There are more specific instruments, focusing on aspects of quality of life that are affected by skin disease. These, include the Dermatology Life Quality Index (DLQI), the Skindex 29, the Skindex 17, and the Dermatology Quality of Life Scale (DQOLS) [15-17].

According to the systematic review by Bronsard et al., DLQI is easy to use in clinical practice because of its brevity and simplicity, SF36 is widely used in clinical trials, and Skindex 29 and Skindex 17, although rarely used, are interesting because of their cross-cultural validation [17]. The DLQI and the SF-36 have been previously used to evaluate the QOL on psoriatic patients [7, 18]. The generic queries, such as the SF-36, are useful to show the impact of psoriasis. The SF-36 has showed that the impact of psoriasis was similar or higher than that imposed by many other serious medical conditions. The DLQI has been most widely used in psoriasis trials as a measure to assess the quality of life related to skin disease. It has been shown that the value of clinical research in psoriasis is improved with the DLQI [19], as the DLQI score banding proposes: 0-1 means "no effect on QOL"; 2-5, "small effect"; 6-10, "moderate effect"; 11-20, "very large effect"; 21-30, "extremely large effect". Apparently, a total DLQI higher than 10 represents a skin disease having a very large effect on patient's life, needing intervention, and, from the individual point of view, a DLQI of 5 or less is associated with improved QOL.

There are even more specific measures for psoriasis. For instance, scores that include psychological impact along with the severity of the skin lesions are the Salford Psoriasis Index and the Psoriasis Disability Index (20). Psoriasis-specific studies of QOL are the psoriasis index of QOL (PSORIQOL), a 25-item instrument [21], and the Impact of Psoriasis

Questionnaire (IPSO) [22]. Another psoriasis-specific QOL evaluation is the Psoriasis Quality of Life Questionnaire [19].

The evaluation of the quality of life of psoriatic patients clarified the multidimensional nature of the disease assessment and outcome, which should include the evaluation of disease associated discomfort, level of disability, and social disruption [8]. It is important to define the severity of psoriasis, but it is also important to identify psoriasis that severely affects the quality of life.

Psychosocial Burden and Quality of Life in Psoriasis

A number of psychiatric/psychological comorbidities have been observed in psoriatic patients [6]. Psoriasis deeply affects the well-being of the patient and has emotional and social consequences [5]. Thus, to define psoriasis as only a skin problem is a very restrictive approach.

The diagnosis of psoriasis itself has a psychological burden, as nearly half of the patients feel depression and anxiety at the time of diagnosis of psoriasis [23]. Patients with psoriasis often report feelings of self-consciousness, helpless, embarrassment, anger and frustration, and suffer social isolation and stigmatization [24-26]. According to Hrehorów et al., the majority of psoriatic patients felt that they were stigmatized by psoriasis, referring that anticipation of rejection and feelings of guilt and shame were the major stigmatization aspects [27]. Moreover, the level of stigmatization correlated with pruritus intensity, stress prior to exacerbation, depressive symptoms and QOL [27].

As referred, psoriatic patients present a variety of psychological problems, including poor self-esteem, sexual dysfunction, anxiety and depression [28]. Indeed, according to Friedewald et al., about 35% of psoriatic patients report symptoms of depression [29], and according to Mease and Menter about 80% of patients refer that the disease has a negative impact on their lives for a variety of reasons, including the physical symptoms, upsetting physical appearance, frustration, anger, anxiety, depression, and in alcohol drinking habits [30]. Chronic alcohol abuse may exacerbate psoriasis and the impairment in health -related, social and occupational functioning, contributing to reduce even more the QOL.

Gupta et al. reported that 9.7% of psoriasis patients showed death wish and 5.5% acute suicidal ideation [31]. Sampogna et al., observed that the problems most frequently experienced by psoriatic patients were shame, anger, worry, difficulties in daily activities and social life, and that all those problems were associated with psoriasis severity and with depression or anxiety [32]. According to the NPF survey data 2003-2011 performed in United States, 88% of 5,604 psoriasis patients reported that the disease affects their overall emotional wellbeing, and 82% reported that psoriasis interferes with their enjoyment of life; a high level of anger and frustration was felt by psoriasis patients, and the conciliation of psoriatic lesions with clothing, because they felt self-conscious and helpless, was reported. For all aspects of emotional wellbeing, patients with severe psoriasis reported a greater emotional impact than patients with mild psoriasis [33]. Clinical improvement contributes to decrease the frequency of psychiatric disturbances, but many patients still suffer psychological comorbidities after physical improvement [34].

Psoriasis is a persistent, disfiguring and stigmatizing disease; therefore, clinicians need to be aware of the emotional and psychological impact of psoriasis in the patient.

Nowadays, the T-helper (Th)1 pathway and the Th17/interleukin(IL)-23 axis are known to be crucial in psoriasis pathogenesis, and raised levels of several pro-inflammatory cytokines were found in psoriasis, especially in the moderate and severe forms. Pro-inflammatory cytokines, such as tumor necrosis factor -alpha, IL-1, IL-18 and IL-6, known to be raised in psoriasis, have been found to be significantly increased in patients with major depression [35-37]. It seems that inflammatory cytokines can interact with pathophysiologic domains relevant to depression, including neurotransmitter metabolism, neuroendocrine function, and synaptic plasticity [37].

Psoriasis is known to be associated with cardiovascular disease, and major depression seems to be a significant predictor of cardiovascular disease events. Depression may be an independent risk factor for death, after suffering an acute myocardial infarction [38], and it may increase the risk for coronary artery disease [39]. A positive association between depressive symptoms and raised serum levels of inflammatory markers was also reported [40]. Acute or chronic psychological stress may induce a chronic inflammatory process that may culminate in atherosclerosis [41].

It is known that in psoriatic patients, psychological stress, by itself, can play a role in the exacerbation of psoriasis, and that higher stress reactivity has been associated with the onset of psoriasis at an earlier age [6, 42]. Indeed, 31% of the patients reported the onset of psoriasis in periods of increased everyday life stress, and 71% of patients reported worsening of the symptomatology during stressful life episodes [43, 44]. The importance of stress in psoriasis has been further highlighted by the negative impact of psychological distress on the treatment outcome of psoriatic patients. For instance, the level of stress may prolong the time needed for psoralen plus ultraviolet light A (PUVA) to clear the symptoms of psoriasis [45]. Accordingly, stress reduction by stress management, relaxation or cognitive techniques shortened the time to clear psoriasis symptoms by PUVA improving the outcome of the treatment of psoriasis [46, 47]. An interesting finding is the increase in the catecholamine levels after stress exposure in psoriatic patients [48], pointing to a hyper responsive sympatho-adrenomedullary system in psoriasis.

The relevance of stress in psoriasis is broadly accepted, however, the underlying mechanisms, of how psychological distress exacerbates or triggers psoriasis, are poorly understood. It is known that psychological stress has the potential to regulate the immune response, and there is emerging evidence that abnormal neuroendocrine response to stress may contribute to the pathogenesis of chronic autoimmune diseases [49].

Psoriatic patients often manifest not only a profound psychosocial disability, but also a significant impairment of QOL [6, 7]. The lack of understanding by the family members may increase the level of anxiety in the patient; the QOL of relatives and partners of patients can also be significantly affected [50].

Sexual impairment seems to be frequent in psoriasis patients with severe disease and is usually linked to psychological problems [51].

A low level of awareness and understanding of the disease by people without psoriasis has been reported, suggesting that a lack of sensitivity may contribute to the social burdens of sufferers [52].

Some authors believe that QOL is more determined by how an individual mentally copes with the disease than by the amount of skin affected [29, 53]. Others refer that the impact of the disease in QOL seems to be greater in patients with more extensive skin involvement [54]. According to our data, the health -related QOL is more affected in the severer forms of psoriasis, as evaluated by PASI [55]. Clinicians need to try also to perceive the severity of psoriasis from the patient's point of view. From the patient's perspective, psoriasis is usually considered as severe, if it causes embarrassment or anxiety, pruritus or soreness; if it affects relationships, everyday activities, working, studying or sport activities, or if there is joint involvement.

Relationship between Quality of Life in Psoriasis and Ageing

The onset of psoriasis vulgaris is usually in the first or second decade of life, and 75% of the cases develop psoriasis before 46 years of age [56]. The age of onset is slightly earlier in women than in men. It seems that psoriasis onset is bimodal, with a peak at 16-22 and the other peak at 57-60 years of age. The age of the first presentation of the disease may substantially determine the individual quality of life; apparently, younger patients are more susceptible to impairment of their life course. Social, psychological, and physical factors are important determinants for QOL impairment or protection. Personality, coping mechanisms, social support, and treatment or therapy may act as positive factors and mitigate these damaging effects [57].

Data is controversial about the relationship of age and gender with quality of life in psoriasis. Gupta et al. reported that the impact of psoriasis in impairment of QOL was higher in the 18 to 45 year age range, affecting the socialization of both sexes equally, and that men face greater work-related stress es with the disease [58]. Young et al., reported that the impact of psoriasis seems to be severer for young adults (18-24 years old), particularly, for women, singles, patients with visible psoriasis, patients who developed psoriasis in early childhood, patients who have a negative state of mind as a result of psoriasis, or patients who have experienced additional problems due to psoriasis [52]. The Korte et al. systematic review of the literature, suggest that higher ages of the patients are associated with slightly lower levels of physical functioning and slightly higher levels of psychological functioning and quality of life [59]. However, Sampogna et al., comparing the quality of life in patients under 65 years with patients with 65 or more years of age, reported that, according to Skindex 29 scores, QOL was more impaired and psychological distress was more pronounced in older patients [60]. In the older group, the impairment in QOL was more significant in older women, suffering from anxiety or depression [60]. In another study of 936 patients, that used the Skindex-29 questionnaire, shame, worry and annoyance were more frequent in women than in men, and shame and anger were associated with a low level of education [32].

A cross-sectional study performed on 305 inpatients with 65 or more years of age, clinical severity increased with age and psychological distress was higher in patients with more than 70 years of age. Even though, QOL showed an improvement in older age groups [61]. Elderly patients, besides psoriasis, may have other medical, social and economic comorbidities that can further negatively affect their overall QOL.

Psoriasis, Avoidance Behaviours and Loss of Productivity

It is known that the stress caused by living with psoriasis can be manifested as avoidance behaviour s, and it has considerable and deleterious economic consequences for patients. Patients with severe psoriasis have significant impairment of work productivity [62-64], particularly, due to an increase in patient absenteeism. Finlay et al., reported that 59.3%, of 369 patients with severe psoriasis, lost an average of 26 days of work because of the disease [40], and more than 30%, of those who were not working, blamed psoriasis by their work status [65]. Schmitt and Ford reported that patients missed about 6.6% of their working per month, due to psoriasis [66]. According to the NPF survey data 2003-2011, 92% of the patients who were not working, cited psoriasis and /or psoriatic arthritis as the sole reasons for not working; 49% of the patients who were working, reported that they have missed some work days due to psoriasis or psoriatic arthritis treatment. In a typical month, among those who missed work days, 62% missed 5 days or less, 6.6% missed 6–10 days, and 31% missed more than 10 days [33]. Sampogna et al. reported that impairment in work and even in hobbies was higher in patients with palmoplantar psoriasis and in those with psoriatic arthritis [32]. Indeed, impairment on QOL seems to be higher in palmoplantar, pustular and arthritis psoriasis [67]. The two main contributors to stress in patients with psoriasis are engaging in avoidance behaviour and the belief that they are being evaluated on the basis of their skin disease, which may lead to low grade persistent stress. It has been reported that psoriatic patients present a reduction in physical and mental functioning comparable to that observed in patients with cancer, arthritis, hypertension, heart disease and depression [68]. Furthermore, the general health status of the patient may be enhanced by other diseases associated with psoriasis, creating a substantial impact on QOL [69].

Impact of Psoriasis Therapies in Quality of Life

Psoriasis imposes a significant economic burden, as it is a choice disease often associated with several comorbidities, and with a poor QOL. The choice of treatment for psoriasis depends on many factors, including the severity of the disease, the skin type, the response to previous psoriatic treatments, the patient's age, the clinical history and the effect on the patient's quality of life. Considering these factors, clinicians usually decides for the most successful treatment. A variety of therapeutic approaches are available, ranging from topical agents, for milder and limited forms of psoriasis, to phototherapy, photochemotherapy and systemic agents, for moderate and severe psoriasis. In the recent years, several new treatment options, such as the biological agents, have been introduced for treatment of psoriasis.

In a survey of patients with severe forms of psoriasis, 79% reported that psoriasis had a negative impact on their lives, 40% felt frustration with recurrent treatments, and 32% did not perceive their treatment to be sufficiently aggressive [70]. The treatment contentment seems to vary across treatment therapies. According to Callis Duffin et al., overall satisfaction scores are highest for patients receiving biologic therapies, combined biologic and methotrexate therapies and phototherapy; satisfaction scores were lowest for those receiving only topical therapies or acitretin [71]. However, data comparing the effectiveness and the improvement in quality of life of biologic agents, systemic agents, phototherapy, and other therapies, are limited.

A study by our group showed that patients submitted to topical therapy, present few improvements on health -related QOL, suggesting that in patients with milder forms of psoriasis and with few skin symptoms, the QOL is less affected by the disease. Narrow-band UVB (NB-UVB) and PUVA treatments seem to be effective in improving the health-related QOL. Nonetheless, considering the SF-36 score, NB-UVB when compared to PUVA, seems to present more significant improvements, suggesting that PUVA therapy has a less evident impact in QOL of patients. Psoriasis treatment with methotrexate or ciclosporin have been associated with satisfactory disease control, improved quality of life and tolerable side-effects [72, 73]; ciclosporin showed to be more effective than methotrexate in a short-term perspective [72].

Considering the DLQI score, the biological agents, etanercept, efalizumab and alefacept, improve health -related QOL when compared with placebo [74]. According to Ragnarson Tennvall et al., [75] patients treated with biological drugs during a 12 month period were more satisfied with their treatment, experienced fewer psoriasis -related problems and experienced less severe problems. Moderate disease-related problems were most common in patients receiving only topical treatment and in patients who had been treated with systemic agents and/or biological drugs for less than 12 months [75]. The costs for treatment of psoriasis with biological drugs are high but their contribution to improve QOL, especially among those patients who are currently not treated efficiently due to under-treatment, might reduce inpatient care and result in improved patient outcome. Indeed, according to Schmitt and Ford, the indirect costs of productivity loss exceed the direct cost s, which may justify the use of these expensive medications [66].

Psychological sequelae of the disease can impair the response to treatment, as patients with pathological levels of anxiety are less likely to respond to therapy [45]. Thus, stress in the form of pathological worry has a deleterious effect on response to therapy. Psychological intervention may, therefore, play an important role in the management of psoriasis. Useful ways of coping with decreased quality of life due to psoriasis may include sharing their experiences with other psoriasis patients and seeking support groups. Other patients who suffer from more mental health consequences of psoriasis may need to seek professional, psychiatric help to cope with this disease.

Conclusion

Psoriasis has physical, but also psychological, social and economic consequences on patients. Moreover, it has a significant emotional impact on patients, which may not be entirely related to the extent of skin disease. Clinicians must be aware of the important role that psychosocial burden has in patient perception of disease severity, quality of life, and disease course; thus, the psychosocial evaluation and quality of life measurement should be considered when assessing psoriasis severity and treatment efficacy. Indeed, the psychosocial burden found in psoriasis requires a multidisciplinary approach, with involvement of dermatologists, psychiatrists, psychologists among others, in order to achieve an optimal outcome. This multidisciplinary approach with the correct psychological intervention may contribute to reduce the level of stress, help the patient to learn how to have emotional control and adequate self-esteem, contributing to the acceptance of the disease and to improve the QOL of psoriasis patients.

References

[1] Iizuka H, Takahashi H, Ishida-Yamamoto A. Psoriatic architecture constructed by epidermal remodeling. *Journal of dermatological science.* 2004 Aug;35(2):93-9.

[2] Gottlieb AB. Psoriasis: emerging therapeutic strategies. *Nat. Rev. Drug Discov.* 2005 Jan;4(1):19-34.

[3] Krueger JG, Bowcock A. Psoriasis pathophysiology: current concepts of pathogenesis. *Annals of the rheumatic diseases.* 2005 Mar;64 Suppl 2:ii30-6.

[4] Salomon J, Szepietowski JC, Proniewicz A. Psoriatic nails: a prospective clinical study. *J. Cutan Med. Surg.* 2003 Jul-Aug;7(4):317-21.

[5] Jobling R, Naldi L. Assessing the impact of psoriasis and the relevance of qualitative research. *The Journal of investigative dermatology.* 2006 Jul;126(7):1438-40.

[6] Gupta MA, Gupta AK. Psychiatric and psychological co-morbidity in patients with dermatologic disorders: epidemiology and management. *American journal of clinical dermatology.* 2003;4(12):833-42.

[7] Reich K, Griffiths CE. The relationship between quality of life and skin clearance in moderate-to-severe psoriasis: lessons learnt from clinical trials with infliximab. *Archives of dermatological research.* 2008 Nov;300(10):537-44.

[8] Naldi L, Gambini D. The clinical spectrum of psoriasis. *Clinics in dermatology.* 2007 Nov-Dec;25(6):510-8.

[9] Frederiksson T PU. Severe psoriasis - oral therapy with a new retinoid. *Dermatologica.* 1978;157:238-44.

[10] Berth-Jones J, Grotzinger K, Rainville C, Pham B, Huang J, Daly S, et al., A study examining inter- and intrarater reliability of three scales for measuring severity of psoriasis: Psoriasis Area and Severity Index, Physician's Global Assessment and Lattice System Physician's Global Assessment. *The British journal of dermatology.* 2006 Oct;155(4):707-13.

[11] Gottlieb AB, Chaudhari U, Baker DG, Perate M, Dooley LT. The National Psoriasis Foundation Psoriasis Score (NPF-PS) system versus the Psoriasis Area Severity Index (PASI) and Physician's Global Assessment (PGA): a comparison. *J. Drugs Dermatol.* 2003 Jun;2(3):260-6.

[12] Bushnell DM, Martin ML, McCarrier K, Gordon K, Chiou CF, Huang X, et al., Validation of the Psoriasis Symptom Inventory (PSI), a patient-reported outcome measure to assess psoriasis symptom severity. *The Journal of dermatological treatment.* 2013 Oct;24(5):356-60.

[13] Ware JE, Jr., Sherbourne CD. The MOS 36-item short-form health survey (SF-36). I. Conceptual framework and item selection. *Med. Care.* 1992 Jun;30(6):473-83.

[14] Brazier J, Jones N, Kind P. Testing the validity of the Euroqol and comparing it with the SF-36 health survey questionnaire. *Qual. Life Res.* 1993 Jun;2(3):169-80.

[15] Finlay AY, Khan GK. Dermatology Life Quality Index (DLQI)--a simple practical measure for routine clinical use. *Clinical and experimental dermatology.* 1994 May;19(3):210-6.

[16] Chren MM, Lasek RJ, Flocke SA, Zyzanski SJ. Improved discriminative and evaluative capability of a refined version of Skindex, a quality-of-life instrument for patients with skin diseases. *Arch. Dermatol.* 1997 Nov;133(11):1433-40.

[17] Bronsard V, Paul C, Prey S, Puzenat E, Gourraud PA, Aractingi S, et al., What are the best outcome measures for assessing quality of life in plaque type psoriasis? A systematic review of the literature. *Journal of the European Academy of Dermatology and Venereology:* JEADV. 2010 Apr;24 Suppl 2:17-22.

[18] Feldman SR, Gottlieb AB, Bala M, Wu Y, Eisenberg D, Guzzo C, et al., Infliximab improves health -related quality of life in the presence of comorbidities among patients with moderate-to-severe psoriasis. *The British journal of dermatology.* 2008 Sep;159(3):704-10.

[19] Finlay AY. Current severe psoriasis and the rule of tens. *The British journal of dermatology.* 2005 May;152(5):861-7.

[20] Kirby B, Fortune DG, Bhushan M, Chalmers RJ, Griffiths CE. The Salford Psoriasis Index: an holistic measure of psoriasis severity. *The British journal of dermatology.* 2000 Apr;142(4):728-32.

[21] McKenna SP, Cook SA, Whalley D, Doward LC, Richards HL, Griffiths CE, et al., Development of the PSORIQoL, a psoriasis -specific measure of quality of life designed for use in clinical practice and trials. *The British journal of dermatology.* 2003 Aug;149(2):323-31.

[22] Nijsten T, Unaeze J, Stern RS. Refinement and reduction of the Impact of Psoriasis Questionnaire: classical test theory vs. Rasch analysis. *The British journal of dermatology.* 2006 Apr;154(4):692-700.

[23] Fried RG, Friedman S, Paradis C, Hatch M, Lynfield Y, Duncanson C, et al., Trivial or terrible? The psychosocial impact of psoriasis. *Int J Dermatol.* 1995 Feb;34(2):101-5.

[24] Koo J. Population-based epidemiologic study of psoriasis with emphasis on quality of life assessment. *Dermatologic clinics.* 1996 Jul;14(3):485-96.

[25] Gupta MA, Gupta AK, Watteel GN. Perceived deprivation of social touch in psoriasis is associated with greater psychologic morbidity: an index of the stigma experience in dermatologic disorders. *Cutis; cutaneous medicine for the practitioner.* 1998 Jun;61(6):339-42.

[26] Schmid-Ott G, Jaeger B, Kuensebeck HW, Ott R, Lamprecht F. Dimensions of stigmatization in patients with psoriasis in a "Questionnaire on Experience with Skin Complaints'. *Dermatology.* 1996;193(4):304-10.

[27] Hrehorow E, Salomon J, Matusiak L, Reich A, Szepietowski JC. Patients with psoriasis feel stigmatized. *Acta dermato-venereologica.* 2012 Jan;92(1):67-72.

[28] Russo PA, Ilchef R, Cooper AJ. Psychiatric morbidity in psoriasis: a review. *The Australasian journal of dermatology.* 2004 Aug;45(3):155-9; quiz 60-1.

[29] Friedewald VE, Jr., Cather JC, Gordon KB, Kavanaugh A, Ridker PM, Roberts WC. The editor's roundtable: psoriasis, inflammation, and coronary artery disease. *Am. J. Cardiol.* 2008 Apr 15;101(8):1119-26.

[30] Mease PJ, Menter MA. Quality-of-life issues in psoriasis and psoriatic arthritis: outcome measures and therapies from a dermatological perspective. *Journal of the American Academy of Dermatology*. 2006 Apr;54(4):685-704.
[31] Gupta MA, Schork NJ, Gupta AK, Kirkby S, Ellis CN. Suicidal ideation in psoriasis. *Int. J. Dermatol.* 1993 Mar;32(3):188-90.
[32] Sampogna F, Tabolli S, Abeni D. Living with psoriasis: prevalence of shame, anger, worry, and problems in daily activities and social life. *Acta dermato-venereologica.* 2012 May;92(3):299-303.
[33] Armstrong AW, Schupp C, Wu J, Bebo B. Quality of life and work productivity impairment among psoriasis patients: findings from the National Psoriasis Foundation survey data 2003-2011. *PloS one.* 2012;7(12):e52935.
[34] Sampogna F, Tabolli S, Abeni D. The impact of changes in clinical severity on psychiatric morbidity in patients with psoriasis: a follow-up study. *The British journal of dermatology.* 2007 Sep;157(3):508-13.
[35] Kim YK, Na KS, Shin KH, Jung HY, Choi SH, Kim JB. Cytokine imbalance in the pathophysiology of major depressive disorder. *Progress in neuro-psychopharmacology & biological psychiatry.* 2007 Jun 30;31(5):1044-53.
[36] Khairova RA, Machado-Vieira R, Du J, Manji HK. A potential role for pro-inflammatory cytokines in regulating synaptic plasticity in major depressive disorder. *Int. J. Neuropsychopharmacol.* 2009 May;12(4):561-78.
[37] Shelton RC, Miller AH. Eating ourselves to death (and despair): the contribution of adiposity and inflammation to depression. *Progress in neurobiology.* 2010 Aug;91(4):275-99.
[38] Carney RM, Blumenthal JA, Catellier D, Freedland KE, Berkman LF, Watkins LL, et al., Depression as a risk factor for mortality after acute myocardial infarction. *Am. J. Cardiol.* 2003 Dec 1;92(11):1277-81.
[39] Barth J, Schumacher M, Herrmann-Lingen C. Depression as a risk factor for mortality in patients with coronary heart disease: a meta-analysis. *Psychosom. Med.* 2004 Nov-Dec;66(6):802-13.
[40] Stewart JC, Janicki-Deverts D, Muldoon MF, Kamarck TW. Depressive symptoms moderate the influence of hostility on serum interleukin-6 and C-reactive protein. *Psychosom. Med.* 2008 Feb;70(2):197-204.
[41] Black PH, Garbutt LD. Stress, inflammation and cardiovascular disease. *J. Psychosom. Res.* 2002 Jan;52(1):1-23.
[42] Naldi L, Chatenoud L, Linder D, Belloni Fortina A, Peserico A, Virgili AR, et al., Cigarette smoking, body mass index, and stressful life events as risk factors for psoriasis: results from an Italian case-control study. *The Journal of investigative dermatology.* 2005 Jul;125(1):61-7.
[43] Griffiths CE, Richards HL. Psychological influences in psoriasis. *Clinical and experimental dermatology.* 2001 Jun;26(4):338-42.
[44] Zachariae R, Zachariae H, Blomqvist K, Davidsson S, Molin L, Mork C, et al., Self-reported stress reactivity and psoriasis -related stress of Nordic psoriasis sufferers. *Journal of the European Academy of Dermatology and Venereology*: JEADV. 2004 Jan;18(1):27-36.
[45] Fortune DG, Richards HL, Kirby B, McElhone K, Markham T, Rogers S, et al., Psychological distress impairs clearance of psoriasis in patients treated with photochemotherapy. *Arch. Dermatol.* 2003 Jun;139(6):752-6.

[46] Kabat-Zinn J, Wheeler E, Light T, Skillings A, Scharf MJ, Cropley TG, et al., Influence of a mindfulness meditation-based stress reduction intervention on rates of skin clearing in patients with moderate to severe psoriasis undergoing phototherapy (UVB) and photochemotherapy (PUVA). *Psychosom. Med.* 1998 Sep-Oct;60(5):625-32.
[47] Fortune DG, Richards HL, Kirby B, Bowcock S, Main CJ, Griffiths CE. A cognitive-behavioural symptom management programme as an adjunct in psoriasis therapy. *The British journal of dermatology.* 2002 Mar;146(3):458-65.
[48] Buske-Kirschbaum A, Ebrecht M, Kern S, Hellhammer DH. Endocrine stress responses in TH1-mediated chronic inflammatory skin disease (psoriasis vulgaris)--do they parallel stress-induced endocrine changes in TH2-mediated inflammatory dermatoses (atopic dermatitis)? *Psychoneuroendocrinology.* 2006 May;31(4):439-46.
[49] Jorgensen C, Bressot N, Bologna C, Sany J. Dysregulation of the hypothalamo-pituitary axis in rheumatoid arthritis. *J. Rheumatol.* 1995 Oct;22(10):1829-33.
[50] Eghlileb AM, Davies EE, Finlay AY. Psoriasis has a major secondary impact on the lives of family members and partners. *The British journal of dermatology.* 2007 Jun;156(6):1245-50.
[51] Sampogna F, Gisondi P, Tabolli S, Abeni D. Impairment of sexual life in patients with psoriasis. *Dermatology.* 2007;214(2):144-50.
[52] Young M. The psychological and social burdens of psoriasis. *Dermatol Nurs.* 2005 Feb;17(1):15-9.
[53] Stern RS, Nijsten T, Feldman SR, Margolis DJ, Rolstad T. Psoriasis is common, carries a substantial burden even when not extensive, and is associated with widespread treatment dissatisfaction. The journal of investigative dermatology Symposium proceedings / the Society for Investigative Dermatology, Inc [and] *European Society for Dermatological Research.* 2004 Mar;9(2):136-9.
[54] Gelfand JM, Feldman SR, Stern RS, Thomas J, Rolstad T, Margolis DJ. Determinants of quality of life in patients with psoriasis: a study from the US population. *Journal of the American Academy of Dermatology.* 2004 Nov;51(5):704-8.
[55] Coimbra S, Oliveira H, Reis F, Belo L, Carvalho A, Figueiredo A, et al., Health-related quality of life in Portuguese psoriatic patients: relation with Psoriasis Area and Severity Index and different types of classical psoriatic treatment. *The Journal of dermatology.* 2011 Aug;38(8):816-9.
[56] Nevitt GJ, Hutchinson PE. Psoriasis in the community: prevalence, severity and patients' beliefs and attitudes towards the disease. *The British journal of dermatology.* 1996 Oct;135(4):533-7.
[57] Mattei PL, Corey KC, Kimball AB. Cumulative life course impairment: evidence for psoriasis. *Current problems in dermatology.* 2013;44:82-90.
[58] Gupta MA, Gupta AK. Age and gender differences in the impact of psoriasis on quality of life. *Int. J. Dermatol.* 1995 Oct;34(10):700-3.
[59] de Korte J, Sprangers MA, Mombers FM, Bos JD. Quality of life in patients with psoriasis: a systematic literature review. The journal of investigative dermatology Symposium proceedings / the Society for Investigative Dermatology, Inc [and] *European Society for Dermatological Research.* 2004 Mar;9(2):140-7.
[60] Sampogna F, Chren MM, Melchi CF, Pasquini P, Tabolli S, Abeni D. Age, gender, quality of life and psychological distress in patients hospitalized with psoriasis. *The British journal of dermatology.* 2006 Feb;154(2):325-31.

[61] Sampogna F, Tabolli S, Mastroeni S, Di Pietro C, Fortes C, Abeni D. Quality of life impairment and psychological distress in elderly patients with psoriasis. Dermatology. 2007;215(4):341-7.

[62] Fowler JF, Duh MS, Rovba L, Buteau S, Pinheiro L, Lobo F, et al., The impact of psoriasis on health care costs and patient work loss. *Journal of the American Academy of Dermatology.* 2008 Nov;59(5):772-80.

[63] Horn EJ, Fox KM, Patel V, Chiou CF, Dann F, Lebwohl M. Association of patient-reported psoriasis severity with income and employment. *Journal of the American Academy of Dermatology.* 2007 Dec;57(6):963-71.

[64] Pearce DJ, Singh S, Balkrishnan R, Kulkarni A, Fleischer AB, Feldman SR. The negative impact of psoriasis on the workplace. *The Journal of dermatological treatment.* 2006;17(1):24-8.

[65] Finlay AY, Coles EC. The effect of severe psoriasis on the quality of life of 369 patients. *The British journal of dermatology.* 1995 Feb;132(2):236-44.

[66] Schmitt JM, Ford DE. Work limitations and productivity loss are associated with health -related quality of life but not with clinical severity in patients with psoriasis. *Dermatology.* 2006;213(2):102-10.

[67] Sampogna F, Tabolli S, Soderfeldt B, Axtelius B, Aparo U, Abeni D. Measuring quality of life of patients with different clinical types of psoriasis using the SF-36. *The British journal of dermatology.* 2006 May;154(5):844-9.

[68] Rapp SR, Feldman SR, Exum ML, Fleischer AB, Jr., Reboussin DM. Psoriasis causes as much disability as other major medical diseases. *Journal of the American Academy of Dermatology.* 1999 Sep;41(3 Pt 1):401-7.

[69] Kimball AB, Jacobson C, Weiss S, Vreeland MG, Wu Y. The psychosocial burden of psoriasis. *American journal of clinical dermatology.* 2005;6(6):383-92.

[70] Krueger G, Koo J, Lebwohl M, Menter A, Stern RS, Rolstad T. The impact of psoriasis on quality of life: results of a 1998 National Psoriasis Foundation patient-membership survey. *Arch. Dermatol.* 2001 Mar;137(3):280-4.

[71] Callis Duffin K, Yeung H, Takeshita J, Krueger GG, Robertson AD, Troxel AB, et al., Patient Satisfaction with Treatments for Moderate-to-Severe Plaque Psoriasis in Clinical Practice. *The British journal of dermatology.* 2013 Nov 22.

[72] Flytstrom I, Stenberg B, Svensson A, Bergbrant IM. Methotrexate vs. ciclosporin in psoriasis: effectiveness, quality of life and safety. A randomized controlled trial. The *British journal of dermatology.* 2008 Jan;158(1):116-21.

[73] Heydendael VM, Spuls PI, Opmeer BC, de Borgie CA, Reitsma JB, Goldschmidt WF, et al., Methotrexate versus cyclosporine in moderate-to-severe chronic plaque psoriasis. *The New England journal of medicine.* 2003 Aug 14;349(7):658-65.

[74] Reich K, Sinclair R, Roberts G, Griffiths CE, Tabberer M, Barker J. Comparative effects of biological therapies on the severity of skin symptoms and health -related quality of life in patients with plaque -type psoriasis: a meta-analysis. *Current medical research and opinion.* 2008 May;24(5):1237-54.

[75] Ragnarson Tennvall G, Hjortsberg C, Bjarnason A, Gniadecki R, Heikkila H, Jemec GB, et al., Treatment patterns, treatment satisfaction, severity of disease problems, and quality of life in patients with psoriasis in three Nordic countries. *Acta dermato-venereologica.* 2013 Jul 6;93(4):442-5.

Part IV. Miscellaneous

In: Geriatric Psychodermatology
Editors: Mohammad Jafferany and Katlein França

ISBN: 978-1-63463-853-1

Chapter 16

Psychodermato-Oncology: Skin Cancers in the Elderly

Katlein França, M.D., MSc and Keyvan Nouri, M.D.*

Introduction

The skin is the largest organ of the body and has several important functions. It helps to control body temperature; covers and protects internal organs; prevents loss of fluids; and protects the body against infection, chemicals, and UV rays. [1]

Skin cancer is the most common form of all cancers. According to the American Cancer Society, more than 3.5 million cases of basal cell carcinoma (BCC) and squamous cell carcinoma (SCC) are found in United States each year. [2]

The incidence of BCC increases with advancing age. Factors such as excessive, chronic sun exposure, genetics, fair complexion, exposure to ionizing radiation indoors tanning, fair complexion, prior exposure to ionizing radiation and exposure to chemical carcinogens are significant risks factors. [2, 3] Squamous cell carcinoma is also more prevalent between elderly. The incidence of SCC among whites is 100 to 150 per 100,000 persons per year. [3,4] The age-specific incidence among persons older than 75 years is approximately 10 times that rate. [2, 3, 4]

Melanoma, the most dangerous type of skin cancer, accounts for more than 9,700 of the nearly 13,000 skin cancer deaths each year. [2] The risk of melanoma diagnosis increases significantly with age. Nearly 50% of all melanoma deaths occur in middle-aged and older white men. [5, 6]

Many dermatologic conditions can cause psychologic problems. Their high visibility and easy accessibility makes the skin a direct gateway to behavioral problems. [7,8] Skin cancer is the only type of cancer that is directly visible to the patient from its early stages and as such serves as a constant reminder of its presence. [9] The psychological impact of skin cancer is an upcoming topic of study part of the psychodermato-oncology subspecialty. [10] This

* Corresponding author: Katlein França. Email: k.franca@med.miami.edu

chapter will present the psychological aspects related to the skin cancer diagnosis in geriatric population.

Melanoma Skin Cancer

The most dangerous form of skin cancer, these cancerous growths develop when unrepaired DNA damage of skin cells (caused by ultraviolet radiation from sun exposure or tanning beds and genetic factors) triggers mutations (i.e., genetic defect s) that lead skin cells to multiply rapidly and form malignant tumors. These tumors originate in the pigment-producing melanocytes in the basal layer of the epidermis. (SCF) Melanoma is the leading cause of death from skin disease, however, it can be cured if diagnosed and treated in early stages. Early detection of thin cutaneous melanoma is the best means of reducing mortality. [11] The possibility of recurrence, metastasis, and mortality levels related to this type of skin cancer is responsible for psychological distress reported and studied in several patients.

Brandberg and colleagues evaluated psychologic and psychosomatic reactions to malignant melanoma, comparing patients with tumor thickness <-0.8 mm versus > 0.8 mm, and recurrent versus non-recurrent patients. All patients were interviewed at their first post-surgery follow-up; a questionnaire containing items concerning nevi, sleeping problems, and psychosomatic complains as well as a Hospital Anxiety and depression scale were completed during a 7- and 13- month follow-up visit. The results showed that patients with a more unfavorable prognosis (tumor thickness > 0.8 mm) reported more sleeping problems than those with a more favorable prognosis (<- 0.8 mm). Women had higher levels of problems than men. Interestingly, amongst patients with an unfavorable prognosis, those with recurrence within 2 years showed lower levels of anxiety at the first visit compared with those free from recurrence after 2 years. [12] The quality of life, emotional status and coping styles were investigated by Vurnek and colleagues. Thirty-one patients were studied and the authors concluded that melanoma has a medium influence on patients' psychological status and quality of life. Coping styles have been shown to have a significant influence on patients' quality of life and their emotional reaction to the illness. [13] Another study that also investigated the quality of life of melanoma patients, found that factors related to the tumor, as well as gender, age, and employment status, were not found to be predictive of quality of life in their sample. Quality of life scores were lower in the functional well-being domain in patients with metastases. They also found that married patients are able to count on greater comfort and emotional support to help them deal with the diagnosis of melanoma. Additionally, patients with a family history of melanoma had significantly higher quality of life scores, while those with poor education levels had lower scores. [14]

A study compared the emotional reactions in patients with melanoma and patients with other dermatological conditions. The authors used a self-report test of mental health developed by the Rand Corporation and previously applied to large segments of general public to measure psychological status. The emotional well being in melanoma patients was approximately equal to the general public and strikingly superior to other dermatology patients. An explanation for this finding would be a diminished self-esteem among non-melanoma dermatology patients and intensified utilization of behavioral therapy and similar resources among melanoma patients. [15] Considering the psychological adjustment to melanoma and differences between genders, women demonstrated more distress, less secondary cognitive appraisal and were more secure in attachment styles while men showed higher secondary appraisal and were more dismissing-avoidant in attachment. Attachment styles are the way you relate to others in the context of intimate relationships. No between-group differences were found in mental well being, subjective functioning, and primary cognitive appraisal or in the global measure of hardiness. [16]

Melanoma patients can present different degrees of psychological distress. Common reactions to melanoma are anxiety, depression and deterioration. The psychological impact can be long lasting and affect the quality of life. [13] Early detection and treatment of melanoma is mandatory to reduce the disease mortality.

Non-Melanoma Skin Cancer

Non-melanoma skin cancer (NMSK) is a group of skin cancers that affect the upper layers of skin. Basal cell carcinoma and squamous cell carcinoma are the most common types. Although considered less aggressive than melanoma and with a higher cure rate, these types of cancers can cause disfigurement. (Figure 1) Individuals may lose part of their nose, an eye or ear if this invasive skin cancer is not detected and treated early. [17] A study involving a hundred patients with NMSC of the head and neck and concluded that this population exhibits lower self-esteem than individuals without cancer. [18] Several factors may contribute to psychological distress in these patients. Subjective beliefs regarding skin cancer, its treatment, prognosis, social support and ability to cope with the situation may play a role in determining the stress response in this population. [19] A study conducted by *Antoszewski* and colleagues with 123 patients showed that many patients delay the treatment because they do not want to undergo surgery, especially elderly population. They also fear that the neoplasm could spread after surgical excision. [20]

The psychological concerns in non-melanoma skin cancer patients are less focused on mortality than melanoma patients. [21] Issues relating to disfigurement, discomfort and illness perception should be focused on by doctors who treat this population. [22]

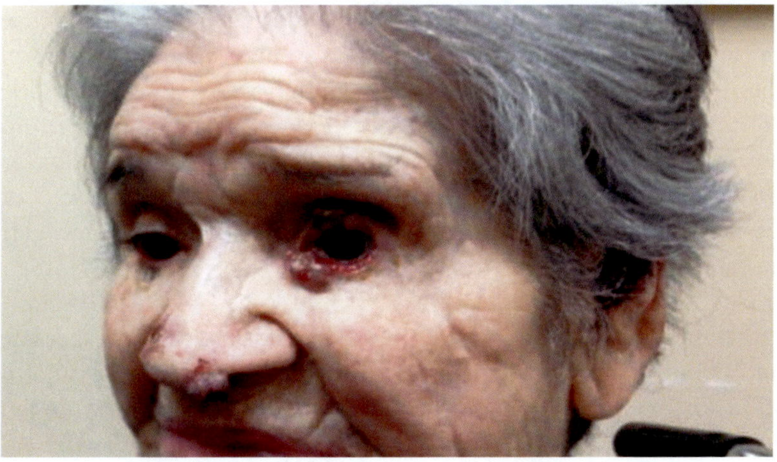

Figure 1. Multiple basal cell carcinomas causing facial disfigurement.

Doctor-Patient Relationship in Cutaneous Oncology

Over the course of a career, a dermatologist may have to disclose unfavorable medical information to patients and families. Breaking bad news can be particularly stressful especially if there are limited prospects for successful treatment. [23, 26]

Research data conducted by Picardi and Sampogna et al. suggests that patients and dermatologists evaluate aspects of quality of life differently; furthermore, detection of psychiatric disorders by dermatologists is inadequate. [24, 25] These authors suggest that dermatologists should probably be more alert to the possibility of psychiatric co-morbidities in their patients. [24, 25]

Allocating more space to this issue in training programs for dermatologists would favor a shift in their conceptual models of skin disease. [24] Another recommended strategy for physicians would be to create a plan, determining the patient's values and wishes to participate in decision-making, as well as a strategy to manage the patient's distress when receiving the diagnosis. [23, 27] The doctor-patient relationship must be based on empathy, ethics, and compassion; hence the dermatologist must encourage the patients to participate in all steps of the treatment plan. [26, 28]

Psychologic Approach to Patients with Skin Cancer

The identification of patients who need psychologic and psychosocial intervention is essential to relieve their distress and to sustain their coping strategy. Dermatologists and nurses should be trained to carefully identify patients with special needs. [29] Pyscho-education should be available to all patients. Several studies mention the value of providing early help to melanoma patients. Different types of approaches can be used to minimize to psychologic distress in this population, such as psychotherapy, educational techniques, behavioral or skills training, and the design of a supportive care program for patients and families. Boesen and colleagues performed a study with 262 patients with primary cutaneous melanoma. These patients were randomly assigned to either control or intervention groups. Patients in the intervention group were offered six weekly sessions of 2 hours of psychoeducation consisting of health education, enhancement of problem-solving skills, stress management, and psychological help. The patients in the intervention group showed significantly less fatigue, greater vigor, and lower total mood disturbance compared with controls; additionally, they used significantly more active-behavioral and active-cognitive coping than the patients in the control group. [30]

Different modalities of psychotherapy may be used, such as psychodynamic, supportive-expressive, relaxation, cognitive-behavioral, and dialectical behavioral therapies. Hypnosis may also be an option for these patients. [31] The choice of the best psychologic approach will depend on factors such as age and preference of the patient, diagnosis, family support, and financial constraints. [29,30]

Conclusion

Receiving a diagnosis of any type of cancer can be a traumatic experience that may trigger significant psychological distress. Skin cancer is the only type of cancer that is visible to the patient and may cause lower self-esteem, depression, and anxiety. Dermatologists should be trained to carefully diagnose these high risk patients. The doctor-patient communication in dermatology should be emphasized in treatment and care of skin cancer patients. Many healthcare professionals in other specialties such as surgical oncology are using a biopsychosocial assessment to analyze the psychological, behavioral, emotional, cognitive, and social factors which impact how patients cope with their diagnosis and treatment; this may be employed in the dermatology setting through gathering relevant information by a dermatologist, social worker, mental health professional, or other healthcare provider to determine coping skills and psychologic status of patients with skin cancer. Allocating more space to this issue in training programs for dermatologists would be an alternative to improve patient care.

References

[1] Marion Richardson. Available: http://www.nursingtimes.net/nursing -practice-clinical-research/understanding-the-structure -and-function-of-the-skin /205222.article. Access 14 may, 2014

[2] American Cancer Society. Skin Cancer Facts. http://www.cancer.org/Cancer /CancerCauses/SunandUVExposure/skin -cancer-facts. Access 14 may, 2014

[3] Tung, R. Vidimos A. Nonmelanoma Skin Cancer Available: http://www.cleveland clinicmeded.com/medicalpubs/diseasemanagement/dermatology /nonmelanoma-skin - cancer / Access: may, 12 2014

[4] Johnson TM1, Rowe DE, Nelson BR, Swanson NA. Squamous cell carcinoma of the skin (excluding the lip and oral mucosa). *J Am Acad Dermatol.* 26: 1992; 467-484.

[5] Geller AC, Swetter SM, Brooks K, Demierre MF, Yaroch AL. Screening, early detection, and trends for melanoma: current status (2000-2006) and future directions. *J Am Acad Dermatol.* 2007;57:555–72. 573–6. quiz.

[6] Coups EJ1, Geller AC, Weinstock MA, Heckman CJ, Manne SL. Prevalence and correlates of skin cancer screening among middle-aged and older white adults in the United States. *Am J Med.* 2010 May;123(5):439-45. doi: 10.1016/j.amjmed. 2009.10.014.

[7] Daniel Todkil. Surgical and Emotional Scars of Skin Cancer Available: (http://www.bsds.org.uk/awards/undergraduate/BSDS_essay_Dan_Todkill.pdf). Access june 28, 2012

[8] Van Moffaert M. Psychodermatology: an overview. *Psychother Psychosom.* 1992;58(3-4):125-36.

[9] Moussas GI, Papadopoulou AG, Christodoulaki AG, Karkanias AP. [Psychological and psychiatric problems in cancer patients: Relationship to the localization of the disease]. *Psychiatrike.* 2012 Jan-Mar;23(1):46-60.

[10] Taube KM. Psycho-oncology in dermatology. *Hautarzt.* 2013 Jun;64(6):424-8. doi: 10.1007/s00105-012-2496-7.

[11] Skin cancer foundation. Skin Cancer facts. Available: http://www.skincancer.org/skin -cancer-information/skin-cancer-facts#melanoma. Access may, 28 2014.

[12] Brandberg Y, Månsson-Brahme E, Ringborg U, Sjödén PO. Psychological reactions in patients with malignant melanoma. *Eur J Cancer.* 1995;31A(2):157-62.

[13] Vurnek M, Buljan M, Situm M. Psychological status and coping with illness in patients with malignant melanoma. *Coll Antropol.* 2007 Jan;31 Suppl 1:53-6.

[14] Barbato MT, Bakos L, Bakos RM, Prieb R, Andrade CD. Predictors of quality of life in patients with skin melanoma at the dermatology department of the Porto Alegre Teaching Hospital. *An Bras Dermatol.* 2011 Apr;86(2):249-56.

[15] Cassileth BR, Lusk EJ, Tenaglia AN. A psychological comparison of patients with malignant melanoma and other dermatologic disorders. *J Am Acad Dermatol.* 1982 Dec;7(6):742-6.

[16] Hamama-Raz Y. Does psychological adjustment of melanoma survivors differs between genders? *Psychooncology.* 2012 Mar;21(3):255-63. doi: 10.1002/pon.1889. Epub 2010 Dec 19.

[17] No author listed. Detection and treatment of nonmelanoma skin cancer prevent disfigurement and death. *Cutis.* 1999 Jun;63(6):344.

[18] Carvalho, Marcelo Prado de et al. Auto-estima em pacientes com carcinomas de pele. *Rev. Col. Bras. Cir.* [online]. 2007, vol.34, n.6, pp. 361-366.

[19] Hamama-Raz Y., Solomon Z., Schachter J., et al: Objective and subjective stressors and the psychological adjustment of melanoma survivors. *Psycho-Oncol* 2007; 16:287-294.

[20] Antoszewski B, Kasielska A, Fijałkowska M. Face skin neoplasms--reasons for delayed treatment. *Pol Przegl Chir.* 2011 Jul;83(7):361-6.

[21] Rhee J.S., Loberiza F.R., Matthews B.A., et al. Quality of life assessment in nonmelanoma cervicofacial skin cancer. *Laryngoscope* 2003; 113(2):215-220.

[22] Walter F. Baile, Robert Buckman, Renato Lenzi, Gary Glober, Estela A. Beale[a] and Andrzej P. Kudelka SPIKES—A Six-Step Protocol for Delivering Bad News: Application to the Patient with Cancer. *The Oncologist.* August 2000 vol. 5 no. 4 302-311

[23] Walter F. Baile, Robert Buckman, Renato Lenzi, Gary Glober, Estela A. Beale[a] and Andrzej P. Kudelka SPIKES—A Six-Step Protocol for Delivering Bad News: Application to the Patient with Cancer. *The Oncologist.* August 2000 vol. 5 no. 4 302-311

[24] Picardi A, Abeni D, Melchi CF, Puddu P, Pasquini P. Psychiatric morbidity in dermatological outpatients: an issue to be recognized. *Br J Dermatol.* 2000; 143: 920–921.

[25] Sampogna F, Picardi A, Melchi CF, Pasquini P, Abeni D. The impact of skin diseases on patients: comparing dermatologists' opinions with research data collected on their patients. *Br J Dermatol* 2003; 148: 989–995.

[26] Haas JS, Cook EF, Puopolo AL, Burstin HR, Cleary PD, Brennan TA. Is the professional satisfaction of general internists associated with patient satisfaction? *J Gen Intern Med* 2000;15: 122–128.

[27] Wessely SC, Lewis GH. The classification of psychiatric morbidity in attenders at a dermatology clinic. *Br J Psychiatry* 1989;155: 686–691.

[28] Poot F. Doctor-patient relations in dermatology: obligations and rights for a mutual satisfaction. *J Eur Acad Dermatol Venereol.* 2009 Nov;23(11):1233-9. Epub 2009 May 19.

[29] Strittmatter G, Tilkorn M, Mawick R. How to identify patients in need of psychological intervention. *Recent Results Cancer Res.* 2002;160:353-61.

[30] Boesen EH, Ross L, Frederiksen K, Thomsen BL, Dahlstrøm K, Schmidt G, Naested J, Krag C, Johansen C. Psychoeducational intervention for patients with cutaneous malignant melanoma: a replication study. *J Clin Oncol.* 2005 Feb 20;23(6):1270-7.

[31] Philip D Shenefelt, MD, MS; Chief Editor: Dirk M Elston, MD Hypnosis - Applications in Dermatology and Dermatologic Surgery. Available: http://emedicine.medscape.com/article/1097553-overview. Access may 27, 2014

In: Geriatric Psychodermatology
Editors: Mohammad Jafferany and Katlein França

ISBN: 978-1-63463-853-1

Chapter 17

Psychodermatological Side Effects of Chemotherapy

Katlein França, M.D., MSc*

Introduction

Cancers are diseases caused by the uncontrolled division of cells in the body. [1] Among people over 65 years old, the incidence of developing cancer increases for most cancers when compared with younger individuals. [2, 3, 4] The mortality rate caused by cancer is also higher among geriatric patients. [2, 5, 6] These groups of patients usually experience age - related comorbid conditions that may impact on the survival rates and cancer prognosis. [6, 7] There are several types of cancer and they can occur in almost any organ. The causes of cancers are variable and include: radiation, obesity, genetics, and toxins, among others. [1] Chemotherapy agents are used to treat cancers. [8]

These drugs are used alone or in combination and side effects such as nausea, vomiting, hair loss and skin rashes can occur [8, 9]. These side effects are not only physical debilitating, but also psychologically devastating for any individual. More than one hundred chemotherapy drugs are available on the market and several cutaneous reactions to these drugs are described in literature.

Research focuses on creation of new drugs with fewer side effects. [8] This chapter will present the most common cutaneous reactions that cause psychological distress to patients undergoing chemotherapy. These reactions vary on frequency and severity and can cause severe cosmetic disfigurement, psychological distress and increase morbidity. [10]

* Corresponding author: Katlein França: Email: k.franca@med.miami.edu

Skin Toxicity of Chemotherapic Agents

Skin, hair and nails are sites particularly susceptible to action of chemotherapic agents and consequently manifest innumerous reactions when exposed to these drugs. [11] This section will review the most common cutaneous reactions of chemotherapeutic agents and will discuss how they psychologically impact patients.

Alopecia

Alopecia is the most common dermatological side effect of chemotherapeutic drugs and can cause serious psychological distress, especially in female patients. [12] There is an estimate that 65% of patients undergoing chemotherapy will have hair loss. [13] (Figure 1)

There are many chemotherapeutic drugs that induce alopecia. (Table 1) Although the severity of alopecia depends on the chemotherapeutic agent used, treatment protocol and association of drugs. [13] If more than one drug is used the alopecia tends to be more severe. [13, 14]

Table 1. Chemotherapeutic drugs that induce alopecia [13, 15]

Class of chemotherapeutic agents	Examples of drugs	Frequencies of chemotherapy-induced hair loss
Antimicrotubule agents	paclitaxel, docetaxel, vincristine, vinblastine, etoposide, teniposide	> 80%
Topoisomerase inhibitors	doxorubicin, daunorubicin,	60-100%
Alkylators	cyclophosphamide, ifosfamide, temozolomide	> 60%
Antimetabolites	5-fluorouracil, gemcitabine, methotrexate	10-50%

Hair loss can cause severe psychological distress and impact individual perception of body image, self-esteem and appearance. [16] It also can be stigma of having cancer. [14, 15] Women are specially affected. A review study published in 2001 showed that 47% of women consider hair loss to be the most traumatic experience of chemotherapy and 8% would decline this treatment due to the fear of presenting hair loss. [12]

Different approaches are described in literature in order to minimize the psychological impact of alopecia. The use of scarves, hats and wigs are the most common methods used by geriatric patients in order to improve their self-esteem and avoid social stigma. (Figure 2)

Scalp cooling is an effective method that aims the reduction of hair loss. It should be done during the infusion. It is a cost -effective method and should be offered to all patients undergoing chemotherapy. [16, 17, 18] The perspective of losing less hair can make the patients more confident to be treated and improve their quality of life. Some authors believe that the purchase of wigs is unnecessary if scalp-cooling method is performed. [17, 18] A study performed with 84 patients who purchased a wig showed that only 52 actually wore it and they just did it for less than six months. [17]

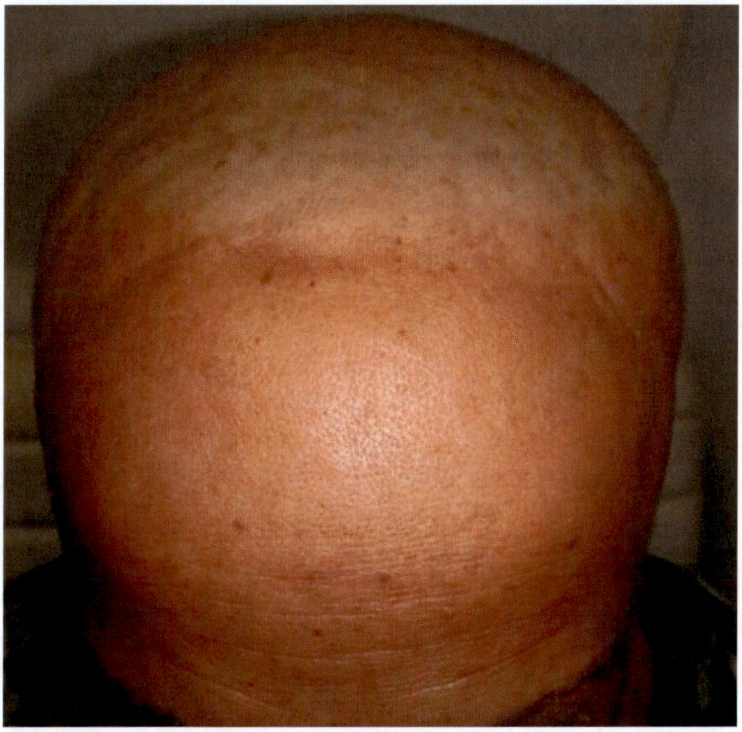

Figure 1. Chemotherapy induced alopecia in a male patient.

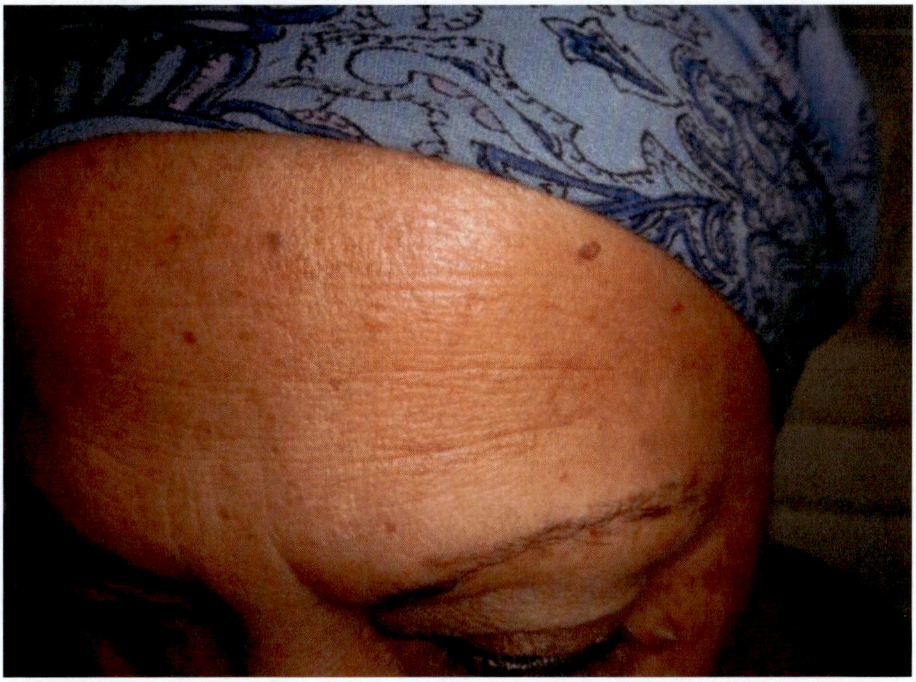

Figure 2. A female patient with chemotherapy induced alopecia wearing a headscarf.

Topical minoxidil and the immunomodulator AS101 are considered and effective therapies for accelerating regrowth after the chemotherapy treatment, but have little or no effect on preventing the chemotherapy induced alopecia. [14, 20] There are experimental studies to the development of drugs to improve the hair loss in patients undergoing chemotherapy. These include: antioxidants, drug-specific antibodies, cytokines and growth factor s, inhibitors of apoptosis, among others. [20]

In the past decade there was in increased number of reports of permanent chemotherapy induced alopecia. [21] This is a delicate situation that can cause or worsen depression symptoms. These patients should receive adequate psychological support and develop strategies and methods to cope with the permanent alopecia.

Helen Roe, from the North Cumbria University Hospitals wrote an interesting paper about advice and support for patients with chemotherapy induced alopecia. She emphasizes that the patients should receive up-to-date verbal and written information to prepare them for losing the hair. Health professionals should also help them to preserve their self-image and minimize the psychological consequences of hair loss while receiving chemotherapy; as well as preparing them for the hair re-growth following completion of chemotherapy. [22]

Nail Changes

Nails are important skin appendages that serve as protection for the tips of fingers and toes. [23] Healthy nails are important for a good body image and any nail abnormalities may impact patient's self-esteem, relationships and work ability. [24] A variety of nail changes can occur as side effects of chemotherapy. The most common drugs associated with nail changes are vincristine, hydroxyurea, etoposide, cyclophosphamide, bleomycin, dacarbazine, 5-fluoraxil and methotrexate. [25, 26] These nail changes occur due to the toxicity to the nail bed, matrix, digital blood vessels and periungueal tissues. [23, 25] The most findings are dystrophies, hemorrhages, onycholysis discoloration, leukonykia, paronychia, Beau's lines among others. [25, 26, 27] These nail changes are usually asymptomatic and resolve after the treatment, but may psychologically impact patients and affect their quality of life.

Patients undergoing chemotherapy should receive orientation to keep good nail hygiene, to avoid cutting the cuticles and use moisturizer.

Several studies suggest that patients undergoing treatment with taxanes may benefit of the use of frozen gloves or socks. [28] Taxanes such as docetaxel and paclitaxel are used for the treatment several types of cancers, including breast cancer. [28, 29] Minisi and colleagues reported in a study that more that 40% of patients treated with taxanes developed nail changes. [30] The gloves and socks should be used during the infusion. [28] It is considered a safe intervention by the majority of the authors, but the effectiveness of the method is still controversial. [28]

Mucositis

Oral mucositis is a frequent complication associated with chemotherapy and radiotherapy. [31] The degree of the lesions depends on several factors such as age, gender, type of medication, underlying systemic disease and tissue specific factors. [32] The most common symptom experienced by patients is dry lips, but the most significant problem is ulcerated mucosa. Pain on swallowing is considered the most distressful symptom. [33] Treatment is palliative and includes nutritional support, topical anesthetics for pain control and controlling of bleeding. [34] Mucositis can severally impact patient's quality of life and well being. [35]

Hand Foot Syndrome

Hand foot syndrome is a cutaneous toxicity that usually occurs 2 to 12 days after the chemotherapy infusion. [36, 37] Symptoms are palmar and plantar dysesthesia, tin gling, burning pain, erythema, edematous swelling, blistering and ulceration. [36, 38, 39] The symptoms usually solves weeks after the drug withdrawal. [36]

Considering the impact in quality of life that these patients may experience, Sibaud and colleagues created a quality of life scale named HFS-14. This scale was specifically developed for patients with hand and foot syndrome. It is an interesting tool to measure the quality of life impairment. [40]

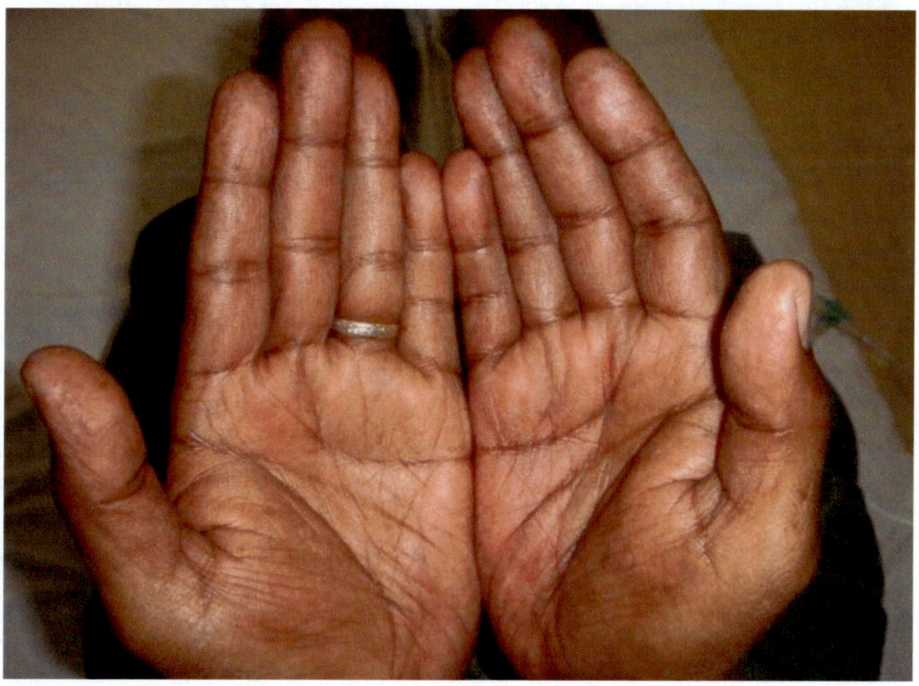

Figure 3. Hand Foot syndrome: palmar erythema.

Acneiform Eruption

Acneiform eruption is also known as folliculitis. [41] This reaction begins as a facial and upper trunk erythema. [41] In contrast with acne there are no comedones and pustules are sterile. [41] Drugs involved with acneiform eruptions are actinomycin D, geftinib and cetuximab. [42, 43, 44, 45] These lesions can cause a psychological impairment, especially if located in the face. Treatment options include: topical retinoid, oral and topical antibiotics and benzoyl peroxide. [41]

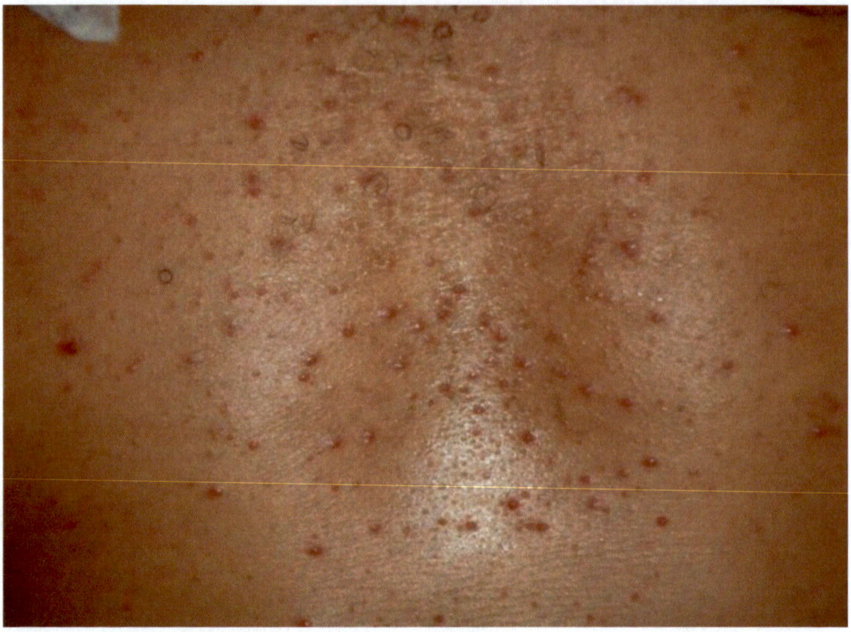

Figure 4. Cetuximab induced Acneiform eruption on the back.

Conclusion

Geriatric patients undergoing chemotherapy may experience different degrees of cutaneous reactions. The appropriate management of chemotherapy side effects in this population can be challenging. Chemotherapy induced alopecia causes serious psychological distress, especially for female patients. Nail changes, mucositis, hand foot syndrome and other skin rashes are common side effects of chemotherapy agents used by geriatric population. Patients should be carefully prepared and informed about all the steps of the treatment. Psychological support is necessary before, during and after the treatment. A good doctor-patient relationship is also extremely important to minimize the psychological distress and discomfort caused by the diagnosis and treatment.

References

[1] Thun M. J., Jemal A. *Epidemiology of cancer.* In Goldman L., Schafer A. I., eds. Cecil Medicine. 24th ed. Philadelphia, Pa: Saunders Elsevier; 2011: chap 183.

[2] Kyale E., Ekundayo J., Zhang Y., Akhter S., Aban I., Love T. E., Ritchie C., Ahmed A. History of Cancer and Mortality in Community-Dwelling Older Adults. *Cancer Epidemiol.* Feb 2011; 35(1): 30-36.

[3] Yancik R. Population aging and cancer: a cross-national concern. *Cancer J.* 2005; 11:437-441.

[4] Yancik R., Ries L. A. Cancer in older persons: an international issue in an aging world. *Semin Oncol.* 2004; 31:128-136.

[5] Wingo P. A., Ries L. A., Parker S. L., Heath C. W. Jr. Long-term cancer patient survival in the United States. *Cancer Epidemiol Biomarkers Prev.* 1998; 7:271-282.

[6] Albano J. D., Ward E., Jemal A. et al., Cancer mortality in the United States by education level and race. *J Natl Cancer Inst.* 2007; 99:1384-1394.

[7] Yancik R., Wesley M. N., Ries L. A. et al., Comorbidity and age as predictors of risk for early mortality of male and female colon carcinoma patients: A population -based study. *Cancer.* 1998; 82:2123-2134.

[8] *American Cancer Society. Chemotherapy Principles.* Available: www.cancer.org/ treatment. Access: Feb, 02, 2014.

[9] Lindley C. 1., McCune J. S., Thomason T. E., Lauder D., Sauls A., Adkins S., Sawyer W. T. Perception of chemotherapy side effects cancer versus noncancer patients. *Cancer Pract.* 1999 Mar-Apr; 7(2):59-65.

[10] Bast R. C. Jr., Kufe D. W., Pollock R. E. et al., editors. Hamilton (ON): *BC Decker;* 2000.

[11] Apisarnthanarax N., Duvic M. *Dermatologic Complications of Cancer Chemotherapy.* In: Bast R. C. Jr., Kufe D. W., Pollock R. E. et al., editors. Holland-Frei Cancer Medicine. 5th edition. Hamilton (ON): BC Decker; 2000. Chapter 144.

[12] McGarvey E. L., Baum L. D., Pinkerton R. C. et al., Psychological sequelae and alopecia among women with cancer. *Cancer Pract* 9(6):283-9 (2001 Nov-Dec).

[13] Trüeb R. M. Chemotherapy-induced hair loss. *Skin Therapy Lett.* 2010 Jul-Aug; 15(7):5-7.

[14] Trueb R. M. Chemotherapy-induced alopecia. *Semin Cutan Med Surg* 28(1):11-4 (2009 Mar).

[15] Chung S., Low S. K., Zembutsu H., Takahashi A., Kubo M., Sasa M., Nakamura Y. A genome -wide association study of chemotherapy -induced alopecia in breast cancer patients. *Breast Cancer Res.* 2013; 15(5):R81.

[16] Munstedt K., Manthey N., Sachsse S. et al., Changes in self-concept and body image during alopecia induced cancer chemotherapy. *Support Care Cancer* 5(2):139-43 (1997 Mar).

[17] Van den Hurk C. J., van den Akker-van Marle M. E., Breed W. P., van de Poll-Franse L. V., Nortier J. W., Coebergh J. W. Impact of scalp cooling on chemotherapy -induced alopecia, wig use and hair growth of patients with cancer. *Eur J Oncol Nurs.* 2013 Oct; 17(5):536-40. doi: 10.1016/j.ejon.2013.02.004. Epub 2013 Apr 6.

[18] Van den Hurk C. J., van den Akker-van Marle M. E., Breed W. P., van de Poll-Franse L. V., Nortier J. W., Coebergh J. W. Cost-effectiveness analysis of scalp cooling to reduce chemotherapy -induced alopecia. *Acta Oncol.* 2014 Jan; 53(1):80-7. doi: 10.3109/ 0284186X.2013.794955. Epub 2013 Sep 23.

[19] Ekwall E. M. 1., Nygren L. M., Gustafsson A. O., Sorbe B. G. Determination of the most effective cooling temperature for the prevention of chemotherapy -induced alopecia. *Mol Clin Oncol.* 2013 Nov; 1(6):1065-1071. Epub 2013 Sep 6.

[20] Yeager C. E. 1., Olsen E. A. Treatment of chemotherapy -induced alopecia. *Dermatol Ther.* 2011 Jul-Aug; 24(4):432-42. doi: 10.1111/j.1529-8019.2011.01430.x.

[21] Wang J. 1., Lu Z., Au J. L. Protection against chemotherapy -induced alopecia. *Pharm Res.* 2006 Nov; 23(11):2505-14.

[22] Roe H. Chemotherapy-induced alopecia: advice and support for hair loss. *Br J Nurs.* 2011 May 27-Jun 9; 20(10):S4-11.

[23] De Berker D. Nail anatomy. *Clin Dermatol.* 2013 Sep-Oct; 31(5):509-15. doi: 10.1016/j.clindermatol.2013.06.006.

[24] Reich A. 1., Szepietowski J. C. Health-related quality of life in patients with nail disorders. *Am J Clin Dermatol.* 2011 Oct 1; 12(5):313-20. doi: 10.2165/11592120-000000000-00000.

[25] Gupta A., Parakh A., Dubey A. P. Chemotherapy induced nail changes. *Indian J Dermatol.* 2008; 53:204-205.

[26] Dasanu C. A., Vaillant J. G., Alexandrescu D. T. Distinct patterns of chromonychia, Beau's lines and melanoderma seen with vincristine, adriamycin, dexamethasone for multiple myeloma. *Dermatol Online J.* 2006; 12:10.

[27] Dasanu C. A., Alexandrescu D. T., Wiernik P. H. *Recognizing nail and skin changes associated with chemotherapy.* Resident and staff physician. 2006. p. 52.

[28] Gilbar P. 1., Hain A., Peereboom V. M. Nail toxicity induced by cancer chemotherapy. *J Oncol Pharm Pract.* 2009 Sep; 15(3):143-55. doi: 10.1177/1078155208100450. Epub 2009 Jan 26.

[29] McCarthy A. L. 1., Shaban R. Z., Gillespie K., Vick J. Cryotherapy for docetaxel -induced hand and nail toxicity: Randomized control trial. *Support Care Cancer.* 2014 May; 22(5):1375-83. doi: 10.1007/s00520-013-2095-x. Epub 2013 Dec 22.

[30] Minisini A. M., Tosti A., Sobrero A. F., Mansutti M., Piraccini B. M., Sacco C., Puglisi F. Taxane-induced nail changes: incidence, clinical presentation and outcome. *Ann Oncol.* 2003; 14(2):333-337. doi: 10.1093/annonc/mdg050.

[31] Saadeh C. E. Chemotherapy- and radiotherapy -induced oral mucositis: Review of preventive strategies and treatment. *Pharmacotherapy.* 2005 Apr; 25(4):540-54.

[32] Kushner J. A. 1., Lawrence H. P., Shoval I., Kiss T. L., Devins G. M., Lee L., Tenenbaum HC Development and validation of a Patient-Reported Oral Mucositis Symptom (PROMS) scale. *J Can Dent Assoc.* 2008 Feb; 74(1):59.

[33] Chen H. M. Patients' experiences and perceptions of chemotherapy -induced oral mucositis in a day unit. *Cancer Nurs.* 2008 Sep-Oct; 31(5):363-9. doi: 10.1097/01.NCC.0000305762.89109.29.

[34] Lalla R. V., Sonis S. T., Peterson D. E. Management of oral mucositis in patients who have cancer. *Dent Clin North Am.* 2008; 52:61-77.

[35] Borbasi S. 1., Cameron K., Quested B., Olver I., To B., Evans D. More than a sore mouth: patients' experience of oral mucositis. *Oncol Nurs Forum.* 2002 Aug; 29(7):1051-7.

[36] Degen A., Alter M., Schenck F., Satzger I., Völker B., Kapp A., Gutzmer R. Review The hand-foot-syndrome associated with medical tumor therapy: Classification and management. *J Dtsch Dermatol Ges.* 2010 Sep; 8(9):652-61.

[37] Qiao J. Fang H Hand-foot syndrome related to chemotherapy. *CMAJ.* Oct 16, 2012; 184(15): E818. doi: 10.1503/cmaj.111309.

[38] Lipworth A. D., Robert C., Zhu A. X. Hand-foot syndrome (hand-foot skin reaction, palmar-plantar erythrodysesthesia): Focus on sorafenib and sunitinib. *Oncology* 2009; 77:257-71.

[39] Webster-Gandy J. D., How C., Harrold K. Review Palmar-plantar erythrodysesthesia (PPE): a literature review with commentary on experience in a cancer centre. *Eur J Oncol Nurs.* 2007 Jul; 11(3):238-46.

[40] Sibaud V. 1., Dalenc F., Chevreau C., Roché H., Delord J. P., Mourey L., Lacaze J. L., Rahhali N., Taïeb C. HFS-14, a specific quality of life scale developed for patients suffering from hand-foot syndrome. *Oncologist.* 2011; 16(10):1469-78. doi: 10.1634/theoncologist.2011-0033. Epub 2011 Sep 30.

[41] Dessinioti C. 1., Antoniou C., Katsambas A. Acneiform eruptions. *Clin Dermatol.* 2014 Jan-Feb; 32(1):24-34. doi: 10.1016/j.clindermatol.2013.05.023.

[42] Walon L. 1., Gilbeau C., Lachapelle J. M. (Acneiform eruptions induced by cetuximab). *Ann Dermatol Venereol.* 2003 Apr; 130(4):443-6.

[43] Cotena C. 1., Gisondi P., Colato C., Girolomoni G. Acneiform eruption induced by cetuximab. *Acta Dermatovenerol Croat.* 2007; 15(4):246-8.

[44] Warthan M. M. 1., Jumper C. A., Smith J. L. Acneiform eruption induced by Iressa (gefitinib) tablets used to treat non-small cell lung cancer. *J Drugs Dermatol.* 2004 Sep-Oct; 3(5):569-70.

[45] DeWitt C. A. 1., Siroy A. E., Stone S. P. Acneiform eruptions associated with epidermal growth factor receptor-targeted chemotherapy. *J Am Acad Dermatol.* 2007 Mar; 56(3):500-5. Epub 2006 Dec 12.

In: Geriatric Psychodermatology
Editors: Mohammad Jafferany and Katlein França

ISBN: 978-1-63463-853-1

Chapter 18

Systemic Diseases with Psychocutaneous Involvement in the Geriatric Population

Zeba Hasan Hafeez[*], M.D.*

Introduction

Physicians can examine the skin to detect internal disease. A careful evaluation of skin lesions can be valuable in diagnosing systemic diseases. The cutaneous signs and comorbid psychiatric conditions associated with Diabetes Mellitus, thyroid disease and internal malignancies and their clinical management are discussed here.

Diabetes Mellitus

The prevalence of diabetes is increasing significantly. The Centers for Disease Control and Prevention conservatively estimates that 12% of Americans will have diabetes by 2050 [1]. It has been estimated that in high risk individuals (65–74 years), diabetes will triple, and in those aged greater than 75 years, the number of diabetic patients will increase to five times its current level. Elderly diabetes patients often have multiple medical problems and increased life expectancy implies that a greater number individuals are likely to suffer impaired quality of life because of diabetes-related complications. Approximately 20% of the elderly have mental illness such as anxiety, severe cognitive impairment, and depression; [2] 8–20% of community -dwelling elderly people can be diagnosed with major depression which tends to increase with age. Older adults have the highest rate of suicide; individuals above 85 years of age have been noted to have twice the national rate of suicide. [2]

[*] Corresponding author: Zeba Hasan Hafeez. Email: zebahafeez@hotmail.com.

Depression is also associated with physical and cognitive decline. [3] Age-related physical changes such as declining physical capacity, decreased muscle mass, visual and auditory acuity, bone strength, and joint flexibility, all contributing to functional, and cognitive decline can be more pronounced in diabetic patients.[4, 5]

The complications associated with diabetes such as diabetic retinopathy, neuropathy, may worsen with age. The elderly are more prone to hypoglycemic episodes due to polypharmacy and the increased potential for drug interaction s; metabolic changes that can affect the processing of oral diabetes drugs; hormonal changes that make it harder for them to identify when their blood glucose is too low. Changes in appetite and missed meals can be contributing factors. Medication regimens become difficult to follow in the setting of cognitive impairment.

Some common psychosocial challenges of aging also can affect both diabetes and depression. The elderly must often deal with multiple losses of family and friends, role transitions such as retirement, and fears about mortality. A longitudinal study that examined the separate and combined effects of depression and diabetes among elderly Mexican Americans concluded that both these factors predicted higher mortality, disability, complications and earlier onset of negative health outcomes. [6] Depression may relate to impaired glycemic control [7] and this predicts an adverse course of depression. [8,9] Another study based on a population aged >50 in West Ireland, concluded that patients with type 2 DM are more likely to suffer from severe depression, and that increased rates of depression observed in these patients are at least partially associated with their burden of illnesses. [10]

Cutaneous Changes Associated with Diabetes

Diabetes mellitus can be complicated by a variety of cutaneous manifestations. Good metabolic control may prevent some of these manifestations and support improvement. Most glucose-lowering drugs also have cutaneous side effects. It is important to be able to recognize these signs such that appropriate treatment can be provided.

Diabetic neuropathy affects sensory and motor nerves and the autonomic nervous system. Numbness, tin gling, aching, burning, restless legs and burning feet are frequent complaints. Autonomic neuropathy may result in decreased or absent sweating of the lower extremity with compensatory sweating of the other areas of the body.

In a diabetic patient, vitiligo can be a possible warning sign for association with autoimmune disease s. There is a dearth of information about the epidemiology of vitiligo in the elderly. In a retrospective study about the presentation of vitiligo in the elderly, the data of patients with vitiligo having onset of disease after the age of 50 showed the following results. Of the 182 patients, 87 were males and 95 were females. The mean age of onset was 55 ± 2.3 years. Vitiligo vulgaris was the most common (83.5%) followed by focal (5.5%), segmental (4.4%), acrofacial (3.8%), mucosal (2.2%), and universal (0.5%). The most common site of onset was the head and neck (24.2%) followed by the upper limbs (23%), trunk (22%), lower limbs (17.6%), oral/genital mucosae (7.1%), and flexures (6%). Associated autoimmune autoimmune/endocrine disorders were present in 39 (21.4%) of the patients. [12]

Table 1. Skin lesions comorbid with type 1 Diabetes Mellitus [11]

Clinical Lesions	Comments
Periungual telangiectasia	Linear telangiectasia due to loss of capillary loops and dilation of remaining capillaries. Nail fold erythema, fingertip tenderness.
Necrobiosis lipoidica	Non-scaly plaques, yellow atrophic center, surface telangiectasia, erythematous or violaceous border, mainly in pretibial region. Women predominantly affected. Treated with topical steroids, intra-lesional steroids at active border, or systemic steroids (rarely)
Bullosis diabeticorum	Asymptomatic, non-inflamed bullae on dorsa and sides of lower legs. Men predominantly affected. Treatment is symptomatic and conservative (aspiration or compresses)
Lichen ruber planus	Flat, polygonal, erythematous lesions on the skin.; white stripes with a reticular pattern in the mouth. Cutaneous involvement mainly seen. on wrists and dorsa of feet and lower legs. Women and men equally affected. Treated with topical corticosteroids, with or without topical cyclosporine
Vitiligo	Skin depigmentation. More common in type 1 diabetes. Treatment involves avoidance of sun exposure, use of sunscreens, cosmetic treatment if desired.

Table 2. Cutaneous changes comorbid with type 2 Diabetes Mellitus (11)

Clinical Lesions	Comments
Acrochordons (skin tags)	Small, pedunculated, soft lesions, most often on eyelids, neck, and axillae. May be a marker of impaired glucose tolerance/ diabetes. Treatment not necessary, but can be removed with grade 1 scissors, cryotherapy, electrodessication.
Yellow Nails	Yellow discoloration prominent on distal end of the hallux nail. Occasionally seen in the elderly or in onychomycosis
Diabetic thick skin	Asymptomatic; Fingers and hands most often affected. Appearance ranges from pebbling over the knuckles to diabetic hand syndrome. May represent diabetic scleredema, with peau d'orange appearance, commonly seen on back of the neck and upper back. No known effective treatment
Acanthosis nigricans	Velvety-looking hyperpigmented plaques, mainly in body folds. Can be comorbid with high levels of circulating insulin. Ointments with salicylic or retinoic acid can be applied to relieve symptoms
Diabetic dermopathy (shin spots)	Atrophic, scarring, hyperpigmented macules on the extensor surface of lower legs. Not specific for diabetes; 20% of nondiabetics can have similar lesions. Men predominantly affected; mean age is 50 years. Treatment not required.
Eruptive xanthoma	Yellow papules with an erythematous halo, seen on extensor surfaces and buttocks. Associated with high levels of triglyceride-rich lipoproteins. Resolves with normalization of carbohydrate and lipid metabolism.
Acquired perforating dermatosis	Dome-shaped papules and nodules with hyperkeratotic plug. Can occur on limbs, trunk, dorsal surface of hands. Seen in patients with kidney failure and or type 2 diabetes, less commonly with type 1 diabetes. Treatment: Avoid trauma; psoralen-ultraviolet A light, ultraviolet B light, topical and systemic retinoids, topical and intralesional steroids, oral antihistamines, cryotherapy
Calciphylaxis	Initially presents as localized redness and tenderness, later as subcutaneous nodules and necrotizing skin ulcers. Usually occurs in vascular regions with thicker subcutaneous adipose tissue. Seen predominently in patients with kidney failure. Outcome is poor; analgesics needed for the relief o f ischemic pain
Granuloma annulare	Oval or ring-shaped lesions with a raised border of skin- colored or erythematous papules. Mainly on dorsal surfaces of hands and arms. No clear association with diabetes has been established although it has been hypothesized. Treatment: sporadic success reported with steroids.

Cutaneous Reactions to Insulin

Impurities in insulin preparations, such as cow or pig proteins, the insulin molecule itself, preservatives, or additives cause allergic reaction s. Human recombinant insulin has decreased the incidence of insulin allergy, such that this is reported in less than 1% of diabetic patients treated with insulin [13].

Immediate-local reactions, mediated by immunoglobulin E (IgE), can present as erythema, which may become urticarial. Immediate reaction may progress to generalized erythema and urticaria. Anaphylaxis is unusual. Delayed hypersensitivity reactions are the most common. They usually appear about 2 weeks after the start of insulin therapy as an itchy nodule at the site of injection. Biphasic reactions are rare (an immediate and a delayed local reaction), often with a generalized illness resembling serum sickness (Arthus-immune complex reactions). [13]. Other local complications of insulin injections include keloids, hyperkeratotic papules, purpura, and localized pigmentation. [11]

For localized immediate allergic reactions switching to a more purified insulin is indicated. [11] Allergic reactions can be managed with antihistamines, addition of glucocorticoids to insulin, discontinuation of therapy, desensitization therapy, or a change in the insulin delivery system. [13, 14]. IgE-mediated anaphylaxis can be managed by temporary reduction in dose. Serum sickness is treated with corticosteroids. [15]

Cutaneous Effects of Oral Hypoglycemics

About 1% and 5% of patients taking first-generation sulfonylureas (chlorpropamide, tolbutamide) develop cutaneous reactions within the first 2 months of therapy. The most common reactions are maculopapular eruptions that often resolve with discontinuation of the medication. Generalized erythema, urticaria, lichenoid eruptions, erythema exsudativum multiforme, exfoliative dermatitis, erythema nodosum, and photosensitivity reactions can occur.

Chlorpropamide can induce an alcohol flush in 10% to 30% of patients (redness and warmth, headache, tachycardia, and occasionally dyspnea) about 15 minutes after alcohol consumption. The symptoms usually disappear after an hour. This reaction pattern is autosomal-dominant. [13]Second-generation sulfonylureas, (glipizide and glimepiride) have also been associated with cutaneous reactions.Common reactions associated with glipizide are photosensitivity, rash, urticaria, and pruritus. These are reported less often with glimepiride. [11].

Metformin, a biguanide derivative can cause a psoriatiform drug eruption, [16] erythema exsudativum multiforme, [17] and leukocytoclastic vasculitis, [18, 19], erythema, exanthema, pruritus,and urticaria. [20]. Acarbose-induced generalized erythema multiforme, [21], acute generalized exanthematous pustulosis have been reported [22].Edema has been reported as an adverse cutaneous effect of rosiglitazone and pioglitzaone [20].

Thyroid Disease in the Elderly

Many changes in thyroid function occur with aging. Thyroid physiology and microscopic anatomy are altered, and the rate at which thyroid hormone is secreted and cleared is reduced. Hypothyroidism is more likely to develop in the elderly compared to young adults, and the manifestations are often less typical, making it more difficult to diagnose thyroid disease in an older patient. [23, 24]

Microscopic and Physiologic Changes in the aging Thyroid Gland

The interfollicular connective tissue increases; the size and colloid content of the follicles decreases. The glandular epithelium undergoes atrophy and the lining cells become flattened and reduced in size. The thyroid 's uptake of iodine (as ^{131}I) somewhat declines, as well as the secretion and rate of degradation of T4. Despite the reduced T_4 output, the elderly remain euthyroid because this lower T_4 level is matched by a reduction in T_4 turnover and need for thyroid hormone. [25] The levels of thyroid-stimulating hormone (TSH) do not change with normal aging, although the amplitude of nocturnal TSH secretion does decrease somewhat with age. [26, 27] Elevated levels of TSH, however, are common in this population which could reflect a true increase in the prevalence of hypothyroidism with aging. Studies have confirmed that TSH levels rise with age, especially amongst women. [26, 28]. Elevated TSH is not a normal accompaniment of old age and indicates subclinical hypothyroidism (increased incidence in the elderly).

Thyroiditis

Patches of thyroiditis may be the precursor of Hashimoto thyroiditis which is a more diffuse, chronic form of thyroid inflammation that can preceed hypothyroidism. Postmortem examination of the thyroid glands of women older than 60 years revealed thyroiditis in 45% of cases, whereas autopsy studies of women younger than 40 indicated that 22% had thyroiditis. [29] A rising incidence of thyroiditis was seen in the autopsy specimens of men older than 60 years. However, the incidence of thyroiditis among men is lower than women at every age. The number of circulating antithyroid antibodies also increase with aging in women. In an English community survey, antithyroglobulin antibodies were found among 7.4% of women older than 74; the overall incidence for females of all ages was 3%. The incidence of antimicrosomal (antithyroid peroxidase, or anti-TPO) antibodies was 8.8% among women older than 75, compared with 7.6% among the overall female population. [28]

The clinical manifestations of hypothyroidism in elderly patients can differ significantly compared with younger persons, and may present as follows: Unexplained elevations in plasma cholesterol or triglyceride levels, (due to reduced uptake of lipids by tissues deficient in thyroid hormone), congestive heart failure (especially if there is evidence of restrictive cardiomyopathy), fecal impaction (caused by decreased gastrointestinal motility) [30], macrocytic anemia (secondary to hypothyroidism itself or from associated pernicious anemia), vague arthritic complaints (may be the presenting symptoms of hypothyroidism). [31]

Thyroid Hormone Replacement Therapy

The TSH level is believed to be the most sensitive indicator of the body's true thyroid status. Most endocrinologists recommend initiating replacement thyroid hormone therapy whenever the TSH level is above the normal range, even if the free T_4 level is still normal. Significant cardiac diseases are more likely to be comorbid in the older hypothyroid patient; and replacing thyroid hormone too vigorously can precipitate angina pectoris, rhythm disturbances, or even a myocardial infarction. For the older patient with non-emergent hypothyroidism, the most conservative approach is to start with levothyroxine, 25 μg daily for 1 to 2 weeks, followed by 50 μg daily for another 1 to 2 weeks, and then 100 μg daily. Thyroid function is checked after 6 weeks on the 100 μg/daily dosing schedule, given that thyroxine has a long half-life (6.6 days). If the free T_4 value is still not in the normal range, the daily dose of levothyroxine may be increased to 125 μg. The usual replacement dosage for younger adults is 100 to 150 μg/d, but geriatric patients generally need a lower dose. In one group of elderly hypothyroid patients, the average replacement dose was 118 μg/d (compared with 158 μg/d given to younger patients). [32]

Cutaneous Signs of Hypothyroidism. Synonyms (Myxoedema, Hypothyreosis)

Skin changes include pale, cold, scaly, wrinkled skin, xerosis, asteatitic eczema, itching, ivory yellow discoloration, edema of hands, face, eyelids, purpura and ecchymoses, punctate telangiectases (vascular dilatations) on arms and fingertips, delayed wound healing, palmoplanter keratoderma, absence of sweating, xanthomatosis (secondary to hyperlipidemia). Nails become brittle and striated, nail growth is slow. Hair changes include coarse, sparse scalp hair, loss of pubic, axillary and facial hair, madarosis (loss of lateral eyebrows), Oral changes include large tongue, oral candidosis, gingival swelling (congenital hypothyroidism) [33].

Hyperthyroidism

The clinical presentation of hyperthyroidism or thyrotoxicosis (eg weight loss, increased appetite, muscle weakness, palpitations, rapid pulse, and exophthalmos), is generally more prominent in younger patients, and less distinct in the elderly. The hyperthyroid state can cause congestive heart failure in an elderly patient. In 1924 Levine and Sturgis, [34] coined the term "masked hyperthyroidism" to describe elderly hyperthyroid patients who presented with congestive heart failure, and the diagnosis of hyperthyroidism, (the underlying cause of the heart failure), was initially overlooked.

Treatment of Hyperthyroidism

Radioiodine is the standard treatment for hyperthyroidism in an elderly patient. Antithyroid drugs (propylthiouracil or methimazole) can be effective, but have a potential for side effects and have been associated with a high recurrence rate. [35]

Cutaneous Signs in Hyperthyroidism

Skin becomes soft, smooth, velvety with increased temperature, palmer erythema, focal flushing, increased sweating, pruritus, hyperpigmentation. Pretibial myxedema and vitiligo are associated with autoimmune thyroid disease. Nail changes include fast nail growth, soft nails, koilonychias, distal onycholysis (plummer's nails). Thyroid acropachy (clubbing of the fingers and toes in graves disease, associated with soft tissue swelling and with periosteal new bone form ation). Hair become fine, thin, diffuse alopecia. [36]

Psychiatric Symptoms Associated With Thyroid Disease

Psychiatric manifestations of hypothyroidism are common among the elderly. Although classically referred to as "myxedema madness," frank psychosis is uncommon, and clinical depression is more frequent. Other age -related presenting symptoms of hypothyroidism include syncopy, seizures, and impaired cerebellar function.

It was noted that only 16% of 124 elderly hyperthyroid patients had increased nervousness (the earliest and somewhat consistent manifestation of the disease in younger patients), indicating their altered response to hyperthyroidism. [37]

According to a study of 192 patients admitted to the psychogeriatric acute ward, the basal TSH was decreased in 16% and increased in 2% of patients. Only three patients had manifest hyperthyroidism and one patient had marginal hypothyroidism. Regardless of their psychiatric diagnosis, patients with hyperthyroidism showed psychomotor agitation, whereas those with latent and marginal hypothyroidism suffered from lack of impulse. These symptoms improved after treatment with carbimazol or levothyroxine, respectively, and psychotropic drugs. [38]

Thyroid Disease and Dementia

Thyroid disease can be a reversible cause of dementia, in both hypo and hyperthyroid states. Thyroid hormone has multiple effects on the brain during early development and advanced aging, postulated to be mediated through direct effects on gene transcription and via neurochemical abnormalities. Changes have been localized to the frontal lobe and hippocampus. [39] Changes in blood flow to the brain have been associated with abnormal levels of thyroid hormone. A 69-year-old man developed hypothyroidism induced dementia as a result of I-131 therapy and an overdose of methimazole. Tc-99m HMPAO SPECT revealed diffuse cerebral hypoperfusion. However, these findings of brain SPECT normalized with the disappearance of symptoms when the euthyroid state was restored. A 25% or 26% reduction of the mean cerebral blood flow was documented during dementia, indicating that SPECT brain imaging revealed reversible hypoperfusion that correlated with reversible hypothyroid dementia. [40] Overt hypothyroidism has been closely associated with dementia. Impaired cognitive function, affecting memory, attention/concentration, and visuospatiatal ability have been described. The degree to which replacement with thyroxine reverses this cognitive decline can be variable. The association between subclinical hypothyroidism and dementia is less clear. Several studies have shown that individuals with elevated TSH, but normal T4 and T3 may have impaired neurocognitive function. [41, 42, 43]

Hyperthyroidism, although less commonly identified, can lead to cognitive changes in the elderly similar to dementia. According to one hospital based study, 33% of patients with hyperthyroidism had evidence of dementia. [44] Treatment may be effective in improving these cognitive changes to some extent. [45]

Cutaneous Signs in Internal Malignancy

Skin lesions can provide clues to internal malignancy or indicate a need for its screening. These skin changes can be referred to as dermadromes of internal malignancy or syndroma dermato-tumorale. Paraneoplastic dermatoses are the most important in the early stage of internal malignancy and include dermatomyositis, figurate erythemas, erythroderma and a number of bullous dermatoses (e.g., bullous pemphigoid, pemphigus vulgaris and dermatitis herpetiformis, sweet's syndrome, pruritus, prurigo, acanthosis nigricans, Leser-Trélat sign, alopecia mucinosa, acquired ichthyosis, Bazex' syndrome, hypertrichosis aquisita lanuginosa). [46]

There are indirect cutaneous markers of internal malignancy (markers of exposure to carcinogens, cancers of the skin related to immunosuppression). These include the following; Brown staining of fingers of a smoker in bronchogenic carcinoma. Arsenic can cause circular, brown keratosis of the palms and soles, diffuse pigmentation with rain drop areas of paler normal skin. Bowens disease on the covered parts. Radiation dermatitis as a result of radiation therapy.

Carcinoma has been noted to be the most common cancer that metastasizes to the skin, and includes lung cancer in men and breast cancer in women. Cutaneous metastasis of epithelial origin are alopecia neoplastica, pulsatile nodules, Sister Mary Joseph's nodules, morpheaform, and cellulitis -like lesions. Histologically, these lesions can reveal adenocarcinoma, squamous cell carcinoma, or anaplastic carcinoma and provide clues to the organ of origin. Lymphocytic leukemia is the commonest form of leukemia having cutaneous metastasis in elderly men. Acute myeloid leukemia that has two peaks in occurrence (early childhood and later adulthood), [47] involves the mucous membrane s. [48] Multiple myeloma would be the likely diagnosis in an elderly patient having bone pain, anemia, elevated blood calcium level, and renal failure with purplish or skin-colored nodules and plaques on the trunk. Biopsy of lesions will most likely reveal atypical plasma cells and blood immunoelectrophoresis will reveal a characteristic monoclonal gammopathy. [48] Kaposi's sarcoma, a multifocal vascular malignancy, has a wide spectrum of clinical presentation s.

Patients who are immunocompromised are more predisposed to a disseminated, fulminant course associated with opportunistic infection. [48]

The specific signs of internal malignancy seem to be less common than nonspecific ones. A study of 750 patients with proven internal malignancy (treated at a cancer chemotherapy center in South India), documented that 65% were males and 35% were females. The most common age group affected was in fifth and sixth decades of life. Of the 750 patients with internal malignancy, skin changes were seen in 52 (6.93%) patients. Cutaneous metastases (specific lesions) were seen in 20 patients (2.66%): contiguous in 6 (0.8%), and non-contiguous in 14 (1.86%). Nonspecific skin changes were seen in 32 patients (4.26%). None of the patients presented with more than one type of skin lesions. Herpes zoster was the most common nonspecific lesion observed, followed by generalized pruritus, multiple eruptive seborrheic keratoses, bullous disorder, erythroderma, flushing, purpura, pyoderma gangrenosum, insect bite allergy and lichenoid dermatitis. [49]

Psychiatric Symptoms Associated with Internal Malignancy

It has been postulated that by 2030, 20% of the United States population will be over the age of 65. Sixty percent of new cancer diagnoses and 70% of cancer deaths occur in people over the age of 65. There will be been an expected 67% increase in cancer incidence among older adults compared with an 11% increase for younger adults from 2010–2030 [50]. Rates of major depression are estimated to be 38% whereas those of depressive spectrum disorders have been found to be as high as 58% [51]. In a review of psychiatric problems in cancer patients, [52], the incidence of depression in cancer patients was estimated to be between 20–25% and increased with higher levels of disability, advanced illness and pain [52]. Another study documented that out of 201 recently diagnosed cancer patients, 15% met the criteria for Major Depression [53]. It has also been noted that although many cancer patients do not meet the criteria for Major Depression, subsyndromal symptoms are highly prevalent and likely require treatment [54, 55].

Depression in cancer patients can be under-diagnosed and under-treated. [56, 57]). In a large study of over 1100 cancer patients, it was found that oncologists had difficulty identifying patient's depression on the Zung Self-Rating Depression Scale [58]. Physicians correctly identified nearly 80% of patients without depression, but only 33% of patients with mild to moderate depression and only 13% of those with severe depression. [58].

In another study of distress in 245 older cancer patients, it was noted that more than 40% of older patients with cancer had a distress thermometer score of 4 or greater [59]. In a survey of 448 practicing oncologists, it was documented that the clincians estimated that over one-third of their patients experienced psychological distress needing intervention. However, only about 47% reported making a referral and starting psychiatric medications (mainly selective serotonin reuptake inhibitors and benzodiazepines). [60]

Depression is associated with decreased quality of life, interpersonal difficulties, sleep disturbance, [61] and correlates with rapid deterioration, more metastasis and pain compared with non-depressed cancer patients. Several recent studies have concluded that suicidal ideations and suicide among older cancer patients is higher than in patients with other medical illnesses [63, 64,65] and a notable increase in suicide in older patients with cancer has been reported [66]. Therefore in addition to the assessment of depressive symptoms, a thorough suicide assessment must be conducted.

Diagnosis of Depression in the Elderly Cancer Patients

The two main symptoms include depressed mood and anhedonia. [66] Additional symptoms that help differentiate depressive from cancer symptoms are weight loss or gain, insomnia or hypersomnia, psychomotor agitation or retardation, fatigue, feelings of worthlessness or inappropriate guilt, decreased concentration, recurrent thoughts of death or suicide.

The following symptoms differentiate symptoms of cancer and depressive symptoms in older cancer patients: general malaise or dissatisfaction rather than ‘loss of interest’ and ‘sad mood’; aches and pains as opposed to cancer or tumor specific pain are commonly reported; diffuse somatic complaints rather than specific complaints associated with treatment side effects; hopelessness with perception of little purpose to treatments compared with most patients with cancer who are somewhat hopeful about the upcoming treatments and potential outcome; insomnia, mood variation throughout the day; change/loss of sexual interest, feelings of worthlessness or inappropriate guilt, decreased concentration, recurrent thoughts of death or suicide [66].

Delirium in Cancer Patients

Delirium is the most common and grave neuropsychiatric complication in patients with advanced cancer [67]. It is frequently underdiagnosed in the clinical setting [68] is associated with increased mortality, and is often multifactorial in etiology. The diagnosis of delirium can be challenging as it is often associated with symptoms of depressed or anxious mood, behavioral disturbance, hallucinations, delusions, sleep-wake disturbances, and a characteristic waxing-waning pattern of impairment. As the cognitive disturbance in delirium can be subtle, clinicians may focus on the psychiatric disturbance. In conditions, such as delirium tremens (from alcohol, benzodiazepine, or barbiturate withdrawal), these neuropsychiatric symptoms are more prominent. An electroencephalogram will show a pattern of diffuse slowing of electrical activity.

Three delirium assessment tools used in clinical practice include the Confusion Assessment Method (CAM) [69], the Memorial Delirium Assessment Scale (MDAS) [70]and the Nursing Delirium Screening Scale (NuDESC) [71].

According to the cholinergic hypothesis a deficiency of acetylcholine and an excess of dopamine are implicated [72]. Other neurotransmitters include glutamate, serotonin, cortisol, and endogenous opioids [73]. Additionally cytokines, especially interleukin (IL)-1, IL-6, and IL-8, and also interferon and tumor necrosis factor [74, 75]. Transient thalamic dysfunction has been proposed as a mechanism for drug-induced delirium [76].

Medications that contribute to delirium [77, 78, 79, 80, 81] include opioids, benzodiazepines, anticholinergics, tricyclic antidepressant s, selective serotonin reuptake inhibitor s, neuroleptics, nonbenzodiazepine hypnotics, antineoplastic agents, Corticosteroids, antihistamines, H2 blockers, antibiotics (quinolones), metoclopramide, anticonvulsants, certain antivirals. In a prospective cohort study in 261 cancer hospital inpatients, it was found that the risk for delirium doubled if the daily dose equivalent (DDE) s.c. morphine was >90 mg/day or if the DDE of lorazepam was >2 mg/day. A DDE >15 mg/day of oral dexamethasone led to a 2.7 higher risk for the development of delirium, but no association with anticholinergics was found in that study. [77]

Medications used for the symptomatic treatment of delirium in advanced cancer patients include conventional neuroleptics, [82] (Haloperidol, Chlorpromazine). Atypical antipsychotics [82, 83] (Olanzapine, Risperidone, Quetiapine, Aripiprazole). Emerging drugs that are not currently recommended for the routine management of delirium include Methyl-phenidatehydrochloride, [84] Modafinil, [85] Melatonin, [86] Ramelteon87] Cholinesterase inhibitors, [88, 89] Cholinomimetics, [90] Valproate [91] Dexmedetomidine, [92] and Ondansetron. [93]

Nonpharmacological measures such as minimizing noise, excessive light, and excessive darkness; Essential items visible and within reach; Simple, and concise communication; Glasses, hearing aid, dentures where needed; Explanation of each intervention prior to instituting care; Orient patient frequently; Clock and calendar should be visible from the bed; Presence of familiar objects. [73]

Anxiety in Elderly Cancer Patients

Anxiety is not well studied in the geriatric cancer population. In patients with cancer the prevalence of anxiety ranges from 21% to 28%. [94] It is commonly experienced by cancer patients, is often seen at crisis points such the initial diagnosis, or following relapse after treatment. Anxiety can also be a component of pain, deliurim and depression. Persistant symptoms of anxiety that significantly impair functioning should prompt further evaluation. These can be be grouped into both cognitive, somatic symptoms. The former include fear of death, loss of control, thoughts of impending doom, overgeneralizing and catastrophizing. The somatic symptoms usually manifest as panic attacks and can present as tachycardia, shortness of breath, gastrointestinal upset, nausea, trembling, and dizziness [95, 96].

Several factors may interact to contribute to anxiety. Pain is closely associated with anxiety and agitation; and when it is adequately controlled there is usually a marked reduction in anxiety. Respiratory ailments such as lung cancer, or respiratory distress can present with anxiety and restlessness. An acute event such as a pulmonary embolus may also present as anxiety. These symptoms respond initially to an anxiolytic medication, but the anxiety ultimately responds to proper medical intervention. Sepsis, endocrine abnormalities, hypoglycemia, hypercalcemia, and hormone secreting tumors may all be associated with anxiety symptoms. Depression, anxiety, and panic attacks can occur in patients with pancreatic cancer. [97] Anxiety can also be associated with several medications (steroids, antiemetics e.g., prochlorperazine and metoclopramide, withdrawal from alcohol or benzodiazepines). [98]

A patient could have a preexisting anxiety disorder or may develop an anxiety disorder after a cancer diagnosis. The latter can include generalized anxiety disorder, panic disorder, post traumatic stress disorder. Phobias such as a fear of needles and claustrophobia can develop in individuals who undergo multiple tests or procedures.. Anxiety symptoms can occur as an anticipatory response to a repeated aversive treatment such as chemothrerapy. [95, 99]

Dementia in Cancer Patients

This syndrome has developed secondary to cancer treatment. For example dementia has been noted to develop following radio therapy of brain tumors when administered alone or in combination with nitrosourea- based chemotherapy [100]. Cognitive impairment in cancer patients is of great impotancc in relation to issues of capacity and decision making [101], and requires further evaluation. A diagnosis of dementia does not automatically determine lack of capacity. When a patient is assessed as lacking capacity, a health care proxy should be determined. Given the potentially poor quality of life for an older cancer patient with dementia, aggressive treatment should be carefully considered. With the exception of endocrine and metabloic abnormalites most dementias are not reversible. Acetylcholinestrase inhibitors like donepezil or the N-methyl-D-Aspartate antagonist, memantine can be prescribed to slow the progression of dementia and postpone the need for nursing home placement. Additionally neuroleptics may need to be used to control behavioral or psychotic symptoms that can develop in advancing dementia.

Treatment of Depression in the Elderly and Medically Ill Patients

The selection of an antidepressant should ideally be based on the best side effect profile and lowest risk of drug-drug interaction s. The selective serotonin reuptake inhibitors (SSRIs) and the newer antidepressants bupleprion, mirtazapine, and venlafaxine a selective norepinephrine reuptake inhibitor (SNRI) are all relatively safe in the elderly. They have lower anticholinergic effects and are thus well tolerated by patients with cardiovascular disease. [102] Common side effects of SSRIs include nausea, dry mouth, insomnia, somnolence, agitation, diarrhea, excessive sweating, and, less commonly, sexual dysfunction. [103]. In the elderly, there is also an increased risk of developing hyponatremia secondary to a syndrome of inappropriate antidiuretic hormone secretion. This is seen in approximately 10% of patients taking antidepressants, and is associated particularly with SSRIs and venlafaxine. [104] The sodium levels should be checked one month after starting an SSRIs, especially in patients taking other medications such as diuretics that can predispose to developing hyponatremia. Sodium levels should also be checked if symptoms of hyponatremia such as fatigue, malaise, and delirium occur. There is also an increased risk of gastrointestinal bleeding associated with SSRIs, especially in patients with peptic ulcer disease or those taking anti-inflammatory medications. [102]

SSRIs are processed through the liver and affect the P450 isoenzyme system. Fluoxetine is generally not recommended for use in the elderly because of its long half-life and prominent effects on P450 isoenzyme system. Paroxetine is also typically not recommended in the elderly as it has the highest anticholinergic effect of all the SSRIs, similar to that of the tricyclics desipramine and nortriptyline. [105] Fluoxetine, paroxetine, and fluvoxamine have higher risks of drug-drug interaction s. [102]

The SSRIs considered to have the best safety profile in the elderly are citalopram, escitalopram, and sertraline. [106]. These have the lowest potential for drug-drug interactions based on their cytochrome P-450 interactions. Venlafaxine, mirtazapine, and bupropion are also considered to have a good safety profile in terms of drug-drug interactions. [106] In August 2011, the U.S. Food and Drug Administration (FDA) issued a drug safety communication that citalopram should not be used at dosages greater than 40 mg per day (or greater than 20 mg per day for patients 60 and older) as it could cause abnormal heart rhythms with higher doses. However, clinical studies using citalopram in patients with cardiac disease and in older patients have not confirmed this. Demethylcitalopram, the major metabolite of citalopram, is subsequently metabolized to the minor metabolite didemethylcitalopram (DDCT). High DDCT concentrations have been associated with QT interval prolongation in beagle dogs. Therapeutic drug monitoring study data suggest that routine or even high oral doses of citalopram would unlikely reach cardiotoxic concentrations of the DDCT metabolite. Various studies suggest that the citalopram dose limitations described in the safety announcement does not have strong clinical justification [107] [108].

Tricyclic antidepressants should not be considered first-line agents for older adults given their potential for side effects, including postural hypotension, which can contribute to falls and fractures, cardiac conduction abnormalities, and anticholinergic effects (delirium, urinary retention, dry mouth, and constipation). [102] Many medical conditions seen in the elderly, (dementia, Parkinson disease, and cardiovascular problems) can be worsened by a tricyclic antidepressant. If a tricyclic is chosen as a second-line medication, then nortriptyline and desipramine are the best choices given that they are less anticholinergic. [106] Also, it is recommended that an ECG and postural blood pressure reading be obtained before starting a patient on a tricyclic antidepressant and after increasing the dose. [105]. Blood levels should be monitored as levels can be high despite low doses because some patients can be slow metabolizers. Monoamine oxidase inhibitors (MAOIs) are not considered first or even second-line agents for depression in the elderly, given their side effect profile, high rates of drug-drug interactions and with certain foods. Nefazodone has received a black box warning from the FDA for cases of hepatic failure and has had decreased usage.

Increased risk of side effects from antidepressant use in the elderly exists due to changes in hepatic metabolism associated with aging, concurrent medical conditions, and drug-drug interaction s. Therefore the starting dose should be half that prescribed for a younger adult such that side effects are minimized. [105] It may not be necessary to titrate upwards very slowly in all individuals; the goal should be to increase the dose as tolerated at 1- to 2-week intervals in order to reach an average therapeutic dose more quickly. [109] Although this dose is generally lower than that prescribed for younger adults, there is much individual variability and some patients may require a higher than average therapeutic dose. [105] If there is no significant improvement after 2 to 4 weeks on an average therapeutic dose, further increases should be made until there is either a clinical improvement, intolerable side effects, or the maximum suggested dose is reached. It is also important to monitor for any worsening of depression, emergence of agitation or anxiety, as well as suicide risk, especially in the early stages of treatment. However, there has been no evidence of increased suicidal ideation due to antidepressant use in the elderly [110]. If there is no improvement after 4 weeks or unsatisfactory results after 8 weeks on the maximum recommended or tolerated dose of an antidepressant, then it should be changed.

Stopping some medications suddenly (especially venlafaxine and paroxetine) can precipitate a withdrawal syndrome (anxiety, insomnia, and flu-like symptoms). This can be prevented with gradual tapering. [111]. Generally, a 7 to 10-day tapering period is recommended for all antidepressants.

Placebo-controlled studies suggest that duloxetine is an effective treatment for depression in the elderly and generally well tolerated at 60 mg daily. [112, 113] It has been seen that Duloxetine improved cognition, depression, and some pain measures and was safe and well tolerated in elderly patients. [113, 114] Mirtazapine is a sedating antidepressant, is less likely to cause gastrointestinal (GI) distress and often leads to weight gain. All of these side effects can be useful for cancer patients who have insomnia, GI distress, and weight loss. Its orally disintegrating tablet form, (Remeron SolTab), can be offered to patients with swallowing difficulty. Methylphenidate has been used in the medically ill depressed elderly, and was found to be effective in treating depressive symptoms, fatigue, and apathy [115]. It has also been administered to ameliorate opioid-induced somnolence, to augment the analgesic effects of opioids, to treat depression, and to improve cognitive function in patients with cancer. [116]

Tamoxifen which is widely used in the treatment of breast cancer, is a prodrug metabolized mainly by the cytochrome P450 isoform CYP2D6 into the active metabolite endoxifen. SSRIs and SNRIs have been effectively used for the treatment of depression and hot flashes, both of which frequently occur in tamoxifen -treated women. Clinicians should be cautious about using strong inhibitors and/or inducers of cytochrome 2D6 as well as 3A4 concomitantly with tamoxifen. Paroxetine, fluoxetine and bupropion are strong CYP2D6 inhibitors which should be avoided in such patients. Fluvoxamine and nefazodone both inhibit CYP3A, which could potentially affect the metabolism of tamoxifen. Gabapentin (given its lack of interaction with cytochrome P450) is effective in treating tamoxifen-induced hot flashes. Treatment with desvenlafaxine and pregabalin could be considered as well although desvenlafaxine has not yet been studied in this population. [117]

Add-on treatment can be considered which include either an antidepressant of a different class or another agent such as an antipsychotic.[102] Atypical antipsychotics used as add-on therapy in the treatment of depression shows some promise. Recently, three placebo - controlled trials suggested efficacy of adjuvant aripiprazole in older adults with an unsatisfactory response to standard antidepressant treatment, resulting in a significant reduction of depressive symptoms and improvement in remission rates. [118] In an open-label trial of risperidone augmentation in older patients who had failed to remit on a previous antidepressant, remission was achieved in a substantial number of patients and a non significant delay in time to relapse. [119] In older adults, the use of atypical antipsychotics have the risk of causing extrapyramidal symptoms and falls as well as sedation, weight gain, dyslipidemia, and diabetes. There is also a black box warning given their association with an increased risk of death, mainly due to cerebrovascular events, among elderly demented patients compared with placebo. [120] However, atypical antipsychotics may prove to be an effective treatment for severe or refractory depression in the elderly who fail to respond fully to other medications. Atypical antipsychotics in low doses are also recommended for the treatment of psychotic symptoms associated with depression. Overall, rates of recovery from psychotic depression in the elderly are low at 33% with medication alone. [102]

Electroconvulsive therapy (ECT) is a very effective antidepressant treatment that is also safe in elderly patients. Relative contraindications may include CNS masses or severe cardiac problems. ECT can in fact be useful for those patients who cannot tolerate medications, have been refractory to multiple trials of different classes of antidepressants or are acutely suicidal such that a quick improvement in symptoms is required for their safety. It can also be useful in individuals whose cancer or other treatments interact with available antidepressant medication s. In the elderly, a recovery rate of over 80% and a faster and fuller response compared to medications has been noted. [106]

Additionally, better treatment outcomes and fewer side effects than medications have been noted. [102]. In cases of psychotic and severe depression, maintenance ECT treatment is typically combined with an antidepressant, thus the use of an antipsychotic medication is avoided. [102]

In a recent case-control study, falls, cardiovascular factors, confusion, gastrointestinal, pulmonary, and metabolic side effects for "old-old" (>75 years) patient groups treated with either electroconvulsive therapy (ECT) or pharmacotherapy were compared. It was noted that individuals receiving ECT had overall fewer side effects and better treatment outcomes. Authors concluded that ECT appears to be relatively safe and more effective than pharmacotherapy for major depressive disorders in patients who are 75 years of age and older. (121)The main side effect of ECT is short-term memory disturbance. Unilateral ECT is associated with a lower incidence of cognitive effects than bilateral ECT.

Besides medications, other therapies for depression that may be considered include various forms of psychotherapy such as interpersonal psychotherapy and/or cognitive-behavioral therapy, as well as increasing social supports and reducing disability and dependence. [102].

Treatment of Anxiety in Elderly Cancer Patients

Educational and emotional support from primary care team is an important therapeutic strategy. Milder forms of anxiety may benefit with the following or may need to be combined with medications if symptoms are severe and disabling. Several cognitive behavioral interventions such as meditation, guided imagery, progressive relaxation, biofeedback, hypnosis, and reframing negative, irrational thoughts have been helpful. Insight oriented, supportive, and group therapy can reduce anxiety. The use of medications to treat anxiety in the elderly cancer population should be approached carefully. In younger individuals benzodiazepines may be one of the first lines of treatment. However, in the elderly, alternative medications should be tried initially and lower doses of benzodiazapines should be administered if needed. Nonbenzodiazapines such as buspar (15 to 45 mg daily) and antidepressants (SSRIs, tricyclics, SNRIs) have been helpful. [122] Atypical neuroleptics have no effect on respiration, and are less likely to cause confusion compared to benzodiazapines. Most may prolong QT interval to a varying degree. Risperidone (0.25 to 2 mg q 12 hours), Olanzapine (2.5 – 5 mg q 12 hours), and quetiapine (25 mg -100 mg q 12 hours) have been preferred to typicals such as haloperidol, given better tolerance in low doses (decreased risk of akathesia). It is unclear if Ziprasidone and aripiprazole are helpful for anxiety. [122]

References

[1] Narayan KMV, Boyle JP, Geiss LS, Saaddine JD, Thompson TJ: Impact of recent increase in incidence on future diabetes burden. *Diabetes Care* 29: 2114–2116,2006.

[2] Paula M. Trief, PhD. *Depression in Elderly Diabetes Patients,* Diabetes Spectrum April 2007 vol. 20 no. 2 71-75.

[3] Sachs-Ericsson N, Joiner T, Plant EA, Balzer DG: The influence of depression on cognitive decline in community -dwelling elderly persons. *Amer J Ger Psychiatry* 13:402 –408, 2005.

[4] Bruce DG, Casey GP, Grange V, Clarnette RC, Almeida OP, Foster JK, Ives FJ, Davis TM: Cognitive impairment, physical disability, and depressive symptoms in older diabetes patients. *Diabetes Res Clin Pract* 61: 59–67,2003.

[5] Kanaya AM, Barret-Connor E, Gildengorin G, Yaffe K: Change in cognitive function by glucose tolerance status in older adults: a 4-year prospective study of the Rancho Bernardo study cohort. *Arch Intern Med* 164: 1327–1333,2004.

[6] Black SA, Markides KS, Ray LA: Depression predicts increased incidence of adverse health outcomes in older Mexican Americans with type 2 diabetes. *Diabetes Care* 26:2822 –2828, 2003.

[7] Lustman PJ, Anderson RJ, Freedland KE, DeGroot MK, Carney RM, Clouse RE: Depression and poor glycemic control: a meta-analytic review of the literature. *Diabetes Care* 23:934 –942, 2000.

[8] Testa MA, Simonson DC: Health economic benefits and quality of life during improved glycemic control in patients with type 2 diabetes mellitus: a randomized, controlled, double-blind trial. *JAMA* 280:1490 –1496, 1998.

[9] Lustman PJ, Clouse RE: Treatment of depression in diabetes: impact on mood and medical outcome. *Psychom Res* 53:917 –924, 2002.

[10] Foran E, Hannigan A, Glynn L. Prevalence of depression in patients with type 2 diabetes mellitus in Irish primary care and the impact of depression on the control of diabetes. *Ir J Med Sci.* 2014 Apr 11. [Epub ahead of print].

[11] Hattem SV, Bootsma AH, Thio B. *Cleveland Clinic Journal of Medicine*, November 2008 vol. 75 11 772-787.

[12] Dogra S, Parsad D, Handa S, Kanwar AJ. *Late onset vitiligo: a study of 182 patients.* 2005 Mar;44(3):193-6.

[13] Ferringer T, Miller F. Cutaneous manifestations of diabetes mellitus. *Dermatol Clin* 2002; 20:483–492.

[14] Sibbald RG, Schachter RK. The skin and diabetes mellitus. *Int J Dermatol*, 1984; 23:567–584.

[15] Grammer L. Insulin allergy. *Clin Rev Allergy* 1986; 4:189–200.

[16] Koca R, Altinyazar HC, Yenidünya S, Tekin NS. Psoriasiform [sic] drug eruption associated with metformin hydrochloride: a case report. *Dermatol Online J* 2003; 9:11.

[17] Burger DE, Goyal S. Erythema multiforme from metformin. *Ann Pharmacother* 2004; 38:1537.

[18] Klapholz L, Leitersdorf E, Weinrauch L. Leucocytoclastic vasculitis and pneumonitis induced by metformin. *BMJ* (Clin Res Ed) 1986; 293:483.

[19] Ben Salem C, Hmouda H, Slim R, Denguezli M, Belajouza C, Bouraoui K. Rare case of metformin -induced leucocytoclastic vasculitis. *Ann Pharmacother* 2006; 40:1685–1687.

[20] Litt JZ. Litt's Drug Eruption Reference Manual. London: Taylor and Francis, 2001.

[21] Kono T, Hayami M, Kobayashi H, Ishii M, Taniguchi S. Acarbose-induced generalized erythema multiforme. *Lancet* 1999; 354:396–397.

[22] Poszepczynska-Guigné E, Viguier M, Assier H, Pinquier L, Hochedez P, Dubertret L. Acute generalized exanthematous pustulosis induced by drugs with low-digestive absorption: acarbose and nystatin. *Ann Dermatol Venereol* 2003; 130:439–442.

[23] Mariotti S, Franceschi C, Cossarizza A, Pinchera A. The aging thyroid. *Endocr Rev* 1995;16:686-715.

[24] Mokshagundam S, Barzel US. Thyroid disease in the elderly. *J Am Geriatr Soc.* 1993;41:1361-1369.

[25] Gregerman RI, Gaffney GW, Shock NW. Thyrox-ine turnover in euthyroid man with special reference to changes with age. *J Clin Invest.* 1962;41:2065-2074.

[26] Sawin CT, Chopra D, Azizi F, et al. The aging thyroid. Increased prevalence of elevated serum thyrotropin levels in the elderly. *JAMA.* 1979;242: 247-250.

[27] Bahemuka M, Hodkinson HM. Screening for hypothyroidism in elderly inpatients. *Br Med J.* 1975;2: 601-603.

[28] Tunbridge WM, Evered DC, Hall R, et al. The spectrum of thyroid disease in a community: the Whickham survey. *Clin Endocrinol* (Oxf). 1977;7: 481-493.

[29] Williams EG, Doniach I. Post-mortem incidence of focal thyroiditis. *J Pathol Bacteriol.* 1962;83:225-264.

[30] 30)Yaylali O, Kirac S, Yilmaz M, Fulya Akin, Yuksel D, Demirkan N et al. Does Hypothyroidism Affect Gastrointestinal Motility? *Gastroenterol Res Pract.* Volume 2009 (2009): ID 529802; 7 pages.

[31] Melmed S, Hershman JM. The thyroid and aging. In: Korenman SG, ed. Endocrine Aspects of Aging. New York: Elsevier Biomedical; 1982:33-53.

[32] Rosenbaum RL, Barzel US. Levothyroxine replacement dose for primary hypothyroidism decreases with age. *Ann Intern Med.* 1982;96:53-55.

[33] Cox NH, coulson IH, Systemic disease and the Skin. Endocrine Disorders. *Rook's textbook of dermatology,* 8th edition. Ed Burns T, Creathnach S, Cox N, Griffiths, Wiley-Blackwell, UK, 2010. Vol 3, 62.10.

[34] Levine SA, Sturgis CC. Hyperthyroidism masked as heart disease. *Boston Med Surg J.* 1924; 190:233-237.

[35] Rehman SU, Cope DW, Senseney AD, Brzezinski W. Thyroid Disorders in Elderly Patients. *South Med J.* 2005;98(5):543-549.

[36] Cox NH, coulson IH, Systemic disease and the Skin. Endocrine Disorders. Rook's textbook of dermatology, 8th edition. Ed Burns T, Creathnach S, Cox N, Griffiths, Wiley-Blackwell, UK, 2010. Vol 3, 62.7.

[37] Bartels EJ, Kingsley JW. Hyperthyroidism in patients over sixty. *Geriatrics.* 1949;4:333-340.

[38] Wagner H. Thyroid gland disorders in elderly psychiatric patients. *Z Gerontol.* 1992 Sep-Oct;25(5):335-8.

[39] White HK, Hommet EL, Cohen HJ. Medical Causes of Dementia, Part 11:Metabolic, Organ related, Nutritional, Toxic, and Psychiatric. *Priniples and Practice of Geriatric*

Psychiatry; second ed. Editors Agronin ME, Maletta GJ. Lippincott Williams &Wilkin. Philadelphia; 2011:p 370.

[40] Kinuya S, Michigishi T, Tonami N, Aburano T; Tsuji S, Hashimoto T. Reversible Cerebral Hypoperfusion Observed With Tc-99m HMPAO SPECT in Reversible Dementia Caused by Hypothyroidism. *Clinical Nuclear Medicine*: September 1999 - Volume 24 - Issue 9 - pp 666-668.

[41] Monzani F, Del Guerra P, Caraccio N, Pruneti CA, Pucci E, Luisi M, Baschieri L. Subclinical hypothyroidism: neurobehavioral features and beneficial effect of L-thyroxine treatment. *Clin Investig*. 1993 May;71(5):367-71.

[42] Quijano del ser, Delgado C, Martinez ES, et al. Cognitive deficiency in mild hypothyroidism. *Neurologica*; 2000;15;193-198.

[43] McDermott MT, Ridgway EC. Subclinical hypothroidism is mild thyroid failure and should be treated. *J Clin Endocrinol Metab*. 2001;86:4585-4590.

[44] Martin FI, Deam DR. Hyperthyroidism in elderly hospitalized patients. Clinical features and treatment outcomes. *Med J Aust.;* 1996; 164; 200-203.

[45] Fukui T, Hasegawa Y, Takenaka H. Hyperthyroid dementia clinicoradiological findings and response to treatment. *J Neurol Sci*; 2001;184; 81-88.

[46] Ryoho GTK. *Useful cutaneous markers of internal malignancy in the early stage*. 1988 Apr;15(4 Pt 2-3):1564-8.

[47] Deschler B, Lübbert M. Acute myeloid leukemia: epidemiology and etiology. *Cancer*. 2006 Nov 1;107(9):2099-107.

[48] Kaplan RP. Specific cutaneous manifestations of internal malignancy. *Adv Dermatol.* 1986;1:3-42.

[49] Ayyamperumal A, Tharini GK, Ravindran V, Parveen B. Cutaneous Manifestations of Internal Malignancy. *Indian J Dermatol*. 2012, Jul-Aug; 57(4): 260–264.

[50] Smith BD, Smith GL, Hurria A, Hortobagyi GN, Buchholz TA. Future of cancer incidence in the United States: burdens upon an aging, changing nation. *J Clin Oncol.* 2009;27(17):2758–65.

[51] Massie MJ. Prevalence of depression in patients with cancer. *J Natl Cancer Inst Monogr*. 2004;(32):57–71.

[52] Breitbart W. Identifying patients at risk for, and treatment of major psychiatric complications of cancer. *Support Care Cancer*. 1995;3(1):45–60.

[53] Grassi L, Rosti G. Psychosocial morbidity and adjustment to illness among long-term cancer survivors. A six-year follow-up study. *Psychosomatics*. 1996;37(6):523–32.

[54] Sellick SM, Crooks DL. Depression and cancer: an appraisal of the literature for prevalence, detection, and practice guideline development for psychological interventions. *Psychooncology*. 1999;8(4):315–33.

[55] Pasquini M, Biondi M. Depression in cancer patients: a critical review. *Clin Pract Epidemol Ment Health*. 2007;3:2.

[56] Massie MJ, Holland JC. Diagnosis and treatment of depression in the cancer patient. *J Clin Psychiatry*. 1984;45(3 Pt 2):25–9.

[57] Greenberg DB. Barriers to the treatment of depression in cancer patients. *J Natl Cancer Inst Monogr*. 2004;(32):127–35.

[58] Passik SD, Dugan W, McDonald MV, Rosenfeld B, Theobald DE, Edgerton S. Oncologists' recognition of depression in their patients with cancer. *J Clin Oncol.* 1998;16(4):1594–600.

[59] Hurria A, Li D, Hansen K, Patil S, Gupta R, Nelson C, Lichtman SM, Tew WP, Hamlin P, Zuckerman E. Distress in Older Patients With Cancer. *J Clin Oncol.* 2009; 27(26): 4346–4351.

[60] Muriel AC, Hwang VS, Kornblith A, Greer J, Greenberg DB, Temel J, Schapira L, Pirl W. Management of psychosocial distress by oncologists. *Psychiatr Serv.* 2009;60(8):1132–4.

[61] Alexopoulos GS. Depression in the elderly. *Lancet.* 2005;365(9475):1961–70.

[62] Miller M, Mogun H, Azrael D, Hempstead K, Solomon DH. Cancer and the risk of suicide in older Americans. *J Clin Oncol.* 2008;26(29):4720–4.

[63] Walker S, Chen L, Madden R. Deaths due to suicide: the effects of certification and coding practices in Australia. *Aust N Z J Public Health.* 2008;32(2):126–30.

[64] Akechi T, Okamura H, Kugaya A, Nakano T, Nakanishi T, Akizuki N, Yamawaki S, Uchitomi Y. Suicidal ideation in cancer patients with major depression. *Jpn J Clin Oncol.* 2000;30(5):221–4.

[65] Misono S, Weiss NS, Fann JR, Redman M, Yueh B. Incidence of suicide in persons with cancer. *J Clin Oncol.* 2008;26(29):4731–8.

[66] Weinberger MI, Roth AJ, Nelson CJ. Untangling the complexities of depression diagnosis in older cancer patients. *Oncologist.* 2009;14(1):60–6.

[67] Lawlor PG, Bruera ED. Delirium in patients with advanced cancer. *Hematol Oncol Clin North Am* 2002;16:701–714.

[68] Delirium in Inouye SK. Delirium in older persons. *N Engl J Med* 2006;354:1157–1165.

[69] Inouye SK, van Dyck CH, Alessi CA et al. Clarifying confusion: The confusion assessment method. A new method for detection of delirium. *Ann Intern Med* 1990;113:941–948.

[70] Breitbart W, Rosenfeld B, Roth A et al. The Memorial Delirium Assessment Scale. *J Pain Symptom Manage* 1997;13:128 –137.

[71] Gaudreau JD, Gagnon P, Harel F et al. Fast, systematic, and continuous delirium assessment in hospitalized patients: The nursing delirium screening scale. *J Pain Symptom Manage* 2005;29:368 –375.

[72] Trzepacz PT. Is there a final common neural pathway in delirium? Focus on acetylcholine and dopamine. *Semin Clin Neuropsychiatry* 2000;5:132–148.

[73] Shirley H. Bush and Eduardo Bruera The Assessment and Management of Delirium in Cancer Patients. *The Oncologist* 2009, 14:1039-1049.

[74] de Rooij SE, van Munster BC, Korevaar JC et al. Cytokines and acute phase response in delirium. *J Psychosom Res* 2007;62:521–525.

[75] Adamis D, Lunn M, Martin FC et al. Cytokines and IGF-I in delirious and non-delirious acutely ill older medical inpatients. *Age Ageing* 2009;38:326–332.

[76] Gaudreau JD, Gagnon P. Psychotogenic drugs and delirium pathogenesis:The central role of the thalamus. *Med Hypotheses* 2005;64:471– 475.

[77] Gaudreau JD, Gagnon P, Harel F et al. Psychoactive medications and risk of delirium in hospitalized cancer patients. *J Clin Oncol* 2005;23:6712–6718.

[78] Han L, McCusker J, ColeMet al. Use of medications with anticholinergic effect predicts clinical severity of delirium symptoms in older medical inpatients. *Arch Intern Med* 2001;161:1099 –1105.

[79] Morita T, Tei Y, Tsunoda J et al. Underlying pathologies and their associations with clinical features in terminal delirium of cancer patients. *J Pain Symptom Manage* 2001;22:997–1006.

[80] Lawlor PG, Gagnon B, Mancini IL et al. Occurrence, causes, and outcome of delirium in patients with advanced cancer: A prospective study. *Arch Intern Med* 2000;160:786 – 794.

[81] Han L, McCusker J, ColeMet al. Use of medications with anticholinergic effect predicts clinical severity of delirium symptoms in older medical inpatients. *Arch Intern Med* 2001;161:1099 –1105.

[82] Alici-Evcimen Y, Breitbart W. An update on the use of antipsychotics in the treatment of delirium. *Palliat Support Care* 2008;6:177–182.

[83] Boettger S, Breitbart W. Atypical antipsychotics in the management of delirium:A review of the empirical literature. *Palliat Support Care* 2005;3:227–237.

[84] Gagnon B, Low G, Schreier G. Methylphenidate hydrochloride improves cognitive function in patients with advanced cancer and hypoactive delirium:A prospective clinical study. *J Psychiatry Neurosci* 2005;30:100–107.

[85] Breitbart W, Alici Y. Agitation and delirium at the end of life: "We couldn't manage him." *JAMA* 2008;300:2898 –2910.

[86] Hanania M, Kitain E. Melatonin for treatment and prevention of postoperative delirium. *Anesth Analg* 2002;94:338 –339.

[87] Hatta K, Kishi Y, Wada K, Takeuchi T;Preventive Effects of Ramelteon on Delirium. A Randomized Placebo-Controlled Trial. *JAMA Psychiatry* 2014, 71(4):397-403.

[88] Slatkin N, Rhiner M. Treatment of opioid-induced delirium with acetylcholinesterase inhibitor s: A case report. *J Pain Symptom Manage* 2004;27:268 –273.

[89] Overshott R, Karim S, Burns A. Cholinesterase inhibitors for delirium. *Cochrane Database Syst Rev* 2008:(1).

[90] Nakamura K, Kurasawa M, Tanaka Y. Apomorphine-induced hypoattention in rats and reversal of the choice performance impairment by aniracetam. *Eur J Pharmacol* 1998;342:127–138.

[91] Bourgeois JA, Koike AK, Simmons JE et al. Adjunctive valproic acid for delirium and/or agitation on a consultation-liaison service: A report of six cases. *J Neuropsychiatry Clin Neurosci* 2005;17:232–238.

[92] Riker RR, Shehabi Y, BokeschPMet al. Dexmedetomidine vs midazolam for sedation of critically ill patients: A randomized trial. *JAMA* 2009;301:489–499.

[93] Bayindir O, Gu¨den M, Akpinar B et al. Ondansetron hydrochloride for the treatment of delirium after coronary artery surgery. *J Thorac Cardiovasc Surg* 2001;121:176 –177.

[94] Payne DK, Massie MJ:Anxiety in palliative care, in Chochinov HM, Breitbart WS (eds): *Handbook of Psychiatry in palliative medicine,* pp 63-74. New York, Oxford University Press, 2000.

[95] Goy E, Ganzini L: End of Life care in eriatric psychiatry. *Clin Geriatr Med* 19:841-856, 2003.

[96] Barraclough J:ABC of palliative care: Depression, anxiety, and confusion. *Br med J,* 315:1365-1368, 1997.

[97] Passik SD, Roth AJ: Anxiety symptoms and panic attacks preceding pancreatic cancer diagnosis. *Psychooncology* 8:268-272, 1999.

[98] Winell J, Roth A. Psychiatric assessment and symptom management in elderly cancer patients. *Oncology.* 2005 Oct;19(11):1479-90; discussion 1492, 1497, 1501-7.
[99] Jacobsen P, Bovberg D, Redd W: Anticipatory anxiety in women receiving chemotherapy for breast cancer. *Health psychol* 12:469-475, 1993.
[100] Vigliani MC, Duyckaerts C, Hauw JJ, et al: Dementia following treatment of brain tumors with radiotherapy administered alone or in combination with nitrosourea-based chemotherapy: A clincal and pathological study. *J Neurooncol* 41:137-149.
[101] Davis BD, Fernandez F, Adams F, Holmes V, Levy JK, Lewis D, Neidhart J. Diagnosis of dementia in cancer patients. Cognitive impairment in these patients can go unrecognized. *Psychosomatics.* 1987 Apr;28(4):175-9.
[102] Wiese BS. Geriatric depression: The use of antidepressants in the elderly. *BCMJ,* Vol. 53, No. 7, September 2011: 341-347.
[103] Alexopoulos GS, Katz IR, Reynolds CF, et al. Pharmacotherapy of depressive disorders in older patients. *The expert con-sensus guideline series: A postgraduatemedicine special report.* New York:McGraw-Hill; 2001.
[104] Kirby D, Harrigan S, Ames D. Hyponatraemia in elderly psychiatric patients treated with Selective Serotonin Reuptake Inhibitors and venlafaxine: A retrospective controlled study in an inpatient unit. *Int J Geriatr Psychiatry* 2002;17:231-237.
[105] Canadian Coalition for Seniors' Mental Health. National guidelines for seniors' mental health: The assessment and treatment of depression. Toronto, ON: Canadian Coalition for Seniors' Mental Health; 2006.
[106] Baldwin RC, Chiu E, Katona C, et al. *Guidelines on depression in older people*: *Practising the evidence.* London: Martin Dunitz; 2002.
[107] Bird ST, Crentsil V, Temple R, Pinheiro S, Demczar D et al. Cardiac Safety Concerns Remain for Citalopram at Dosages Above 40 mg/Day. *Am J Psychiatry* 2014;171:17-19. doi:10.1176/appi.ajp.2013.13070905.
[108] Howland RH. A critical evaluation of the cardiac toxicity of citalopram: part 2. *J Psychosoc Nurs Ment Health Serv.* 2011 Dec;49(12):13-6.
[109] Roose SP, Sackeim HA, Krishnan KR, et al. Antidepressant pharmacotherapy in the treatment of depression in the very old: A randomized, placebo -controlled trial. *Am J Psychiatry* 2004;161:2050-2059.
[110] Barak Y, Olmer A, Aizenberg D. Antidepressants reduce the risk of suicide among elderly depressed patients. *Neuropsychopharmacology* 2006;31:178-181.
[111] Baldwin DS, Montgomery SA, Nil R, etal. Discontinuation symptoms in depression and anxiety disorder s. *Int J Neuropsychopharmacol* 2005;19:1-12.
[112] Wise TN, Wiltse CG, Iosifescu DV, et al. The safety and tolerability of duloxetine in depressed elderly patients with and without medical comorbidity. *Int J Clin Pract* 2007;61:1283-1293.
[113] Nelson C, Wohlreich MM, Mallinckrodt CH, Detke MJ, Watkin JG, Kennedy JS. Duloxetine for the Treatment of Major Depressive Disorder in Older Patients. *The American Journal of Geriatric Psychiatry*, Volume 13, Issue 3; 227-235.
[114] Raskin J, Wiltse CG, Siegal A, Sheikh J, Xu J, Dinkel JJ, Rotz BT et al. Efficacy of duloxetine on cognition, depression, and pain in elderly patients with major depressive disorder: an 8-week, double-blind, placebo -controlled trial. *Am J Psychiatry.* 2007 Jun;164(6):900-9.

[115] Hardy SE. Methylphenidate for the treatment of depressive symptoms, including fatigue and apathy, in medically ill older adults and terminally ill adults. *Am J Geriatr Pharmacother* 2009;7:34-59.

[116] Rozans MDreisbach A, Lertora JJL, Kahn MJ. *Palliative Uses of Methylphenidate in Patients with Cancer: A Review*. JCO Jan 1, 2002:335-339.

[117] Desmarais JE, Looper KJ. Managing menopausal symptoms and depression in tamoxifen users: implications of drug and medicinal interactions. *Maturitas*. 2010 Dec;67(4):296-308.

[118] Steffens DC, Nelson JC, Eudicone JM, et al. Efficacy and safety of adjunctive aripiprazole in major depressive disorder in older adult patients: A pooled subpopulation analysis. *Int J Geriatr Psychiatry* 2010.

[119] Alexopoulos GS, Canuso CM, Gharabawi GM, et al. Placebo-controlled study of relapse prevention with risperidone augmentation in older patients with resistant depression. *Am J Geriatr Psychiatry* 2008;16:21-30.

[120] Schneider L, Dagerman K, Insel P. Risk of death with atypical antipsychotic drug treatment for dementia: Meta-analysis of randomized placebo -controlled trials. *JAMA* 2005; 294:1934-1943.

[121] Manly DT, Oakley SP, Bloch RM. Electroconvulsive therapy in old-old patients. *Am J Geriatric Psychiatry*, 2000;232-236.

[122] Winell J, Roth AJ. Psychiatric assessment and symptom management in elderly cancer patients. *Oncology* (Williston Park). 2005 Oct;19(11):1479-90; discussion 1492, 1497, 1501-7.

In: Geriatric Psychodermatology
Editors: Mohammad Jafferany and Katlein França

ISBN: 978-1-63463-853-1

Chapter 19

Cosmetic Dermatology for the Elderly

Maria Helena Lesqueves Sandoval**, *M.D.

Introduction

With the aging of the population, the care concerning appearance became an important issue for patients and doctors. The human being is living longer, remaining in the labor market for a longer period of time and having a larger social circle. Statistics show an increase in the number of people above 60 years of age, a fact that causes several changes in senescence. In this chapter, we will not discuss the diseases resulting from the increase of age, but the aspects related to the improvement of appearance that can be obtained with the current cosmetic treatments that will result in the satisfaction of patients in this age range. Maintenance of a youthful appearance and the beauty of the skin are very beneficial for emotional balance, a fact that has already been described in medical literature.

The skin is a powerful component of communication and is the first means of contact with the outside world. Besides its ability to exhibit important manifestations of conflicts and emotions, the skin also expresses well-being, health and mood. Beautiful and healthy skin, treated by a skin expert, allows the patient to reach advanced ages without many wrinkles, scars, blemishes or sagging. The growing interest of scientists, physicians and the pharmaceutical industry led to advances in cosmetic dermatology in the past decades. We report here how the available techniques in the cosmetic dermatology can effectively help men and women to reduce the impact of changes that results from aging.

The main objective of cosmetic Dermatology is to improve the patient's appearance, self-esteem and provide an improvement in their quality of life.

It is necessary to know the patient's previous medical history, allergies, surgeries and current medications. It is very important to establish a good physician-patient relationship by exploring their desires and meeting the real possibilities of the technique. This enables the right conduct.

* Corresponding author: Maria Helena Sandoval. Email: mhlsand@terra.com.br

Another extremely important topic is the psychological state of the patient. Starting a cosmetic treatment on a patient with emotional disorders is a big risk. Our medical skills enable us to distinguish psychiatric problems that should be treated before any aesthetic intervention.

Delaying the chronological age is impossible, but delaying the visual and psychological impact is possible. We have a considerable arsenal within cosmetic Dermatology, and the indication of the treatment will consider the needs and individuality of each patient. The psychological aspect of the patient will guide this indication because their satisfaction requires an understanding of how the procedure will be done and how they will look to themselves and the people that surround them. We should explain in detail the potential benefit that the available treatments can offer so their expectations will meet the real potential result. The patient needs to know what to expect from a treatment.

A point to be demystified concerns the artificial expression that some patients acquire after a cosmetic intervention. The result of an aesthetic treatment depends almost exclusively on the professional who does it. It is extremely important not to over treat.

It is also important to make the patient understands that the aging process happened slowly, and not overnight. Therefore, we should not try to repair all these changes in one single visit; a single procedure may not be enough to correct the changes caused by the time. Today, the combination of therapeutic methods provides an overall improvement in the appearance with the beneficial improvement of the self-esteem of the patient.

Global Aging and Indication of Aesthetic Procedures

Aging occurs both by genetics and environmental factors and lifestyle habits such as smoking, unhealthy diet and lack of exercise. The intrinsic and extrinsic aging is closely related and occurs simultaneously, leading to several epidermal, dermal, muscle and bone changes. The epidermal maturation is abnormal, leading to lower hydration, loss of brightness, uneven tone, wrinkles and skin laxity. The collagen degeneration will cause greater or lesser appearance of wrinkles. Stains and seborrheic keratosis arise from the change of the melanin pigment system and changes in the blood supply of the papillary dermis, causing telangiectasia, micro angiomas and purpura. The fragility of the skin is noticed with a minor trauma, such as the simple act of scratching. The appearance is of skin without elasticity, with wrinkles and expression lines. Bone modification of head, face and neck, also become visible in both sexes around 50 years, being more evident in women.

Several studies have shown that bone remodeling is a key factor in the pathogenesis of facial aging. By understanding these changes and the physiological mechanism of the aging of skin, we can then indicate the best procedure for the degree of aging that the patient has at the time of consultation. The dermatologist should first always ask the patient about what bothers him or her most. Accepting and respecting what ales the patient is an important step to a good relationship and the satisfaction of those who are in need of help and support.

Chemical peels, laser procedures and other technologies, Botulinum Toxin and Dermal Fillers applications, are a group of minimally invasive procedures that can be performed in a Dermatology Clinic, avoiding the inconvenience of unnecessary hospitalizations. When the degree of aging indicates a more aggressive surgical procedure, the professional will evaluate the cost -benefit and discuss the need of hospitalization. Accurate assessment of facial changes is essential since problems in this assessment will lead to errors in treatment indication. Good indication means good results and patient satisfaction.

According to Professor of Dermatology Dr. Luis Carlos Cucé, in his book "Rumos da Cosmiatria", patients' satisfaction regarding cosmiatric treatments generally achieves a rate of 75%. According to his opinion, botulinum toxin pleases 95% of patients and fillers please approximately 65% of patients. It is helpful to relate average satisfaction with improved image and quality of life of those who underwent the treatment.

We emphasize in this context that "Beauty" also involves daily skin care, cleansing, moisturizing, use of anti-aging creams and sun protection. At this stage of life, support and patient education make a lot of difference.

We will describe the clinical signs of aging in relation to the benefit of each indicated treatment.

Photoaging

The photodamage is caused by the accumulation of solar radiation, leading to a transformation of the skin where the heliodermatosis and actinescence are evident. Roughness, color changes, solar lentigines, melanosIs, wrinkles, telangiectasia's, xerosis and actinic keratosis are present. Topical skin care products recommended for daily use are rejuvenating creams that increase the turnover of cells, like the gold standard Retinoic Acid, Retinol and Retinaldehyde, and derivatives of Vitamin A Acid. Creams with Vitamin C, Vitamin E, Ferulic Acid, and Hyaluronic Acid can be associated with moisturizers such as alpha- hydroxy acids, urea, and ceramides of plant origin. This includes a huge arsenal of other products with antioxidants such as Coenzyme Q 10, idebenone, Lipoic Acid, and Flavonoids followed by antiglicants, tensioners, brighteners, etc.

Treatment will depend on the degree of photoaging that can be classified as mild, moderate or severe, according to the level of histopathological lesions. We can use the Intense Pulsed Light, fractional ablative lasers and Chemical peels.

The Intense Pulsed Light (IPL) treats mainly melanosis and telangiectasias. Very common at maturity, the embarrassment is caused by the aggravation of Rosacea in males and particularly females, caused by erythema and burning sensations. In this case the IPL may be one of the first treatment options to reduce telangiectasias, erythema and secondarily will stimulate collagen, promoting well-toned the skin.

Another great indication of IPL is the treatment of melanosis of the hands and arms, associating both non-ablative fractional laser and a superficial chemical peel right after the first procedure to renew the skin surface. A frequent complaint of patients is the emergence of these solar melanosis located on the back of the hands, making the aging process evident and increasing embarrassment. It often causes more discomfort than a wrinkle or furrow in the face. Chest and neck "reddishness" and ageing, usually not improved with conventional techniques, also have good results with the IPL.

Lasers treat more severe wrinkles. There is improvement due to contraction of collagen fibers that compose the supporting tissue of the skin, relieving wrinkles and sagging. Widely used nowadays is the CO2 laser that targets the water in the tissue. This procedure requires knowledge and observation from the practitioner since the correct dosage of power used should consider each specific case and the fact that the elderly skin is thinner and more xerotic.

Chemical peels treat the signs of photoaging. The choice of the peel will depend on the lesions presented. It can be very superficial (only reaches the stratum corneum and granular layer: 0.06 mm), superficials (up to the basal layer: 0.45 mm), medium (up to the papillary dermis: 0.6 mm) and deep (into the medial reticular dermis: 0.8 mm). Medium peels have great indication for actinic keratosis while the deep ones such as the Baker and Gordon Phenol peel treat solar elastosis with impressive results. The indication of this deep peel undergoes a comprehensive explanation from the physician to the patient about the procedure since the recovery is slow and demands attention and dedication after the procedure. In this case, this procedure should be performed in a hospital setting and requires cardiac and renal monitoring.

Case 1

Female patient, born in 1958.

This patient sought the care of a dermatologist in 2004 at age 45, telling the story that "she needed to look younger to keep her job."

At that time, she occupied an important position in a Management Insurance Company and she feared that a younger face, a bright and rested appearance, would replace her experience. She used to work directly with the public and her appearance was important in order to continue working in this company.

I suggested Botulinum Toxin Type A (BTA, IPL sessions and superficial peels following the IPL for the whitening of the face, fillers and facial bio stimulation with Poly -L - Lactic Acid (Sculptra ®) applications.

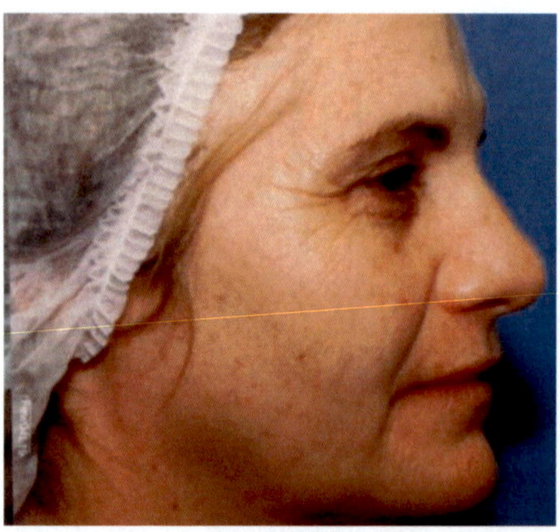

1A - 2004

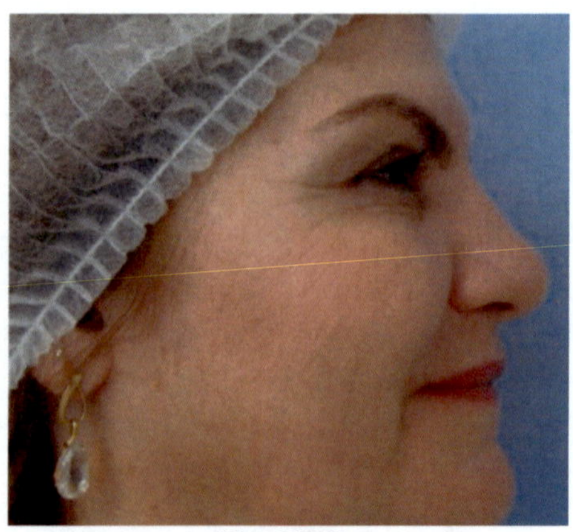

1B - 2012

Before and after treatments

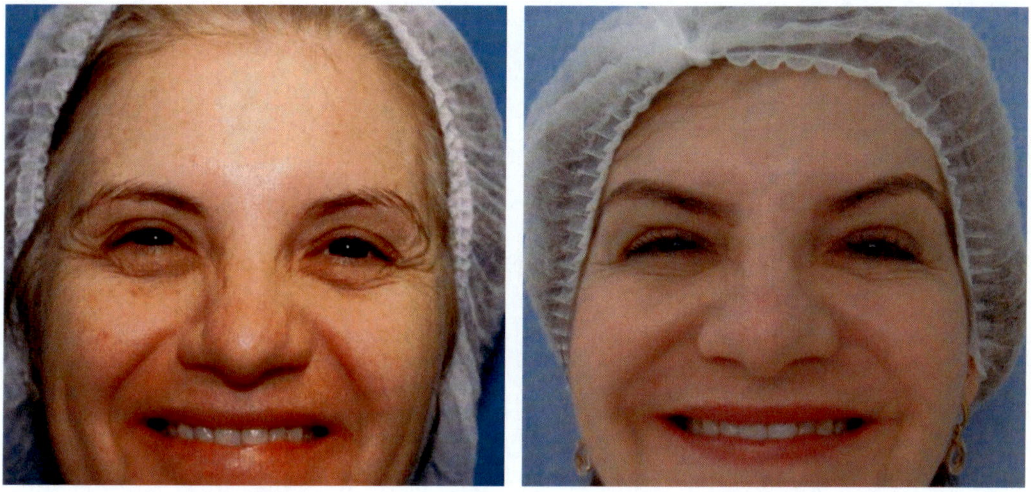

2A - 2004 2B - 2012

Before and after treatments

The pictures show her evolution and improvement. The achievement of good self-esteem occurred after Botulinum toxin sessions since 2004, fillers in eyebrow tails, 10 IPL sessions followed by superficial peels, 2 sessions of erbium glass laser (Star Lux, 1540nm) and 5 applications of Sculptra ® in the face (Dilution 6:1 ml, 1 vial per session) over 8 years. The combination of techniques brought confidence and long term permanence in her job position due her good working skills associated with a good appearance. She got an important promotion and is now assistant to the President of the Company.

Dynamic Wrinkles

The "gold standard" treatment of hyperkinetic wrinkles is undoubtedly Botulinum Toxin Type A (BTA). Wrinkles are caused by movements of the facial muscles. With the application of the substance there is a block in the motor neuromuscular transmission, reducing muscle activity. With aging, these wrinkles become more apparent on the forehead, crow's feet, perioral and glabella region. Other results that add satisfaction to aged patients is the elevation of the eyebrow tail, the elevation of the angle of the mouth and the technique of "Nefertiti", where we apply the toxin in the facial and cervical depressor muscles to improve contour and highlighting in the middle third of the face by the action of muscles that were not blocked.

In 2009, a publication of the Journal of Cosmetic Dermatology showed highly significant evidence that the improvements in forehead wrinkles, glabella and corrugator improved patients with depression. The improvement would be due to the psychological mechanism of this effect, leading to less facial feedback for negative emotions. This would make it difficult to maintain the negative effect of the contraction evolving into a better mood.

Another great use of Botulinum Toxin is for the treatment of facial asymmetry caused by sequelae of paralysis, facial trauma, sequelae of cerebrovascular accident (CVA), blepharospasm etc. Because they are very disabling, both from a functional and aesthetic perspective, facial paralysis is a serious problem of acceptance and low self esteem. The correction of these situations by rebalancing the muscles will cause an improvement in function and aesthetic conditions of the patient. The final result will be a significant improvement in the quality of life translated by a symmetrical smile and a happier aspect.

Case 2

Male patient, born in 1942, presenting an aged face with many wrinkles that never bothered him. He showed great discomfort after sequel of a brain surgery to remove a benign tumor that resulted in a significant unilateral intermittent spasm of all the facial muscles that extends to the left ear. This worsens with stress or when stirring, accompanied by blepharospasm on the same side.

He was referred to the clinic by his daughter for the application of Botulinum Toxin for the treatment of this important facial asymmetry. The toxin was applied throughout the area that had spasms and also on the contralateral side (fewer units) for correction of asymmetry.

After this physical improvement, his psychological improvement was also significant, regaining his joy. He sought out a dentist for a treatment and tooth whitening. He made several international trips with the grandchildren such as trips to Disney World, Spain and skiing in Bariloche. His joy is contagious and he is currently learning English and Spanish.

He continues getting BTA applications. He made a total of seven applications so far, with important correction of facial asymmetry and dramatic reduction of muscle spasms.

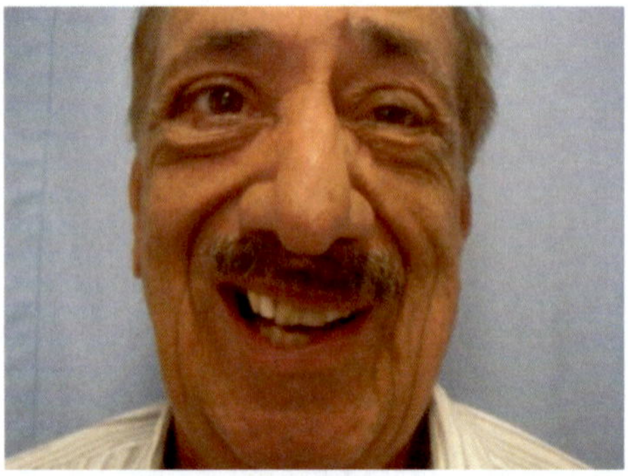

3A - 2011

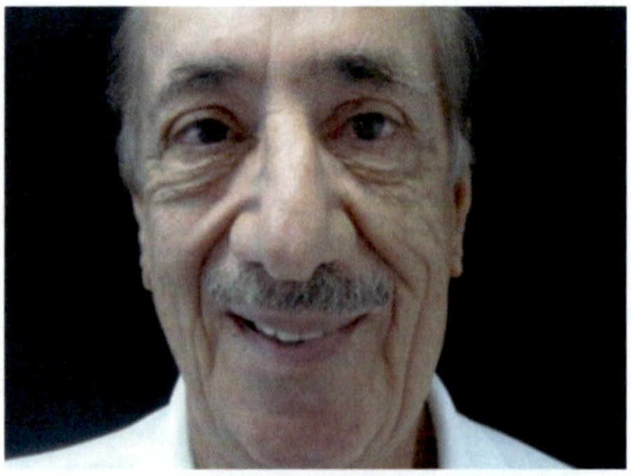

3B - 2014

Photos of the patient before treatment with emphasis on the correction of facial asymmetry

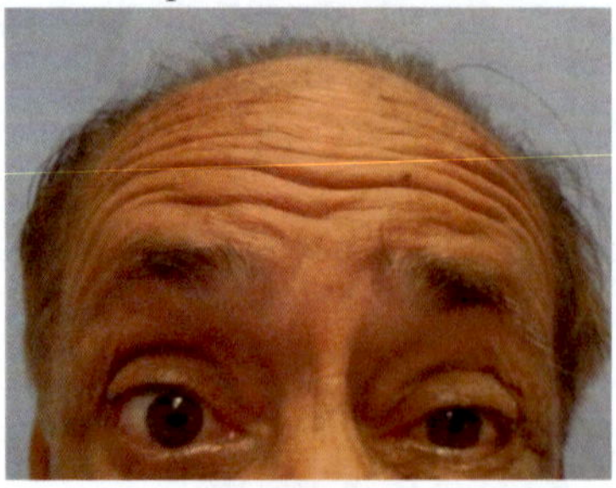

4A - 2011

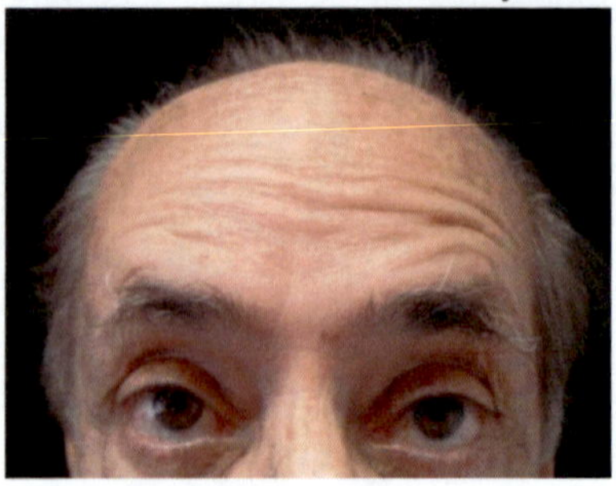

4B - 2014

Pictures of the patient before the treatment showing a reduction of the asymmetry, the blepharospasm and left facial "pulling"

Volume Facial Changes

In the study of the field of facial fillers, the evolution was very significant since the discovery of the first filler until the current volumizing used for subcutaneous or supraperiosteal level. Often, only the volume replacement leads to effective results without the use of other techniques.

It is known that in older people, there is a significant generation of bone remodeling. Knowing this, we will decide which dermal filler will cause improvement, explaining to the patient that not everything is correctable when there is a lack of a “floor” to sustain the filler.

It is essential to examine the entire face valuing facial volume as a whole and avoiding isolated correction of wrinkles or furrows. Treatment should pursue a three-dimensional perspective. Thus, we can improve the nasolabial folds after filling the malar area if there is not much sagging.

There are various fillers on the market, temporary or permanent, other than those considered biostimulators, which are best for sagging. There is a choice for temporary fillers due to the low rate of adverse effects. The most used products are made with hyaluronic acid in its multiple presentations, calcium hydroxyapatite and poly-L-lactic acid. We opt for the last one when we notice a significant loss of tone and sagging. Fillers should be avoided in people who have some kind of allergy to components of the product, autoimmune diseases or who have permanent fillers in place.

Case 3

A male patient, born in 1941.

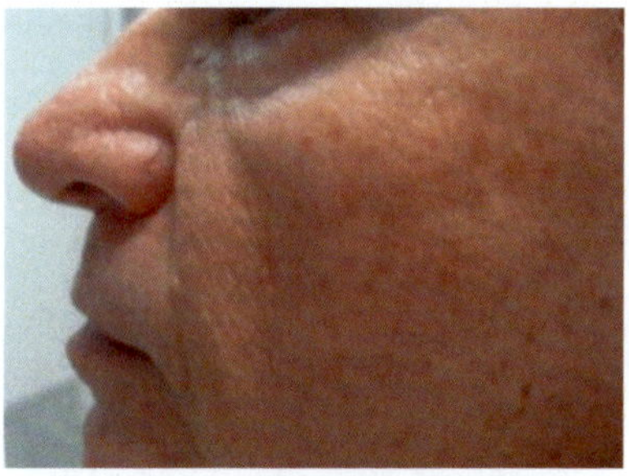

5A - 2010

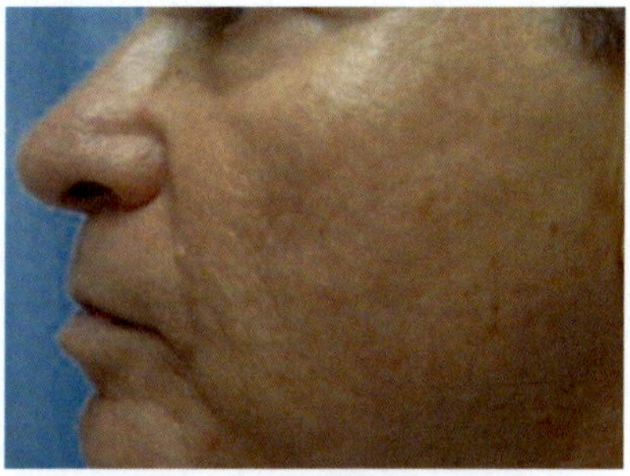

5B - 2012

Before and after treatment, showing the improvement of the skin

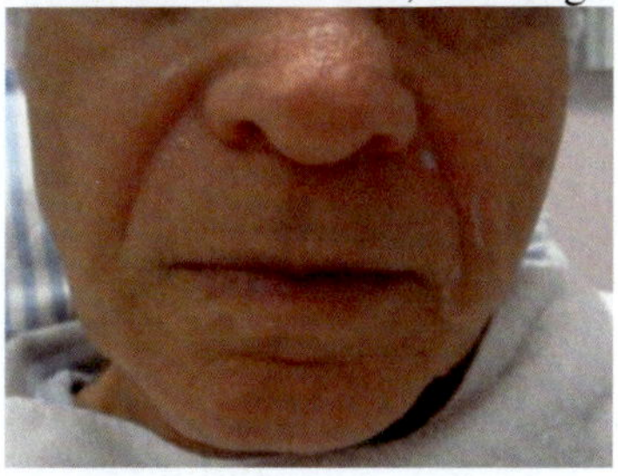

6A - 2010

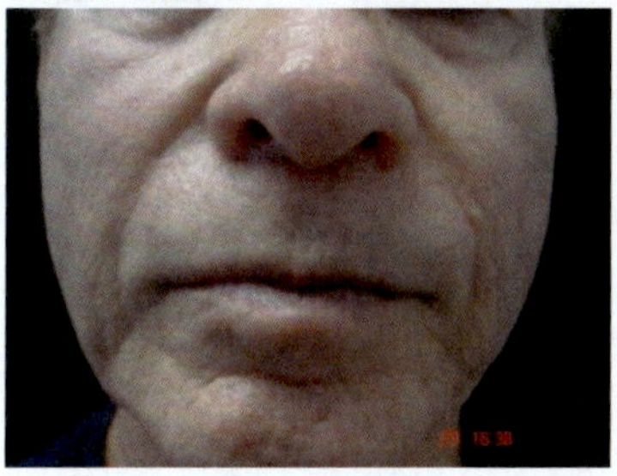

6B - 2013

Before and after treatment. Volumizing of the NLF and medial malar

He sought out a dermatologist after his divorce because he felt aged and discouraged. He already knew some techniques in the field of dermatology as he used to come with his ex-wife to my office. After hearing his complaints and anxieties, I suggested some procedures. I prescribed bleaching of melanosis of the face and hands with IPL followed by superficial peels, non-ablative resurfacing laser (Star Lux 1540 nm erbium glass), facial volumizing and Botulinum Toxin.

The patient started the treatment in 2012, at age 70. On the occasion he had large pores, aging skin, melanosis, pronounced nasolabial folds, atrophy of the medial malar, sebaceous hyperplasia on the nose, and wrinkles on the upper third of the face, marking the skin.

The patient was excited with the results. He intensified his work as a lawyer, continued active in the labor market, improved his relationship with his only child and confessed how much he was pleased to take care of himself, something he had not done before. He is a frequent patient, never missing a scheduled appointment.

Perioral Wrinkles

Most female patients around 60 years present marked wrinkles and a shift of the skin of the perioral region, even if the rest of the facial skin is well cared for. This aspect is caused by the reduction of connective tissue, changes of the dental arch and atrophy of dental alveoli, with a significant worsening if teeth are absent. Another aggravating factor for the appearance of these wrinkles is the photoaging factor of the region, leading to a change in texture and color of this skin. The same is evident in chronic smokers who experience significant change in the perioral region with formation of deep and multiple rhytids.

The dynamic wrinkles can be treated with Botulinum Toxin at low doses (0.5 and 1U pp) of not more than 4U at the top and 2U in the bottom. The application should be done far from the superior lip filter so the erasure of this will not occur. The Hyaluronic Acid Filling with low viscosity improves the volume, leading to a more harmonious appearance of the site. It is best suited for the most distensible rhytids.

In the case of deep rhytids in this region, it should be used the chemical peel of ATA 35% or phenol Baker and Gordon peel, in skin types Fitzpatrick I and II. In the rest of the face, we can opt for a less aggressive procedure.

The thick skin of men is less affected by senescence in this region.

Sagging or Tissue Ptosis

It is one of the most obvious signs of chronological ageing, possibly associated with other disorders that cause this "leftover" skin, like severe acne scars in youth, excessive photoaging, rapid weight loss or bariatric surgery.

This aspect can be mitigated through non-surgical techniques such as radiofrequency, infrared or micro focused Ultrasound (Ulthera ®). There are many surgical procedures for the different areas. The techniques that may be used include a simple Dermabrasion until surgeries such as Blepharoplasty, Rhytidectomy, Browlift, S-lifting and Minilifting. Surgical procedures should be performed in hospitals or equipped clinics.

Subcutaneous Tissue Atrophy of Hands

The aging of the hands involves some fairly visible mechanisms, especially in women after menopause, such as volume loss, change in skin texture, and dermal thinning with loss of adipose tissue and muscles. This results in greater visibility of vessels and tendons, besides the appearance of actinic keratosis and melanosis, causing aesthetic disorder.

In addition to treatments to improve the skin quality, which have already been mentioned above, the dermal filling with volumizing complete the improvements.

The most commonly used products for return of the volume are: hyaluronic acid, calcium hydroxyapatite and poly-L-lactic acid, all temporary products that should not cause sensory or motor dysfunction in hands.

Evaluation of Patient

The rejuvenation techniques should in general be offered to healthy, well informed patients with realistic expectations.

As we discussed elderly patients in this chapter, it is important to remember to investigate smoking, alcohol, allergies to antibiotics, use of analgesics, anxiolytics and investigate their levels of blood pressure, bleeding disorders, hepatitis, diabetes and AIDS. The hypotensive drugs, hypoglycemic or other controlling any chronic disease, should be continued. Medicines that should be suspended include those that may interfere with clotting ten days before the interventions, as acetylsalicylic acid, Vitamin E, Ginkobiloba and non-steroidal anti-inflammatory.

Associated with all these precautions, remember the importance of good nutrition, control of diseases typical of senescence, regular habits of physical exercise and social interaction.

Conclusion

The role of Cosmetic Dermatologists is to frankly explain what patients can expect from the treatment, so their expectations can be effectively achieved.

The procedures in this chapter have the potential to correct minor or major decrepitude (age marks) that when eliminated bring psychological relief and improves quality of life of patients.

The techniques associated potentiate the possibility to produce an overall correction and rejuvenation effect.

This effect is recognized by patients as improved self-esteem and joy of living, free from bothersome marks, even if only perceived by themselves.

References

Cucé, L. C. (2010). *Rumos da Cosmiatria.* 1ed. São Paulo, SP: Grupo Lopso de Comunicação.

Fenske, N. A. & Albers, S. E. (1990). Cosmetic modalities for aging skin: What to tell patients. *Geriatrics,* 45, 59-67.

Gupta, M. A. & Gilchrest, B. A. (2005). Psychosocial Aspects Of Aging Skin. Dermatol *Clin,* 23, 643-648.

Honigman, R. & Castle, D. J. (2006). Aging and Cosmetic Enhancement. *Clinical Interventions in Aging,* 1 (2), 115-119.

Kadunc, B. V. (2013). Avaliação do paciente e indicação de procedimentos no envelhecimento facial. *Programa de Educação Continuada SBD.*

Lewis, M. B. & Bowler, P. J. (2009). Botulinum toxin cosmetic therapy correlates with a more positive mood. *Journal of Cosmetic Dermatology,* 8, 24-26.

Muller, M. C. & Ramos, D. G. (2004). Psicodermatologia: uma Interface entre Psicologia e Dermatologia. *Psicologia Ciência e Profissão,* 24 (3), 76-81.

Ramos-e-Silva, M. & Carneiro, S. C. S. (2007). Elderly skin and its rejuvenation: products and procedures for the aging skin. *Journal of Cosmetic Dermatology,* 6, 40-50.

Rocha, T. N. (2003). Integrative Dermatological Consultation – Contextualizing medical assistance within an integrative perspective. *An bras Dermatol,* 78 (5): 619-624.

Sandoval, M. H. L., & Ayres, E. (2013). *Preenchedores – Guia prático de Técnicas e Produtos.* 1 ed. São Paulo, SP: AC Farmacêutico.

In: Geriatric Psychodermatology
Editors: Mohammad Jafferany and Katlein França
ISBN: 978-1-63463-853-1

Chapter 20

Cutaneous Sensory Syndrome: Chronic Cutaneous Dysesthesia

Eva Wang, BS, John Koo, M.D. and Mohammad Jafferany, M.D.*

Introduction

Cutaneous sensory disorder or chronic cutaneous dysesthesia, also known as hallucinatory dysesthesia is a disorder consisting of 2 parts. The first part is the patient has disagreeable cutaneous sensations e.g., itching, burning, stinging and the second part is the sensation lacks a neurologic, psychiatric, or medical explanation for the dysesthesia [1]. This sensation can affect any body region but tends to develop in areas with greater density of epidermal innervation, most commonly involving the face, scalp, or perineum [2]. Often the associated body parts with cutaneous sensory disorder are termed as vulvodynia, scrotodynia, glossodynia or burning mouth syndrome or stomatodynia. Most of the time there are no apparent dermatologic or medical conditions that explain symptoms and all work up appears negative.

Epidemiology. Chronic cutaneous dysesthesia affects all genders and ages but predominantly affects females with an increased prevalence with age and during perimenopause. [3, 4] Geriatric population is particularly prone.

Classification. Chronic cutaneous dysesthesia are typically referred either by affected anatomy or known pathogenesis.

- Head
    - Glossodynia
    - Stomatodynia or burning mouth syndrome
    - Scalp dysesthesia
    - Trichodynia

* Corresponding author: Mohammad Jafferany, MD. Email: mjafferany@yahoo.com

- Urogenital
  - Vulvodynia
  - Orchiodynia
  - Urodynia
  - Urethral syndrome
  - Phallodynia
  - Prostatodynia
  - Coccygodynia
  - Perineal pain syndrome
  - Anodynia
  - Proctodynia

- Known pathogenesis
  - Erythromelagia
  - Trigeminal neuralgia
  - Postzosteric neuralgia
  - Proctalgia fugax

Pathophysiology

Various neurologic and clinical factors are involved in the pathogenesis of cutaneous sensory syndrome. A better understanding of the pathophysiology of sensation will allow us to better understand therapeutic options for chronic cutaneous dysesthesia. There are two main types of nociceptive afferents—the Aδ fibers and C fibers. The Aδ fibers transmit signals for fast, well-localized sharp pain and temperature. The C fibers transmit signals for slow, diffuse, aching pain, temperature, pressure, and itch. These fibers activate nociceptors in skin. While much research is still being conducted on nociceptive processing, current research shows that nociceptors are activated via TRP (transient receptor potential) and purinergic receptors, which allow Na+ and Ca2+ through the membrane of free nerve endings. The TRP channels can be directly modulated by H+, capsaicin, noxious temperature or force, and the purinergic receptors can be directly modulated by ATP. TRP channels are further potentiated at GPCR receptors by bradykinin, histamine, prostaglandin, serotonin. Once the nociceptors are activated, the peripheral nervous system utilizes substance P and calcitonin gene related peptide to transduce the signal from primary afferent to the anterolateral system. Centrally, the sensation of pain is inhibited by enkaphalinergic interneurons and by glutamate, norepinephrine, and serotonin neurotransmitters. Anxiety and depression are commonly seen in cutaneous sensory syndrome.

Emotional and psychological trauma suffered in life causes grave psychological consequences for an individual and lead to "dissociation " and "conversion" of emotional symptoms into cutaneous somatic symptoms. The dissociation process plays a central role in the development of medically unexplained symptoms and somatization.

Psychiatric factors noted in chronic sensory syndrome are related to somatization phenomenon. Somatization appears to be an important factor in cutaneous sensory syndrome. Somatization is a clinical situation where the patient attributes the somatic symptom to a physical problem but the condition actually is a psychiatric illness that responds to psychiatric treatment. Common dermatologic symptoms associated with somatization in chronic sensory syndrome include cutaneous pain, itching, burning, tin gling and numbness.

Clinical Management

A diagnosis of chronic cutaneous dysesthesia is a clinical diagnosis of exclusion; therefore, a good history and physical is key. A thorough medical, neurologic, and psychiatric work-up should be performed to exclude an organic etiology. Patient should have basic labs and be up to date on cancer screening s. The duration and nature of the dysesthesia should be well-documented, including exacerbating and alleviating qualifiers.

Once diagnosed, physicians should first acknowledge and validate the patient's symptoms and experience. Irritating and possible contributing factors should be avoided. Inquiries into the patient's sleep hygiene are important, as sleep disruptions are known to enhance perception of chronic cutaneous dysesthesia. It is important to identify whether or not the patient has a diagnosable psychiatric comorbidity, most commonly depression and anxiety. If present, the psychiatric comorbidity should be treated regardless if the psychiatric comorbidity is related since psychiatric disease can also enhance the perception of chronic cutaneous dysesthesia.

Pharmacologic management targets molecules involved in sensation of pain both peripherally and centrally. Benefit is seen within 4-6 weeks; resolution is achieved within 2-3 months. While some patients may eventually be tapered off pharmacologic therapy without recurrence of pain, other patients may require long-term pharmacologic therapy. In our clinical experience, it is possible for a patient to continue long-term pharmacologic therapy safely and without waning efficacy. Currently, we see a patient who takes fluoxetine 20mg daily for chronic cutaneous dysesthesia of the buttocks. He has been on this medication for 30 years to date without waning efficacy or side effect.

Pharmacologic therapy for chronic cutaneous dysesthesia targets molecules involved in the pathophysiology of pain. The following pharmacologic therapies are based on clinical experience with this rare disease.

Amongst the above medications, doxepin and paroxetine are typically used when pruritis is the predominant symptom. TCAs, SSRIs, anticonvulsants, and capsaicin are typically used when pain is involved. Antipsychotics have been found to be very effective in cases refractory to treatment. A therapeutic dose can be reached, followed by eventual tapering to a lower maintenance dose or to no medication at all. More studies are needed to elucidate our understanding of chronic cutaneous dysesthesia; however, many available pharmacologic treatments have been show to be successful in the off-label treatment of chronic cutaneous dysesthesia. We encourage physicians to exhibit empathy and patience when treating this very challenging disease.

Drug	FDA indication	Starting dose	Dose used in CCD
Tricyclic Antidepressant (TCA) – blocks serotonin/ NE reuptake; antihistamine			
amitriptyline	MDD	10mg QHS	10-100mg QHS [5, 6]
nortriptyline	MDD	10mg QHS	10-100mg QHS [7]
imipramine	MDD, childhood enuresis	10mg QHS	10-100mg QHS [7]
desipramine	MDD	10mg QHS	10-100mg QHS [7]
clomipramine	OCD	25mg QHS	25-100mg QHS [7]
doxepin	MDD, GAD, insomnia, pruritis due to atopic dermatitis or lichen simplex chronicus	25mg QHS	25-100mg QHS [5], topical 5% cream
Selective Serotonin Reuptake Inhibitor (SSRI) – blocks serotonin reuptake			
paroxetine	MDD, OCD, panic disorder, social phobia, GAD, PTSD, PMDD	20mg daily	20-60mg daily [7]
fluoxetine	MDD, OCD, PMDD, panic disorder, bulimia nervosa	IR: 20mg daily	20-50mg daily [7]
sertraline	MDD, OCD, panic disorder, PTSD, PMDD, social phobia	50mg daily	50-200mg daily [7]
fluvoxamine	OCD, social phobia	50mg QHS	50-150mg BID [7]
citalopram	MDD	20mg daily	20-60mg daily [7]
escitalopram	MDD, GAD	10mg daily	10-20mg daily [7]
Serotonin-Norepinephrine Reuptake Inhibitor (SNRI) – blocks serotonin/ NE reuptake			
duloxetine	MDD, GAD, diabetic neuropathy, fibromyalgia	30mg daily	30-60mg daily [8]
venlafaxine (ER)	MDD, GAD	37.5mg daily	37.5mg-225mg daily [9]
Anticonvulsant – GABA- ergic or inhibit Na+ or Ca2+ channels			
gabapentin	Postherpetic neuralgia, epilepsy	100mg daily	300-2700mg daily [10-14]
pregabalin	Postherpetic neuralgia, neuropathic pain, fibromyalgia	50mg daily	50mg daily-150mg TID [15]
topiramate	Epilepsy, migraine headache	50mg BID	50-150mg BID [16]
carbamazepine	Epilepsy, trigeminal neuralgia	100mg daily	100-2400mg daily [11]
diazepam	GAD, acute alcohol withdrawal, skeletal muscle spasm	2mg BID	2mg BID [17]
clonazepam	Seizure disorder, panic disorder	0.25m BID	0.25-1 mg BID [17-19]
Antipsychotic			
pimozide	Tourette's syndrome	0.5-1mg daily	1-6mg daily [7, 20]
olanzapine	Schizophrenia, Bipolar I disorder	2.5mg QHS	2.5-5mg QHS [21, 22]
Other – TRPV1 receptor desensitization			
capsaicin	Postherpetic neuralgia	0.025% cream daily	0.025-0.075% cream daily-QID or 8% dermal patch [23, 24]

References

[1] Koo J, Gambla C. Cutaneous sensory disorder. *Dermatologic clinics* 1996;14:497-502.

[2] Cotterill JA. Dermatological non-disease. *Dermatology nursing / Dermatology Nurses' Association* 1981;3:315-7.

[3] Bergdahl M, Bergdahl J. Burning mouth syndrome: prevalence and associated factors. *Journal of oral pathology & medicine: official publication of the International Association of Oral Pathologists and the American Academy of Oral Pathology* 1999;28:350-4.

[4] Grushka M. Clinical features of burning mouth syndrome. *Oral surgery, oral medicine, and oral pathology* 1987;63:30-6.

[5] Hoss D, Segal S. Scalp dysesthesia. *Archives of dermatology* 1998;134:327-30.

[6] McKay M. Dysesthetic ("essential") vulvodynia. Treatment with amitriptyline. *The Journal of reproductive medicine* 1993;38:9-13.

[7] Park KK, Koo J. Use of psychotropic drugs in dermatology: unique perspectives of a dermatologist and a psychiatrist. *Clinics in dermatology* 2013;31:92-100.

[8] Nagashima W, Kimura H, Ito M, Tokura T, Arao M, Aleksic B et al. Effectiveness of duloxetine for the treatment of chronic nonorganic orofacial pain. *Clinical neuropharmacology* 2012;35:273-7.

[9] Miranda Sivelo A, Nunez Rodriguez MH. Venlafaxine for depression and glossovulvodynia: a case report. *Primary care companion to the Journal of clinical psychiatry* 2010;12.

[10] Ventolini G, Barhan S, Duke J. Vulvodynia, a step-wise therapeutic prospective cohort study. *Journal of obstetrics and gynaecology: the journal of the Institute of Obstetrics and Gynaecology* 2009;29:648-50.

[11] Martin WJ, Forouzanfar T. The efficacy of anticonvulsants on orofacial pain: a systematic review. *Oral surgery, oral medicine, oral pathology, oral radiology, and endodontics* 2011;111:627-33.

[12] Scheinfeld N. The role of gabapentin in treating diseases with cutaneous manifestations and pain. *International journal of dermatology* 2003;42:491-5.

[13] McGraw T, Kosek P. Erythromelalgia pain managed with gabapentin. *Anesthesiology* 1997;86:988-90.

[14] Spoelstra SK, Borg C, Weijmar Schultz WC. Anticonvulsant pharmacotherapy for generalized and localized vulvodynia: a critical review of the literature. *Journal of psychosomatic obstetrics and gynaecology* 2013;34:133-8.

[15] Jerome L. Pregabalin-induced remission in a 62-year-old woman with a 20-year history of vulvodynia. *Pain research & management: the journal of the Canadian Pain Society = journal de la societe canadienne pour le traitement de la douleur* 2007;12:212-4.

[16] Siniscalchi A, Gallelli L, Marigliano NM, Orlando P, De Sarro G. Use of topiramate for glossodynia. *Pain medicine* (Malden, Mass) 2007;8:531-4.

[17] Barker KE, Batstone MD, Savage NW. Comparison of treatment modalities in burning mouth syndrome. *Australian dental journal* 2009;54:300-5; quiz 96.

[18] Gremeau-Richard C, Woda A, Navez ML, Attal N, Bouhassira D, Gagnieu MC et al. Topical clonazepam in stomatodynia: a randomised placebo -controlled study. *Pain* 2004;108:51-7.

[19] Zakrzewska JM, Forssell H, Glenny AM. Interventions for the treatment of burning mouth syndrome. *The Cochrane database of systematic reviews* 2005:CD002779.

[20] Koblenzer CS, Bostrom P. Chronic cutaneous dysesthesia syndrome: a psychotic phenomenon or a depressive symptom? *Journal of the American Academy of Dermatology* 1994;30:370-4.

[21] Gick CL, Mirowski GW, Kennedy JS, Bymaster FP. Treatment of glossodynia with olanzapine. *Journal of the American Academy of Dermatology* 2004;51:463-5.
[22] Ueda N, Kodama Y, Hori H, Umene W, Sugita A, Nakano H et al. Two cases of burning mouth syndrome treated with olanzapine. *Psychiatry and clinical neurosciences* 2008;62:359-61.
[23] Turini D, Beneforti P, Spinelli M, Malagutti S, Lazzeri M. Heat/burning sensation induced by topical application of capsaicin on perineal cutaneous area: new approach in diagnosis and treatment of chronic prostatitis /chronic pelvic pain syndrome? *Urology* 2006;67:910-3.
[24] Backonja MM, Malan TP, Vanhove GF, Tobias JK. NGX-4010, a high-concentration capsaicin patch, for the treatment of postherpetic neuralgia: a randomized, double-blind, controlled study with an open-label extension. *Pain medicine* (Malden, Mass) 2010;11:600-8.

In: Geriatric Psychodermatology
Editors: Mohammad Jafferany and Katlein França
ISBN: 978-1-63463-853-1

Chapter 21

Dermatological Infections in Geriatric Population

Ruqiya Shama Tareen, M.D.*, and Kinza Tareen, BS

Introduction

With the growing geriatric population in the United States, it is vital for healthcare providers to emphasize focus on geriatric medicine including geriatric dermatology. [1] As the body matures and ages it is more susceptible to develop a dermatological disorder. It is no secret that our skin changes as we age, however while many changes are visible to general observation, such as wrinkles and ages spots, aging skin reflects changes that are not apparent, but attribute to dermatologcial disorders encountered in geriatric population. Aging skin demonstrates changes such as intrinsic loss of epidermal thickness, a decline in number of cell lines including Langerhans cells and melanocytes, as well as a loss of elastic tissues. [1] The loss of collagen leads to less elastic dermal bed resulting in the appearance of wrinkles amplified by a atopic epidermis. [1] Furthermore, dermal density and the vascularity and neural circuitry of the dermis declines as the skin ages. [1] Many conditions commonly encountered in the geriatric population such as atherosclerosis, diabetes mellitus, as well as congestive heart failure can have lasting effects to skin. These diseases cause complications in the peripheral vascular and microcirculatory system of the skin and consequently predispose individuals to a more rapid aging of skin and decrease immune response. Consequently, aging skin exhibits decreased responsiveness to invading organisms reduced ability to heal. [1] These characteristics of aging skin account for the heightened susceptibility of viral, bacterial, fungal, and parasitic infections in the geriatric population.

* Corresponding author: Email: shama.tareen@med.wmich.edu.

Viral Infections

Herpes Zoster

Caused by the varicella zoster virus (VZV), herpes zoster is a relatively common infection occurring in the elderly at a rate of approximately 3-5 cases per 1000 persons per year. [2]. Varicella, or chickenpox, is the primary infection caused by VZV in childhood which usually resolves without any major sequelae. After the resolution of varicella the VZV becomes latent and stays dormant in the ganglia of the autonomic nervous system, dorsal root, and cranial nerve s. Aging causes immunity against VZV to diminish and can result in reactivation of VZV resulting in a Herpes Zoster. [2] The prodromal phase which can be as short as 2 days and as long as a week is marked by paraesthesia, burning or itching sensation, or pain in the affected dermatome. Patients may also suffer from fever, myalgia, and malaise. Eruption soon follows, allowing for the formation of the typical dermatome or dermatomes, usually unilateral and not crossing the midline. The initial erythematous macular lesions give rise to the typical vesicular lesions 1-2 mm in size. The lesions may confluent to make larger lesions, and become hemorrhagic in a matter of days. Eventually, lesions dry out, however a new crop of lesion may occur in same area and it may take 2-4 weeks for the infection to complete its cycle. The major issue associated with herpes zoster is pain. Patients experience severe stinging and burning pain which may persist even after the active lesion is resolved. Post herpetic neuralgia (PHN) affects between 2-9 persons out of 1000 who suffered from herpes zoster. Patients reportedly suffer from daily pain in the affected dermatome for 3-6 months after the resolution of active infection. PHN is a debilitating condition, with severe paroxysmal pain.

Additionally, PHN is most commonly seen when the thoracic dermatomes, particularly T5-T10 are involved, followed by the craniocervical dermatomes. Trigeminal ganglion are involved in 20% of patients and the most commonly involved is the ophthalmic division. [3] Herpes Zoster Opthalamoplegia is a serious condition and a late complication which can cause permanent damage to the affected eye. Some other less common complications are encephalitis, contralateral hemiparesis /hemiplegia, myelitis and more systemic involvement.

Treatment of active infection with antiviral medications like acyclovir 800 mg taken 5 times daily for 7-10 days, may not help with the intensity of pain but may shorten the duration of pain by few days. Famciclovir 500 to 750 mg daily was shown to be effective in reducing pain and promoting cutaneous healing. Corticosteroids like prednisone 40 mg/d for 3 weeks followed by gradual taper when used in conjunction with antiviral medications can cause significant decrease in pain, however has not shown any significant impact on the duration of the acute phase. If pain continues to be severe and does not respond to the standard treatment regimen, non-traditional treatments may be considered. For instance, Epidural injection of methylprednisolone administered once or local anesthetics bupivacaine can help with pain but the effect does not last beyond 1 month. Injection of an anesthetic agent in the stellate ganglion block may produce short-term pain relief but is not employed commonly. [3]

Molluscum Contagiosum (MC)

Molluscum Contagiosum (MC) is a very common and highly contagious infection easily transmitted from person to person in close quarters, and when people use community facilities like shared bathtubs, swimming pools etc. MC presents with a tiny dome shaped skin colored papules ranging from 2-8 mm in size. MC can occur as single or multiple lesions, their pathognomonic feature is when they become umblicated and pearly white in appearance. MC commonly affects areas such as the face, hands, trunk, and genitalia. Some MC lesions can assume a uncharacteristically large size and these large papules are prone to develop secondary bacterial infection s. Topical application of cantharidin such as 0.7% cantharone is safe when applied sparingly and is 95% effective in localized lesions. [4] In larger areas of infection and in cases when response to topical therapy is not optimal, immunomodulatory agents can be used. Tarcolimus is one such therapeutic agent and can be very effective, however it may predispose patients to herpetic infection. Excision and curettage and electrodessication can be employed when lesions are fewer and localized. Oral cimetidine has shown some efficacy especially when molluscum is associated with atopic dermatitis. Cryotherapy with liquid nitrogen application on each lesion for 6-10 seconds is effective and may need to be repeated in 3 weeks. Imiquimod is a relatively new agent that has also shown efficacy however, evidence is still limited. [5]

Bacterial Infections

Impetigo

Geriatric patients with conditions that compromise the immune system are predisposed to the common skin infection impetigo. Such conditions include: diabetes mellitus, B-cell immunodeficiency states, malnutrition, use of steroids and other conditions making skin susceptible to cutaneous infections like contact dermatitis, or other intensely pruritic lesions, like second or third degree burns. [6] Impetigo has a predilection for the face especially around the mouth and nose area. Typical lesions can be bullous or non bullous and possibly a mix presentation can occur within the same area. Historical beta-hemolytic Streptococcus (GABHS) was considered the main causative agent for impetigo especially in non-bullous form but more recently Staphylococcus aureus has emerged as the main causative organism in both bullous and non-bullous forms of impetigo. [7] Bullous impetigo accounts for up to 70% of cases, it usually starts as tiny innocuous papules that coal esces to form small bullae. The bullae rupture easily giving rise to erosions covered with the typical honey colored thick crust. The non-bullous forming impetigo presents with larger bullae up to 2-5 cm in diameter, filled with thin serous fluid, which when rupture leave behind a raw erosive area surrounded with smaller bullae. [7]

Secondary Impetigo: resulting from secondary infection of already present skin lesions like cuts and insect bites or due to excoriation caused by excessive scratching of eczematous, scabies, and other pruritic lesions. Secondary impetigo is especially common in diabetic or immunocompromised patients and typically presents in the non-bullous form and in non typical sites. Topical antibiotic applications is the first line of treatment for small lesions confined to one or two areas. The most commonly used topical antibiotics are mupirocin, bacitracin and fusidic acid. [8] Topical antibiotics like mupirocin and bacitracin were found to be superior to oral erythromycin in treating localized impetigo lesions. However, repeated application for an extended period of time can result in resistance to antibiotics and may cause local skin irritations and possible contact dermatitis. In cases where larger and multiple areas are involved a systemic antibiotic like Amoxicillin/Clavulanate 125/30 mg per ml three times daily and cephalosporin like cefuroxime, cefadroxil, cefaclor, cephalexin and dicloxacillin 90 mg/kg in 2-4 divided doses per day, for 7-10 days are found to be effective in eradicating infection. Erythromycin and clarithromycin for 7-10 days have also been shown to be effective in some cases. [9]

Folliculitis

An infection of hair follicle, folliculitis, usually affects areas where hair are thick and short, such as the nape of neck or in beard area. Folliculitis is classified in types based on the depth of the hair follicle involved, the infecting organism, and the area involved.

Superficial Folliculitis: Caused by Staphylococcus, superficial folliculitis is the most common form and can affect any area of body, however, it is most common in areas with poor hygiene and maceration. Characteristic of the lesion is a small pustule with hair in center and it generally resolves without treatment and leaves no scarring. However when infection becomes recurrent it may require treatment and usually responds to topical antibiotics like mupirocin 2%, clindamycin, or erythromycin. [7]

Deep Folliculitis: A less common form deep folliculitis, occurs when the infecting organism reaches the base of follicle resulting in painful papules and pustules. Since the infection reaches deeper layers of dermis healing is often difficult and may leave scarring. Treatment with oral antibiotics targeting staphylococcus aureus is required especially to avoid scarring. [7]

Gram-Negative Folliculitis: Gram-negative folliculitis is most commonly associated with patients who are being treated with long term antibiotic regimens, which give rise to an opportunity for gram-negative bacteria like Klebsiella, Enterobacter, and Proteus to over populate and infect the hair follicle s. [6]

Hot-Tub Folliculitis: Also known as “spa pool folliculitis,” hot-tub folliculitis is characterized by erythematous itchy papulo-pustules overlying large areas of the trunk, extremities, and other areas of the body exposed to the infected water. Symptoms generally present after few hours or up to 3 days after exposure to a hot-tub, whirlpool, or swimming pool that was not chlorinated properly or if pH of water was suboptimal. Large outbreaks have been reported with use of community water facilities like pools, whirlpools and water slides. [10] Lesions are self-limiting in few days, 1% acetic acid soaks can hasten the dry out process of these lesions. In cases of severe infection fever, malaise, sore throat and lymph adenopathy can occur. [11]

Furunculosis

More commonly known as "boil" furunculosis is a perifollicular erythematous abscess caused by Staphylococcus aureus infection. The commonly affected areas are intertriginous folds, scalp, and other areas in which hair follicles are in abundance. Hyperhidrosis can predispose one to furunculosis and maintaining hygiene of intertriginous areas may be the key to prevent autoinoculation and recurrence. Community acquired methicillin-resistant Staphylococcus aureus (CA-MRSA) has been shown to cause furunculosis. Patients with an immunocompromised status like HIV or inherited immune deficiencies as well as having other conditions lowering immune mechanisms are more susceptible to treatment resistant and recurrent furunculosis. [12] Larger solitary lesions of around 5 cm in diameter respond well to excision and drainage only. For cases in which multiple or much larger lesions are present or where systemic signs of inflammation are present an oral antibiotic like Flucloxacillin is an effective treatment option. Additionally, in most cases Clindamycin can be used in cases of MRSA furunculosis at a dose of 2–8 mg/kg every 6–8 hours. In cases of MRSA furunculosis with systemic infection hospitalization and a course of intravenous antibiotics like Vancomycin is the appropriate form of treatment. [12]

Carbuncle

Carbuncle is characterized by a large erythematous, painful, and indurated mass located within deep subcutaneous tissue. Resulting from chronic non healing furunculosis, a carbuncle is formed when multiple inflamed furuncles in a small area connect with each others by interconnecting abscesses and via subcutaneous tracts ultimately draining the pus on the surface. The favored sites for carbuncles are thighs, back of neck, and trunk where the dermis is quite thick. Deep seated carbuncles are hard, fixed, and feel like a malignant tumor on palpation. Such deep carbuncles when perforated cause deep lesions and heal with scarring. Oral antistaphylococcal antibiotics are only indicated in the treatment of cases of systemic involvement or when concomitant cellulitis is present. [13] Surgical consultation may be indicated for large carbuncles to excise and drain the abscesses and clean some of the tracts.

Cellulitis

A common skin infection seen in geriatric patients, cellulitis, can spread rapidly within the skin layers and subcutaneous tissue s. The infection is usually acquired by entry of the infecting organism through a minor cut, or any other type of break in skin continuity. Although any part of the body can be affected it is most commonly seen on areas of exposed skins like extremities, particularly on lower extremities. The majority of infections are caused by β-hemolytic streptococci, mainly from groups G and A, followed by infection caused by Staphylococcus aureus, and rarely infection have been shown to arise from Gram negative organisms like Proteus Mirabilis, Pseudomonas aeruginosa, and organisms from the Enterobacteriaceae group.

The infection is announced by diffuse erythematous and rapidly progressive lesions with no clear cut margins. These lesions may or may not result in a break in skin where the infection has started. The lesion is accompanied with signs of inflammation, it is warm and tender to touch and also appears red and shiny due to subcutaneous swelling. When cellulitis becomes more pronounced it can induce signs of systemic infection like fever, malaise, pain, lymhangitis, and lymphadenitis. Regional lymphadenitis is chiefly pronounced if the infective organism is Bartonella henselae, and is introduced to the skin by a cat scratch, hence called Cat scratch disease. Orbital cellulitis is especially threatening due to the possibility of rapid spread to adjacent structures which may lead to serious complications including cavernous sinus thrombosis, meningitis, permanent loss of vision, and diplopia. [7] Orbital cellulitis is generally unilateral and often is due to a spread of infection from the infected frontal sinuses. The most common agents involved are Staphylococcus aureus, S epidermidis, and S pyogenes. [14]

Empirical antibiotic treatment with coverage for gram positive bacteria with penicillin, or Flucloxacillin for 10 days is usually effective. Methicillin-resistant penicillin, cephalosporin and amoxicillin-clavulanate and macrolide all are considered effective first line treatment in uncomplicated cases of cellulitis. One must attempt to isolate the organism by skin swab or needle aspiration if empiric treatment fails to show any signs of improvement. [7] Patients who are immunocompromised, or have conditions like diabetes or other serious medical conditions may require hospitalization and intravenous administration of a second or third generation cephalosporin with or without aminoglycoside antibiotics. Periorbital cellulitis should be treated as an emergency, intravenous antibiotics and hospitalization is necessary as well as a consultation with ophthalmologist and ENT due to concomitant sinusitis.[7] Perianal cellulitis can be treated with Amoxicillin 40 mg/kg/day in 3 divided doses, along with topical antibiotic like mupirocin 2% 3 times daily for 10 days. [15]

Erysipelas

Erysipelas represents a very localized infection of the skin and subcutaneous tissues most commonly caused by group B hemolytic streptococcus, and less likely by Staphylococcus Aureus. It usually affects exposed areas of skin like face and extremities. Erysipelas lesions are sharply demarcated erythematous lesions with an advancing margin. The appearance of the lesions may be preceded by a prodromal illness of fever, chills, nausea, vomiting, and arthralgia. [16] In geriatric patients quick spread of infection can also induce a delirious state. Immediate administration of oral antibiotics and at times intravenous antibiotics are indicated for treatment. Other well localized lesions with defined margins like a drug reaction or contact dermatitis may pose a diagnostic challenge but targeted questioning may delineate history of exposure. Anti-streptococcal antibiotics should be employed without delay. First line treatment penicillin given for 7-10 days is usually very effective. In penicillin resistant patients cephalosporin or macrolides can be used. In immunocompromised patients mixed infections with gram positive agents with enterococci can occur requiring a broad spectrum I/V antibiotic such as cephalosporin. Local comforting measures like elevation of extremity, warm compresses and wet saline dressing are effective in reducing swelling, discomfort and pain. [16]

Ecthyma Gangrenosum (EG)

Ecthyma Gangrenosum is a very rare infection especially in the geriatric population, however when present in this age group EG usually results from occlusive vasculitis associated with pseudomonas septicemia. This infection generally presents itself in patients who are immunocompromised, patients who have renal or hepatic failure, malnutrition, and victims of burns who have a high rate of pseudomonas septicemia. The most commonly affected sites are buttocks and anogenital area, but infection can occur any where on the body. [17] The lesion of EG usually begins as a small innocuous macule that becomes purulent and develops into thick walled hemorrhagic bullae, which ultimately becomes a gangrenous ulcer. The pathognomonic feature is a grayish-black eschar surrounded by an almost hemorrhagic ring. Non-pseudomonas ecthyma gangrenosum has also been reported. [17] Clinical diagnosis can be difficult between ecthyma gangrenosum and pyoderma gangrenosum as both lesions appear quite similar. In rare cases pyoderma gangrenosum can be complicated with superimposed ecthyma gangrenosum. [18] At times biopsy and histopathology may be required in order to establish the nature of the lesion, while blood cultures, and cultures of aspirate from the lesion can confirm the pseudomonas aeruginosa. Localized smaller lesions can be treated with topical silver sulfadiazine. However, systemic antibiotics with pseudomonas coverage like B-lactams penicillin including piperacillin-tazobactam, ceftazidime, cefepime, imipenem, or aminoglycosides like gentamicin, or tobramycin are usually the treatment of choice. [19]

Necrotizing Fasciitis (NF)

Necrotizing Fasciitis (NF) is a potentially life threatening skin infection which is highly invasive and rapidly involves all layers of skin and subcutaneous tissues including fat and superficial layer of fascia. NF usually affects patients with lowered immunity and other debilitating conditions like diabetes, trauma or surgery, irradiation, malnutrition, alcoholism, and obesity. [20] NF can be of two types based on the causative organism; type I NF is polymicrobial in origin and both aerobic and anaerobic may be involved. Type II NF is generally caused by a single agent, most likely streptococcus pyogenes but other organisms are also known to be the single causative agent. Infection spreads rapidly and presents with severe systemic signs of infection, including fever, autonomic dysfunction, and other signs of septic shock. [20] Skin becomes dusky and erythematous followed by development of severe edema and hemorrhagic bullae. Initially patient may complain of severe unrelenting pain but it is later replaced by numbness as the advancing infection causes damage to nerve endings. [13] Presence of crepitus in subcutaneous tissue signifies infection with gas producing organism like clostridium or enterobacteriaceae. A diagnostic scoring system has been used to streamline the diagnostic process for early diagnosis of NF known as Laboratory Risk Indicator for Necrotizing Fasciitis (LRINEC) it comprises some basic laboratory test including total WBC, hemoglobin, sodium, glucose, serum creatinine, and C-reactive protein. [13] LRINEC uses a cut off score of 6 for the possibility of NF. Tissue oxygen saturation is also used as a way to identify NF, and a level of less then 70% is indicative of NF in lower extremities. Radiography can also be used to detect gas in subcutaneous tissues and in up to about 13% of cases, gas can be detected confirming NF. However, computed tomography remains a much accurate technique in detecting gas over plain radiographs as it can detect early soft tissue changes like fascial thickening, fat stranding, and dissection along the fascial plains. [21] Ultrasonography has been used more frequently and has shown some efficacy. Additionally, magnetic resonance imaging (MRI) has shown to be highly sensitive in diagnosing NF. [22, 23]. Prompt recognition of NF and isolation of the organism is the key to a smooth recovery and requires a multidimensional approach. Patients need to be hospitalized with surgical and infectious disease consultation, and strict attention must be paid to abiding by strict sterile precautions, hydration, and nutritional status of patient. Emergency surgical exploration and debridement is the key component of treating NF and in some patients multiple debridements may be necessary. Hyperbaric oxygen and intravenous immunoglobulins as adjunctive treatments have shown to hasten the tissue healing process. [21] Immediate treatment with intravenous broad spectrum antibiotics with coverage for MRSA should be started with aim of changing it to a more specific regime once results of culture and sensitivity are available. Continuation of antibiotic regimen may be necessary until no additional surgical debridement is required or the systemic signs of septic shock begin to reverse. [21, 24]

Table 1.

Common Dermatological Infections in Geriatric Population		
Viral	Varicella zoster Varicella Molluscum Contagiosum	
Bacterial	Impetigo Bullous impetigo	
Fungal		
Parasitic	Pediculosis	Pediculosis capitis Pediculosis corporis Pediculosis or Phthirus pubis
	Scabies	Sarcoptes scabiei var hominis

Table 2.

Skin layers/ Structures	Disease	Common sites	Predominate organism	Secondary organism
Epidermis	Impetigo	Face	Staphylococcus Aureus	Streptococcus Pyogenes (GABHS)
	Superficial Folliculitis	Face, scalp,	Staphylococcus Aureus	
	Furunculosis	Face, scalp, axillae	Staphylococcus Aureus	
	Staphylococcal Scalded Skin Syndrome		Staphylococcus Aureus Phage group II	

Skin layers/ Structures	Disease	Common sites	Predominate organism	Secondary organism
Epidermal/ Subepidermal	Toxic Shock Syndrome	whole body	Staphylococcus Aureus	
	Ecthyma	Legs, buttocks	Pseudomonas aeruginosa	Many gram negative and some gram positive organism
Dermis	Carbuncle	Back, thighs	Staphylococcus Aureus	
	Erysipelas	Face	Streptococcus Pyogenes (GABHS)	
	Deep Folliculitis	Scalp	Staphylococcus Aureus	
	Folliculitis Decalvans	Scalp		
Dermis and upper part of subcutaneous tissues	Cellulitis	Legs	Staphylococcus aureus	Streptococcus pyogenes (GABHS)
Deeper Dermis, Subcutaneous Tissues & Fascia	Necrotizing Fasciitis Type I: Mixed aerobic & anaerobic infection	Legs Arms Less commonly; Trunk Perineum Buttocks Head & Neck	Facultative Streptococci, Staphylococci, Enterococci Gram-negative bacilli, such as Escherichia coli, Klebsiella, Pseudomonas, Enterobacter, and Proteus, and Anaerobes, such as Peptostreptococcus, Bactericides, and Clostridium specie	
	Necrotizing Fasciitis Type II: Monomicrobial Ref (Lopez)		Streptococcus pyogenes (GABHS)	Streptococcus Agalactiae & pneumoniae V vulnificus Clostridium Staphylococcus aureus aureus [28,41]. Aeromonas spp– and

Spirochete Infection

Syphilis

Since the advent of penicillin in 1940s syphilis once a common melady has become quite rare. However in late 1980s with the emergence of HIV we have seen a reemergence of primary syphilis. 5 cases per 100,000 of primary infection of syphilis are being diagnosed each year in USA, Canada and Western Europe while in developing countries this rate is much higher. According to World Health Organization approximately 12 million people are infected with syphilis each year globally. [25] Despite the fact that the geriatric population is not on the forefront of the newly diagnosed cases, this population is most vulnerable to the resurgence of tertiary syphilis. Acquired as an asexually transmitted disease in young age the Treponema Pallidum can remain dormant in nerve ganglion for years without causing any problems. Conditions that can compromise the immune system can lead to reactivation of the infection leading to manifestations of tertiary syphilis. Most common cutaneous manifestation of tertiary syphilis is the typical granulomatous gummata which can get deeply ulcerated with resulting scarring. These lesions can not only occur in the skin and mucous membrane s, but can also be encountered in every internal organ including solid organs, bones and nervous system. The most commonly used non-treponemal antigen tests that are highly sensitive are the Venereal Disease Research Laboratory (VDRL) and Rapid Plasma Reagin (RPR) test. These tests can be used to monitor the efficacy of treatment by following serial titers. Test based on identification of treponemal antigen includes Treponema Pallidum Haemaglutination test (TPHHA), Florescent Treponemal Antibody Absorption test (FTA-ABS), and Treponema Palladium Particle Agglutinations tests (TPPA). The treponemal test is more specific and can be useful for screening purposes. The newer immunoassays tests aim to identify presence of anti-treponemal antibodies both IgG and IgM type. The specificity and sensitivity of Enzyme Immunoassays (EIAs) tests depends on the laboratory and ranges between 60-90%. The treatment of choice for tertiary syphilis is benzathine penicillin given once a week at a dose of 2.4 million units, for the duration of 3 consecutive weeks. [26]

Fungal Infections

Candida Albicans

Candidal mucocutaneous infections such as candida albicans, are common in older populations. Conditions predisposing to candidiasis includes malnutrition, use of antibiotics and corticosteroids, and most importantly HIV infection. Furthermore, Diabetes mellitus is often complicated with mucocutaneous candidal infections. [27] Any condition predisposing to defects in immunity especially of cellular immunity can predispose to candidal infections. Candida itself can exert specific immunomodulatory effect on the host's immune response against candida. [28] Candida favors warm and moist intertriginous areas of skin most commonly under breast, abdominal folds, in perineum, and perianal area. Typical rash associated with infection is a smooth, moist, erythematous rash with some discrete satellite lesions just beyond the advancing edge of the infection. Diagnosis is confirmed by identification of pseudohyphae in KOH preparation under direct microscopy. Aeration and attempts to keep the affected area dry by application of a medium which can absorb the moisture is helpful. Use of mild soap with water with gentle cleansing is recommended. In recurring infection using barrier preparations like petroleum, Titanium oxide in paraffin, Zinc oxide cream can provide added protection against infection by providing a breathable environment. Combination of corticosteroid and antifungal preparations should be avoided. Continue use of a topical antifungal agent twice daily for a week after rash is cleared to ensure a decreased likelihood of recurrence. Nystatin, ketoconazole, clotrimazole, econazole, miconazole, oxiconazole, and ciclopirox are all shown to be very effective anti-candidal agents. [28]

Tinea Corporis

Tinea Corporis, or more commonly known as ringworms, represents a dermatophyte infection most commonly seen on the torso of elderly persons. Trichophyton rubrum acquired through direct skin contact is most commonly responsible for infection. Warm and moist environments are ideal for the fungi and elderly persons unable to access daily bathing or who have moderate perspiration may be predisposed to fungal infection. [29] The organism invades the stratum corneum producing hyphae and grows outward in a circular fashion with erythematous slightly raised margins surrounding a clear center producing the typical ringworm round or annular lesions. Potassium hydroxide (KOH) preparation is used for diagnosis and reveals the infectious expanding border is scaly and when scrapped can show hyphae under microscope. [29] Clinical diagnosis can be difficult as differential diagnosis includes other annular scaly lesions like erythema multiforme, nummular dermatitis, pityriasis rosea, pityriasis versicolor, discoid lesions of systemic lupus erythematoses, and drug eruptions. The initial difficulty in accurate diagnosis may lead to treatment with corticosteroid application which can change the morphology of the lesion and it may appears more smooth, shinier, and extremely pruritic whenever the effect of corticosteroids wears off. Application of corticosteroids can cause it to spread even more quickly. This particular lesion and change is known as tinea incognita. [29]

Tinea Cruris

More commonly known as "jock itch", tinea cruris is a superficial fungal infection of inguinal folds, perineal and perianal area. It affects the moist, non aerated areas of skin such as in between skin folds where maceration can provide perfect breeding grounds for certain dermatophytes including Trichophyton rubrum, Mentagrophytes and Epidermophyton floccosum. The infection presents as brown-red plaques with scaly borders and potentially may have a central clearing. [29] At times it is difficult to differentiate between other rashes having predilection for same body areas. Erythrasma which is a chronic intertriginous infection caused by corynebacterium minutissimum can be easily ruled out by wood's light inspection as it gives rise a bright orange hue under wood's light. Other fungal infection like candidal rash can be distinguished by presence of pinkish red smooth lesions without an erythematous border and satellite punctate lesions in adjacent areas. Less commonly other skin condition like psoriasis and seborrheic dermatitis can also cause confusion.

Tinea Pedis

A common condition in athletes, tinea pedis, or athlete's foot, and in some more extensive types of infection in which the entire foot is involved in a pattern of a shoe covering the foot is known as "moccasin foot." Infection produces itchy macerated lesions with fissuring and causing foul smell usually in between toes where skin is moist nurturing dermatophytes. Most common organisms is Tinea rubrum, which affect relatively dry areas of the foot like heels, soles, and sides producing lesions which are somewhat thickened pink plaque like lesions covered with fine silver scales. A common risk factor for infection is the use of community shower stalls, swimming pools, sharing slippers, socks and shoes, wearing shoes for long time, especially when not wearing absorbent socks, and walking bare foot on moist grounds which can harbor fomites. Differential diagnosis includes contact and atopic dermatitis, psoriasis, and candidal infection between toes. Direct microscopy is effective but the majority of infections are diagnosed purely on clinical judgment, although the potassium hydroxide (KOH) preparation can also provide a cheap, quick and up to 88% sensitive method of confirming the diagnosis. Samples collected by scraping the border of the infection with a scalpel are placed on slide with a drop of 10-20% of KOH, typical septate hyphae of dermatophytes are easy to detect under plain microscope. [30] Wood's light Examination is not so useful in dermatophyte infections other then tinea capitis or to rule out erythrasma.

Treatment with topical antifungals is highly effective in most cases of superficial infections limited to a small areas, except in cases of tinea capitis and tinea unguium where systemic antifungal treatment is indicated. Commonly used topical preparations like miconazole, clotrimazole and terbinafine when applied twice daily for 2 weeks produces positive results. Butenafine has the advantage of only having to be applied once daily for 2 weeks with same effectiveness although it cost more. Patient should be advised to apply topical application to about 2 cm of surrounding area to account for the advancing edge of the infection. [30] Combination preparation including antifungal and corticosteroids are widely used, mostly prescribed when diagnosis is not fully established. However concern that such treatment leads to partial resolution and quick relapse of infection or recurrent infections limits their use. One such combination preparation Clotrimazole/betamethasone has shown a 45% failure and a 36% relapse rate. [31]

Onychomycosis

Fungal infections of nails, or onychomycosis, is the most common nail disease encompassing up to 50% of all nail diseases. In recent years we have seen an upward trend in incidence of onychomycosis especially in the US and in other Western countries. Perhaps this increase in prevalence can be related to more people living longer with diseases like diabetes mellitus, immunosuppression, hyperhidrosis, poor peripheral circulation. Some other predisposing factors are increasing age, male gender, trauma to nail, and nail dystrophy due to other reasons. In fact trauma is the most common preceding event to the nail infection. Toenails are more commonly involved compared to fingernails. In fact, it is not uncommon for hand nails to become infected due to scratching affected feet. Dermatophytes are predominantly the offending agent causing overwhelming majority of infection (90%). The most common dermatophyte causing onychomycosis is Trichophyton rubrum followed by Trichophyton mentagrophytes and Epidermophyton floccosum. About 5% infections are due to candidal infection and remaining are caused by non dermatophyte molds like Acremonium, Aspergillus species, Cladosporium carrionii, Fusarium specie, Onycochola Canadensis etc. Diagnosis can be made with taking nail clipping or in case of distal onychomycosis sample from the nail bed and using 15-20% Potassium Hydroxide (KOH) to dissolve the keratin to identify the fungi under direct microscope. Use of the counter stains can help identify some of the pathogens more clearly. However, culture of the organism is the only way one can confirm the specie and genus of the organism. At times cultures are not successful and in that case histopathology with Pperiodic acid -Schiff (PAS). In very rare event nail biopsy may be required to establish the diagnosis with certainty. [32] Topical therapy is usually not effective unless disease in in the early stages and has affected a limited area. Topical treatment like ciclopirox lacquer 8% has been shown to be 5-8% effective in limited disease. Other topical agents that may be employed in treatment include 40% urea gel and topical antifungal agents in the form of lacquer. Treatment with systemic antifungal medications like Terbinafine, Itraconazole and Fluconazole is usually effective. Terbinafine 250 mg daily for 12 weeks has been shown to be up to 74% effective overall. [33] In some recalcitrant cases the duration of treatment is increased to 16 weeks. Itraconazole can be given in fixed dose of 200 mg daily for 6-12 weeks versus pulse dose of 400 mg daily for one week per month for 8-12 weeks. The concern regarding hepatic toxicity and possibility of causing congestive heart failure can limit its use in older patients with hepatic disease or risk factors for developing CHF. Itraconazole is also very active at hepatic P-450 enzyme system where it is a potent inhibitor of CYP2D6 interfering with the metabolism of other medications especially some commonly used one in geriatric population like statins, and benzodiazepines. [33] It has an overall success in achieving mycologic cure in 35% of cases. Fluconazole has high bioavailability and can be given in pulse dose of 150 mg only once a week for as long as the nail grows out. In a large study of patients receiving 150, 300 or 450 mg once a week for as long as 6-7 months the efficacy of treatment was as high as 86 percent. One must be cautious about drug-drug interactions when it is being used with other medications like rifampin, cimetidine, and HCTZ. [33]

Parasitic Infections

Scabies

Scabies affects people of all social class es and people of all ages, but when seen in geriatric population it is more commonly seen in older people living in poorly sanitized, crowded living situations in urban areas. It is caused by the arthropod Sarcoptes scabiei var hominis, a mite that cannot only transmit by skin -to-skin contact but also by contact with contaminated material like bedding or clothing. Once in contact it can survive for up to 36 hours. [34]

The incubation period is long and it takes 3-6 weeks for female mites to burrows itself in the epidermis where it lays eggs. The larva emerges within 2-3 days and it takes 15 days to mature into an adult mite. The initial lesion is a small erythematous papule or burrows which can become a vesicle and pustules and are highly pruritic, which is worse during night when skin is warmer. The burrows are most commonly seen in between the finger webs, along the sides of fingers, flexor aspects of wrist, on the border of hand, and in areola of nipples of female breasts and in genital area in males. Other less likely affected areas include elbows, axilla, and buttocks. Intense itching causes excoriations and breaks in skin leading to secondary infections like impetigo. [35]

Scabies is usually diagnosed through clinical examination and by finding typical burrow lesions in typical sites like between finger webs. When in doubt attempts should be made to extract mite, or eggs from these burrows by gently scraping the burrows and examining the scrapings under light microscope.

Videodermatoscopy can provide high-resolution magnification of skin up to 600 times under incidental light and is a noninvasive and effective diagnostic tool to locate mites and eggs. Other such technologies in use are Epiluminescence microscopy and dermatoscopy has also shown diagnostic accuracy in identifying the typical lesions and mites. [36, 37, 38] However, failure to have such confirmatory evidence does not rule out scabies. The treatment should be started without delay based on clinical judgment. Oral ivermectin generally prescribed in two 12 mg doses is shown to be effective in treatment when topical treatment is not effective or disease is severe and widespread.

Pediculosis

Although commonly seen in children, pediculosis, or head lice can be a common problem in older adults living in places with close contact with peers. Transmission of infestation occurs due to head to head contact mainly by sharing personal items like combs, scarves, hats etc. Head lice can cause significant itching which leads to frequent scratching which in turn may give rise to secondary infections like impetigo in rare cases. Diagnosis can be established by visualizing the live lice and use of a louse comb can aid is diagnosis. Finding of occasional nits especially 1/4th inch far from the skull is not indicative of a current infestation, however, it indicates that there was a previous infestation. Finding multiple nits within a quarter of an inch area from scalp is predictive of active infestation in about one third of cases. [39]

Once the diagnosis is established application of 1% Permethrin, pyrethrins or 0.5% Malathion can be effective. 1% Permethrin is very effective in form of a crème rinse when left in hair for 10 minutes and rinsed. A second application is suggested in 7-10 days. Alternatively treatment on 0, 7, and between 13 to15 day has been proposed. Efficacy has decreased due to development of resistance. Malathion 0.5% is an organophosphate and is applied to dry hair and left for 8-12 hours with good ovicidal activity, repeat application is usually not necessary unless live lice is detected post treatment in that case reapplication on day 7-9 is recommended. Lindane 1% (gamma benzene hexachloride) shampoo can also be used. [40]

Single oral dose of ivermectin 200 μg /kg has shown 74% effectiveness which increased to 95% when dose was repeated at 10 days. [41,42] Confining the spread of infestation is the most effective way of controlling the infection. Floors and furniture should be vacuumed although risk of infestation via this route is minimal especially after 1-2 days. Prophylactic treatment of person sharing the same personal items and bedding is recommended. All clothes, hairbrushes, combs and linens used 2 days prior to treatment should be washed in hot water.

Conclusion

Chronic diseases, including dermatological diseases, are rapidly becoming more prevalent due to the growing population of the elderly. Clinicians should respond to the rising needs of the geriatric population by staying informed. Early detection of diseases of the skin in geriatric population may lead to better treatment and containment of common viral, bacterial, fungal, and parasitic dermatological diseases resulting in easing discomfort and maximizing positive prognosis for geriatric patients.

References

[1] Norman R. Common skin condition in geriatric dermatology. *Annals of Long Term Care.* 2008 Nov; 16(6): 40-45.
[2] Staikov I, Neykov N, Marinovic B, Lipozencic J, Tsankov N. Herpes zoster as a systemic disease. *Clin Dermatol.* 2014 May; 32(3): 424-9.
[3] Opstelten W, Eekhof J, Necen AK, Verheii T. Treatment of herpes zoster. *Can Fam Physician.* 2008 Mar; 54(3): 373-7.
[4] Lam JM. Characterizing viral exanthems. Pediatric Health. 2010; 4(6): 623–635.
[5] Brown J, Janniger CK, Schwartz RA, Silverberg NB. Childhood molluscum contagiosum. *Int J Dermatol.* 2006 Feb; 45(2): 93-99.
[6] Sadick NS. Current aspects of bacterial infections of the skin. *Dermatol Clin.* 1997 Apr;15(2):341-349.
[7] Stulberg DL, Penrod MA, Blatny RA. Common skin infections. *Am Fam Physician.* 2002 Jul;66(1):119-24.
[8] Cole C, Gazewood J. Diagnosis and treatment of Impetigo. *Am Fam Physician* 2007; 75:859-64.
[9] George A, Rubin G. A systematic review and meta- analysis of treatments for impetigo. *Br J Gen Pract* 2003;53:480-7.
[10] Jen I. Pseudomonas folliculitis. *Can Fam Physician.* 1982 Aug;28:1423-5.
[11] Hogan PA. Pseudomonas folliculitis. *Australas J Dermatol.* 1997 May;38(2):93-4.
[12] Antanaskova N, Tomecki KJ. Innovative management of recurrent furunculosis. *Dermatol Clin.* 2010 Jul; 28(3): 479-87.
[13] Lopez FA, Lartchenko S. Skin and soft tissue infections. *Infect Dis Clin North Am.* 2006 Dec;20(4):759-72.
[14] Hauser A, Fogarasi S. Periorbital and orbital cellulitis. *Pediatr Rev.* 2010 Jun;31(6):242-9.
[15] Brilliant LC. Perianal Streptococcal Dermatitis. *Am Fam Physician.* 2000 Jan; 61(2):391-3, 397.
[16] Inghammar M, Rasmussen M, Linder A. Recurrent erysipelas - risk factors and clinical presentation. *BMC Infectious Diseases* 2014, 14:270-76.
[17] Reich HL, Williams FD, Naik NS, Honig PG, Yan AC. Nonpseudomonal ecthyma gangrenosum. *J Am Acad Dermatol.* 2004 May; 50(5 Suppl): 114-7.
[18] Yang CC, Hsieh FS, Lee JY. Pyoderma gangrenosum complicated by ecthyma gangrenosum. *Br J Dermatol.* 2004 May;150(5):1025-6.
[19] Mesaros N, Nordmann P, Plésiat P. Pseudomonas aeruginosa: resistance and therapeutic options at the turn of the new millennium. *Clin Microbiol Infect.* 2007 Jun;13(6):560-78.

[20] Eneli I, Cavles HD. Epidemiology and outcome of necrotizing fasciitis in children: an active surveillance study of the Canadian pediatric surveillance program. *J of Pediatrics.* 2007 Jul; 151(1): 79-84.
[21] Stoneback JW, Hak DJ. Diagnosis and management of necrotizing faciitis. *Orthopedics.* 2011 Mar; 34(3): 196.
[22] Schmidr MR, Kossmann T, Duewell S. Differentiation of necrotizing fasciitis and cellulitis using MR imaging. *AJR Am J Roentgenol.* 1998 Mar; 170(3): 615-20.
[23] Yu JS, Habib P. MR imaging of urgent inflammatory and infectious conditions affecting the soft tissues of the musculoskeletal system. *Emerg Radiol.* 2009 Jul; 16(4): 267-76.
[24] Thompson ML, Martin C. Management of necrotizing fasciitis infections. *Orthoperdics.* 2011 Feb;34(2):111-5.
[25] World Health Organization. The global elimination of congenital syphilis: rationale and strategy for action. http://whqlibdoc.who.int/publications/2007/978924159 5858_ eng.pdf. 3-13.
[26] Pastuszczak M, Wojas-Pelc A. Current standards for diagnosis and treatment of syphilis: selection of some practical issues, based on the European (IUSTI) and U.S. (CDC) guidelines. *Postep Derm Alergol* 2013; 4: 203–10.
[27] Tekeli A, Dolapci I, Emral R, Cesur S. Candida carriage and Candida dubliniensis in oropharyngeal samples of type-1 diabetes mellitus patients. *Mycoses.* 2004 Aug;47(7):315-8.
[28] Segal E. Candida, still number one—what do we know and where are we going from here? *Mycoses.* 2005; 48 Suppl 1:3-11.
[29] Thomas DR, Burkempe NM. Geriatric Dermatology, An Issue of Clinics in Geriatric *Medicine.* Elsevier; 2013.
[30] Berg D, Erickson P. Fungal skin infections in children. New developments and treatments. *Postgrad Med.* 2001 Jul;110(1):83-4, 87-8, 93-4.
[31] Alston J, Cohen BA, Braun M; Persistent and Recurrent Tinea Corporis in Children Treated With Combination Antifungal/ Corticosteroid Agents. *Pediatrics* 2003;111: 201.
[32] Weinberg. Comparison of diagnostic methods in the evaluation of onychomycosis. *J Am Acad Dermatol.* 2003; 49: 193-219.
[33] Gupta AK, Sauder DN, Shear NH. Antifungal agents: an overview part II. *J Am Acad Dermatol.* 1994; 30: 911.
[34] Church RE, Knowelden J. Scabies in Sheffield: a family infestation. *Br Med J.* 1978;1(6115):761-3.
[35] Chosidow O. Scabies clinical practices. *N Engl J Med.* 2006 Apr; 354(16): 1718-27.
[36] Dupuy A, Dehen L, Bourrat E, Lacroix C. Accuracy of standard dermoscopy for diagnosing scabies. *J Am Acad Dermatol.* 2007 Jan;56(1):53-62.
[37] Heukelbach J, Feldmeier H. Scabies. *Lancet.* 2006 May; 367(9524): 1767-74.
[38] Lacaarrubba F, Musumeci ML, Catabiano R. High-Magnification Videodermatoscopy: A New Noninvasive Diagnostic Tool for Scabies in Children. *Pediatric Dermatology* 2001; 18(5): 439-441.
[39] Center for Disease Control and Prevention. 1600 Clifton Rd. Atlanta, GA 30333, USA. http://www.cdc.gov/parasites /lice /head/diagnosis.html. Date accessed06/30/2014
[40] Frankowski BL, Bocchini JA Jr. Head lice. *Pediatrics.* 2010 Aug;126(2):392-403.

[41] Bukhart CN, Bukhart CG. An assessment of topical and oral prescriptions and over-the-couter treatments for head lice. *J Am Acad Dermatol.* 1998 Jul; 38(6) 979-82.

[42] Chosidow O. Scabies and pediculosis. *Lancet.* 200 Mar; 355(9206): 819-26.

In: Geriatric Psychodermatology
Editors: Mohammad Jafferany and Katlein França
ISBN: 978-1-63463-853-1

Chapter 22

Bioethics, Ethics and Medicolegal Aspects in Geriatric Psychodermatology

Reginaldo de França, MSc,* Aparecida Porto França, MSc and Katlein França, M.D., MSc

Introduction

In the life cycle, there are two times when the human being deserves greater attention because of their fragility. These moments are childhood and elderly age (when an individual can suffer of limitation of physical and psychological senses). Without disregarding other pathological conditions that may occur in the course of life, children and the elderly (with limitations), can not by themselves, walk through the paths of existence without support from others, family, society or the state.

Since the beginning of life, human beings have rights. These rights accompany them thought all their existence. As stated by Immanuel Kant [1], dignity is a quality inherent to human beings as moral beings. When they exercise, autonomously, their practical reason, humans constitute distinct human personalities, each of them absolutely individual and irreplaceable. Consequently, dignity is totally inseparable from the autonomy.

The conception of the dignity of the elderly involves many aspects. The right to live with dignity, not be discriminated against receiving an appropriate retirement and especially health assistance.

Elderly people have peculiarities that differentiate them from younger. These peculiarities have to be observed and respected by health professionals responsible for their care in all areas, including psychodermatology. Dermatologic diseases can more deeply affect their self-esteem, causing psychological distress and discomfort.

* Corresponding author: Reginaldo de França. Email: reginaldodefranca@hotmail.com.

The aging process causes visible changes in physical appearance. The elderly may also experience psychological changes that can cause serious damage and impact quality of life. Martinoff explains that psychiatric disorders in elderly patients occur due to the impact of the pejorative concept of aging on an individual that fears the perspective of becoming a useless person and consequently unvalued [2]

The psychological risks change according to the circumstances of life and have different effects, depending on each individual. It is important to identify the processes and mechanisms that influence the life of each person. [3]

An elderly person has a long history of life with conflicts, successes or failures. The future prospects are limited. He has the right to live well within the present.

Physiological Conditions of the Elderly- The Third Age

According to Goldman, the term "third age" was created by the French gerontologist Huet, which the chronological principle matches the retirement time (approximately 60 to 65 years) although changes in this pattern are already happening. [4]

According to the World Health Organization, persons achieve the third age when they achieve 65 years of age. At this time, many anatomical changes happen, such as wrinkling of the skin, decreasing of the oiliness, hair whitens and hair loss, especially in men.

In women the skin becomes drier and saggy by decreased estrogen, which is responsible for the level of hydration and formation of collagen fibers. There is a reduction in the reproductive process of the cells, and cellular elements of the various organs and tissues can not be recovered, affecting the performance of their specific functions.

Sandra Lopes Matos and colleagues, explain that, from the Dermatology perspective, the aging process of the skin occurs in two different ways: [5]

a) Intrinsic aging, senescent, due to the chronological action on the skin and adjacent tissues, universal and inevitable to everyone that ages. The main changes ranging from dehydration, wrinkles and sagging
b) The extrinsic aging due to lifestyle and/ or environmental factors, particularly chronic sun exposure (photo aging) and smoking. Senile changes occur in various degrees, according to the exposure, age, and individual susceptibility. Benign and malignant neoplasms are important examples.

It is clear that such physical transformations generate psychological consequences and affect more significantly the elderly than the young.

However, it should be considered that there is no uniformity of criteria as the pathological symptoms of aging may manifest early or much later. The aging process should not be generalized. Many adults reach to 80 or 90 years-old without showing symptoms of physical or psychological degeneration. Numerous historical conditions influence the aging, so is highly inconvenient to generalize or set standards on chronological age. According to Neri, each organism is characterized by a finite number of behavioral change s, which are increasingly present in a unique way: your individuation or intrinsic aging process that lasts from conception to death.

In this chapter, therefore, the elderly will be considered those with the psychosocial characteristics that match the concept of vulnerability arising from organic and psychological changes as a result of the aging process.

Bioethical Principles

The study of bioethics, an eminent field, brought many controversial, but important discussions, about the relationship of healthcare professionals and their patients.

In fact bioethics is responsible for the study of many moral values and principles. It promotes human dignity and quality of life.

Mario Lopez defines bioethics as "the systematic study of human behavior in the areas of life sciences and health care, considering the moral principles."[7]

This science has four basic principles that will be discussed in this chapter.

Non-Maleficence (Primum Non Nocere)

The doctor has a duty to help the elderly patient, without causing damage. Not only physical, but also psychological damage. Psychodermatology patients are psychologically vulnerable and the medical professional must consider their psychological fragility.

Beneficence

This principle, contained in the Hippocratic Oath, states that the doctor should use the treatment to help the patient, never to harm them.

Jussara de Azambuja Loch states that Beneficence means doing good. [8] This concept means doing what is best for the patient, not only from the technical point of view, but also the ethical point of view. They should use all the knowledge and professional skills in the service of the patient, minimizing risks and maximizing the benefits of the procedure to be performed.

Autonomy

The elderly have their own point of view, thoughts and beliefs. Except for specific exceptions, they have the capacity to make decisions and seek the best for themselves. The health provider has no right to belittle or settle judgments in that the age hinders their reflexes and their judgment. If there are no scientifically proven medical reasons that justify such a suspicion, the elderly are fully possessed with will, even in the most difficult moments. Respecting the autonomy is, as stated by Dalla Saad "to preserve the fundamental rights of the man, accepting the social-ethical pluralism that exists today. This principle is ethically grounded in human dignity." [9] In addition, Kvitko mentions the respect that should be improved in relation to the patient's autonomy. According to this author, an autonomous person is a person able to decide on their personal goals and work towards achieving such deliberations. Respecting autonomy means giving value to people's options and elections, while avoiding obstructing their actions, unless they are clearly over others. Showing a lack of respect for an autonomous agent is to repudiate that person's decisions, to deny a person's freedom to act according to their decisions or withhold information necessary for an individual to make a decision when there are not enough reasons thereto. [10]

It is not the frailty of the elderly that might remove their power to decide. Gandolfo & Ferrari claim that "we call an autonomous person who, regardless of age, freely makes decisions, choose between alternatives presented to them, according to values, beliefs, aspirations and own goals in life, and is able to make action based upon such decisions." [11]

If, however, there is fullness of mental conditions, there is no need to speak of restrictions on the right to opine and decide. And even if they are limited, the manifestations of will allow us to recognize the will of the elderly, and the latter will have to be respected.

Autonomy and Informed Consent

Informed consent is not really a Bioethics principle, but a consequence of the very Autonomy principle. It is a patient's right, despite of any age or social status, however, with the requirement that, one that informs their consent must be in the full exercise of his mental faculties.

The elderly in the fullness of their consciousness are able to assess medical information, consider the possible risks and effects and give their consent. However, in case of presenting restrictions, as in the case of carrying Alzheimer's disease or other cases of senile dementia, the family assumes legal responsibility to the consent. According to Silvia Reyes Gonzales and Estela Reyes Gonzales, "In all cases it is necessary to provide adequate information to patients or their families. The elderly have the right to receive a full and clear communication from the physician, considering their psychological and cultural conditions." [12]

Factors that may pose hindrance to the elderly to manifest themselves in informed consent are indicated by Melba Barrantes-Monge et al. as being: cognitive impairment, disabling chronic illness, loss of self-determination, economic dependence, etc. [13] Salvarezza considers that aging involves a complex social behavior, with historical, cultural, social, psychological and ideological dimensions, based on a set of prejudices, stereotypes and discrimination that apply to the elderly because of their age. [14]

The physician is responsible for evaluating the conditions of the elderly to rationally express their consent and if they do not have the necessary conditions for such a decision, it is important to listen to family members exercising, still, a critical sense of what's best for the patient.

Justice

The concept of justice is abstract and fluid. It originates from the Latin term *iusticia*, which refers to one of the four cardinal virtues (allying themselves with prudence, fortitude and temperance). It is the firm belief of giving to others what they are worth [15] Another way to interpret this concept is that the equals shall be treated with equality.

França makes the following observation:

> In relation to the patient, the concept of justice can not be merely a concept of equality, as the patient does not feel the same level as healthy people. The equality of the patient is linked to the rights that it possesses in the legal systems, however, ensured a privileged status because of their vulnerability.

An elderly patient, when seeking a dermatological treatment, does not want to be treated unfairly, indifferent, being discriminated for his condition because of their age. Clearly as being sick, regardless of being elderly, is also vulnerable, and thus it is fair that receives preferential treatment.

Justice comprises impartiality, adequacy for what is right and ethical, therefore, is fair in the fullness of the term. Often the concept of justice is understood from injustices practiced. That is, when someone has the right to be respected as a human being to see their wills thriving and those who have the power of decision simply deny them unfairly this right to become effective.

The Elderly in the Context of the Human Rights

In international law, there are no specific rules dealing with the protection for the elderly, differently from what happens to children and adolescents. The elderly are considered ordinary human beings, object of protection provided for the man without, however, relying on own instruments of institutional support.

Historically, the United Nations has been the birthplace of the human rights protection instruments. However, when the elderly have no multilateral agreements that place them main focus of what follows that its protection happens by the application of the existing international human rights instruments. The Universal Declaration of Human Rights of 1948, only cites old age in its art. XXV:

> Everyone has the right to a standard of living capable of assuring health and well-being for them and their family, including food, clothing, housing, medical care and necessary social services, and the right to security in the event of unemployment, sickness, family disability, widowhood, old age or other lack of livelihood in circumstances beyond their control.

Due to this gap, the United Nations Population Fund - UNFPA along with the HelpAge International held in Madrid, in April 2002, the Second World Assembly on Aging in order to address the challenges posed by a rapidly aging of the population, adopting the "International Action Plan for the Aging, whose focus was to promote the integration between aging and development, promote health and wellness in this particular phase of life and ensure welcoming environments that encourage autonomy." The Executive Summary, outcome of such meeting, calls for changes in attitudes, policies and practices that ensure the elderly not be seen simply as a recipient of pension plans, but as active participant of the development process, whose rights shall be respected.

The World Medical Association - though without a binding effect as imposing standard - makes conduct recommendations to physicians responsible for treating the elderly, while urging national medical associations to give notice of its contents to its members. According to these recommendations, the physicians' duties include:

- Make every effort to create a relationship of trust with the elderly patients in order to urge them to seek medical attention when necessary, and make them feel comfortable when trusting the physician
- Provide a medical evaluation and treatment for damage caused by abuse or neglect
- Try to establish and maintain a therapeutic relationship with the family (usually the doctor is the only professional who keeps a lasting contact with the patient and the family) and maintain, to the greatest possible extent, the patient's reliability
- Report all suspected cases of elder mistreat or abuse, according to local legislation
- Use a multidisciplinary team comprised of careful medical professions, social work, mental and legal health, whenever possible
- Stimulate the generation and use of support community resources providing in-home services, rest or stress reduction to high-risk families

Some countries have established protective standards for the elderly. It is the case in Brazil which, through Law No. 10,741; 2003 (Elderly Statute), contemplates the age of 60 and above and which expresses: "Aging is a major personal right and its protection is a social right. It is the State's obligation to ensure their aged population to have protection to life and health through the implementation of social policies that enable a healthy and dignified aging. Analyzing the Brazilian standard, Silvia Fernández comments: "It is to say, the law provides a *right to respect* that assumes inviolability of their physical and mental integrity, image, identity, autonomy, ideas, beliefs, possessions, reaffirming the fundamental rights of the person; provides a *guarantee of priority*, comprising public and private preferential attention, privileged allocation of public resources, priority to family care and access to health services." [16]

It becomes apparent that, given the aging of humanity and because of the low fertility rate, it will result in the need for creating mechanisms to protect a population segment that will be soon the majority in many of the western countries.

References

[1] Queiroz VS. A dignidade da pessoa humana no pensamento de Kant. Da fundamentação da metafísica dos costumes à doutrina do direito. Uma reflexão crítica

para os dias atuais. Revista Jus Navegandi. Available: http://jus.com.br/revista/texto /7069/a-dignidade-da-pessoa-humana-no-pensamento-de-kant.

[2] Martinoff, EHS. O direito à felicidade na terceira idade. Direitos Humanos – proteção e promoção. Daniela Buci, José Blanes Sala, José Ribeiro de Campos: coordenadores. São Paulo, Saraiva, 2012. page 219.

[3] Yunez, M. A. M, Szimanski, H. Resiliência: noção, conceitos afins e considerações críticas. In TAVARES, J. (org.). Resiliência e educação. São Paulo: Cortez, 2001.

[4] Goldman, S.N. Velhice e Direitos Sociais. In: Paes, Serafim Paz *et al.* Envelhecer com Cidadania: quem sabe um dia? Rio de Janeiro: CBCISS; ANG/ Seção Rio de Janeiro, 2000.

[5] Matos, S.L *et al.* Prevalência de Dermatoses em Idosos residentes em instituição de longa permanência. Revista da Associação Médica Brasileira, Vol. 54, nº 6, São Paulo, Nov./Dez.2008.

[6] Neri, A. L. Psicologia do envelhecimento: temas selecionados na perspectiva de curso de vida. Campinas, SP: Papirus, 1995.

[7] Lopes, M. Fundamentos da Ciência Médica: a relação paciente-médico. Rio de Janeiro, Medri, 1997.

[8] Azambuja, J. Princípios da Bioética. Available at: http://www.nhu.ufms.br/Bioetica /Textos/Princ%C3%ADpios/PRINC%C3%8DPIOS%20DA%20BIO%C3%89TICA%2 0(3).pdf

[9] Dalla Saad E.R. Bioética aplicada à pesquisa e inovação farmacêutica. Revista Pesquisa e Inovação Farmacêutica nº 1: ago-dez, 2009.

[10] Kyitko, L.A. El consentimiento informado. 1 ed. Ciudadela: Dosyuna Ediciones Argentinas, 2009.

[11] Gandolpho, M.A. Ferrari, M.A.C. (2006, jul./set.). A enfermagem cuidando do idoso: reflexões bioéticas. *In*: *O Mundo da Saúde, 30*(3). São Paulo (ano 30).

[12] González, S.R. et al. Consentimiento Informado en el paciente geriátrico. Hospital Clínico Quirúrgico Universitario Dr. Salvador AllendeCiudad de la Habana CUBA.Año 2003. Available at: http://indexmedico.com/publicaciones/indexmed_journal/edicion7 /cons_inf_ger/reyes_gonzalez.htm.

[13] Barrantes-Monge, M *et al.* Relación Médico-Paciente: Derechos del Adulto Mayor. Acta Bioetich, Vol. 15 nº 2, Santiago (Chile), nov. 2009. Available at: http://www.ncbi.nlm.nih.gov/pmc/articles/PMC2850536/

[14] Salvarezza, L. Psicogeriatría. Teoría y Clínica. Editora Paidós. Buenos Aires, 2002.

[15] Franca, K. A Dermatologia e a Relação Médico-Paciente: Aspectos sociais e Bioéticos. Curitiba: Juruá, 2012.

[16] Fernández, S. Ancianidad, autonomía y vulnerabilidad: Una mirada a la situación jurídica de los adultos mayores desde la reforma proyectada para el Código Civil argentino. Infojus – Sistema argentino de Información Jurídica. Ministerio de Justicia y Derechos Humanos. Presidencia de la Nación. Available at: http://www.infojus.gob.ar /doctrina/dacf120180-fernandez-ancianidad_autonomia_vulnerabilidad_una.htm; jsessionid=1a6plcy8occmsli3opz0x2wol?0

Index

A

B

C

D

R

S

T

V

W

Z